Nature and Treatment of Stuttering:
New directions

Nature and Treatment of Stuttering:
New directions

Edited by

RICHARD F. CURLEE, PhD
University of Arizona
Tucson, Arizona

WILLIAM H. PERKINS, PhD
University of Southern California
Los Angeles, California

 College-Hill Press, San Diego, California

College–Hill Press, Inc.
4284 41st Street
San Diego, CA 92105

Library of Congress Cataloging in Publication Data
Main entry under title:

Nature and treatment of stuttering: New directions

    Bibliography: p.
    Includes index.
    1. Stuttering. I. Curlee, Richard F., 1935-
II. Perkins, William H. (William Hughes), 1923-
[DNLM: 1. Stuttering.   2. Stuttering—Therapy. WM
475 N285]
RC424.N38   1984   616.85'54   83-26337
ISBN 0-933014-71-6

Printed in the United States of America

5-20-86

Contributors

Martin R. Adams, PhD, University of Houston, Houston, TX 77004

Gavin Andrews, MD, The University of New South Wales, Sydney, 2036, AUSTRALIA

Oliver Bloodstein, PhD, Brooklyn College, Brooklyn, NY 11210

Edward G. Conture, PhD, Syracuse University, Syracuse, NY 13210

Janis M. Costello, PhD, University of California at Santa Barbara, Santa Barbara, CA 93106

Richard F. Curlee, PhD, University of Arizona, Tucson, AZ 85721

David A. Daly, EdD, University of Michigan, Ann Arbor, MI 48109

Frances J. Freeman, PhD, University of Texas at Dallas, Dallas, TX 75235

Hugo H. Gregory, PhD, Northwestern University, Evanston, IL 60201

Curt E. Hamre, PhD, Texas Tech University, Lubbock, TX 79413

Pauline Howie, PhD, University of New South Wales, Sydney, 2036, AUSTRALIA

Roger J. Ingham, PhD, Cumberland College of Health Sciences, Lidcombe, New South Wales, 2141, AUSTRALIA

James Jerger, PhD, Baylor College of Medicine, Houston, TX 77030

Ray D. Kent, PhD, University of Wisconsin, Madison, WI 53706

Kenneth K. Kidd, PhD, Yale University School of Medicine, New Haven, CT 06510

Maryellen C. MacDonald, MA, University of California at Los Angeles, Los Angeles, CA 90024

Donald G. MacKay, PhD, University of California at Los Angeles, Los Angeles, CA 90024

Walter H. Moore, Jr., PhD, California State University at Long Beach, Long Beach, CA 90804

William H. Perkins, PhD, University of Southern California, Los Angeles, CA 90007

David Prins, PhD, University of Washington, Seattle, WA 98195

John C. Rosenbek, PhD, William S. Middleton Memorial Veterans Hospital, Madison, WI 53705

David Rosenfield, MD, Baylor College of Medicine, Houston, TX 77030

Marcel E. Wingate, PhD, Washington State University, Pullman, WA 99163

Martin A. Young, PhD, Illinois State University, Normal, IL 61761

Gerald N. Zimmermann, PhD, University of Iowa, Iowa City, IA 52242

Contents

PREFACE

This volume is intended to provide current perspectives of the nature and treatment of stuttering. The literature on this disorder has been vast for years, but in the last decade it has all but exploded in many directions. Consequently, students and clinicians who are interested in stuttering must sift through a proliferation of published information, opinion, and speculation in order to remain current in their understanding of the problem and how to treat it.

We have attempted to present comprehensive coverage of a variety of points of view about stuttering in a fair, balanced manner. We invited only authors whose research or clinical experience permitted them to speak with authority on the topics of their chapters. We also asked these authors to evaluate critically the scientific credibility of the data available on their topic and to synthesize such information in an objective, scholarly, readable fashion. As a result, we believe that we have been extraordinarily successful in obtaining state-of-the-art perspectives of our current knowledge base as well as the directions such perspectives are taking us toward future research and treatment.

Our personal contributions to this text have been limited largely to the selection of topics to be covered and of authors to provide such coverage. In retrospect, and in all modesty, we believe that our latter contributions may have been inspired. We wanted readers to obtain an appreciation of a variety of points of view about stuttering and stutterers, its etiology, and its treatment. We wanted this appreciation to evolve from an exposure to the work and ideas of researchers and clinicians who have shaped our current views. In short, we wanted our readers to get the word straight from the horse's mouth with little editorial chewing. When we did chew, it was to reduce chunks of jargon or difficult-to-understand concepts to more digestible bites for easier comprehension. Consequently, we have tried to sublimate our own biases, yet have insisted that authors clearly differentiate opinion from empirical observation. This reflects our distrust of opinion and unqualified conclusions based on isolated, unreplicated studies that have employed small samples or have lacked satisfactory experimental controls.

This volume contains a challenging collection of ideas about stuttering. Indeed, recent research has furthered our understanding of stuttering and how to go about treating it in a number of significant areas. Nevertheless, many questions and doubts remain. After so many years and so much work, it may seem somewhat discouraging that our knowledge base on stuttering will rarely support unequivocal inferences or conclusions. But such uncertainty accurately reflects the status of our scientific understanding of stuttering and may well be typical of all areas of scientific inquiry during the formative stages of their development. In effect, it is the current state of our art.

We have not attempted to provide exhaustive coverage of the stuttering literature but have included comprehensive coverage of what we believe to be the more important topics. Even this limited coverage may exceed the scope of information an instructor finds appropriate for a single quarter or semester. Accordingly, we have organized the chapters into units of study which instructors can arrange to accommodate the needs of different courses. Obviously, this organizational scheme and the selection of topics to be included reflect our biases about stuttering and about how one can best assimilate the information available on this topic. In general, we grouped those chapters that basically summarized information about stuttering and stutterers into an initial unit of study, then added those that focused on etiological perspectives of stuttering, and ended with those that were most pertinent to therapy.

Information has been gathered, for the most part, through comparisons of groups of stutterers to matched groups of nonstutterers or through within-group comparisons of stutterers while they are stuttering versus while they are speaking fluently. It should not be surprising that authorities differ with regard to which differences cause stuttering, which result from it, and which covary with stuttering or stutterers but are not causally related. Generally speaking, there is substantial overlap in the performance of stutterers and nonstutterers. Even statistically reliable differences between the two groups rarely suggest abnormal or impaired performance except for the fact that stutterers stutter. Furthermore, there is usually less consistency, or greater heterogeneity, of performance among different stutterers or for individual stutterers on the same task than one finds among nonstutterers. Indeed, one cannot generalize from the findings obtained from a group of stutterers to an individual stutterer with certainty. Finally, and most important, the importance of differences found between stutterers and nonstutterers or between fluent and stuttered periods of stutterers is yet to be clearly established.

Compared to the natural sciences, etiological explanations of stuttering should not be viewed as theories, at least in a formal or technical sense. For the most part, theories of stuttering strive not only to meet scientific standards of empirical verification, but also to achieve intuitive plausibility. Indeed, the popularity of some explanations of stuttering likely derive more of their success from meeting the latter criterion than the former. To date, causal explanations have provided somewhat simplified descriptions of stuttering onsets that appeal to human understanding. Such explanations are more qualitative and empirical and less quantitative and theoretical than those in the physical sciences. Still, it should be acknowledged that scientific explanations change and that few current scientific truths in any discipline seem likely to emerge some centuries hence as an eternal verity. The theoretical perspectives presented in this volume include chapters that emphasize environmental factors in the onset of stuttering as well as those that focus on cognitive–motor programming factors. These perspectives fit with our suspicion that a genetically transmitted predisposition, which interacts with environmental factors, holds the most promise for our future understanding of the cause of stuttering.

We have grouped the treatment of stuttering, both for children and adults, into two approaches—those that manage fluency and those that manage stuttering. The former group focuses on training stutterers how to speak more fluently, while the latter emphasizes techniques intended to foster less effortful, more fluent stuttering. This grouping captures, we believe, the primary differences that characterize current treatment procedures used with stutterers. Moreover, it is consistent with some basic philosophical differences that also distinguish these approaches. For example, many clinicians whose treatment procedures emphasize managing fluency usually advocate these techniques as a form of behavior therapy. In contrast, those clinicians who strive to manage stuttering often regard behavioral approaches with genuine distaste. They frequently see behavior therapies as the treatment of superficial symptoms rather than the resolution of problems that cause such symptoms. The fluency managers are likely to reply with similar hostility that these symptoms *are* the problem. Typically, therefore, discussions of stuttering treatment often combine equal amounts of description of a clinician's preferred approach with attacks on different approaches. While there are many claims and much heat generated in such discussions, there is no scientifically credible basis for predicting which therapeutic procedure will be most beneficial for a given stutterer. While complete permanent recoveries from stuttering occur relatively infrequently among adults, a variety of treatment procedures seem to be effective with many stutterers. There is also reason to believe that treatment of children who stutter produces better, longer-lasting results than can be achieved with adults. To our knowledge, however, no approach has been permanently effective with all stutterers. While we believe that the clinical management of stuttering continues to be, at present, more of an art than a science, substantial improvements in therapeutic success will rest with future scientific advances rather than artistic achievement.

Omission of our own concluding statement that attempts to integrate the contributions of other chapters is not by accident or oversight. To be a useful statement would require that it be a responsible statement. To be a responsible statement would require that it encompass the full range of evidence presented in these chapters. Clearly, such a synthesis is needed, but we do not believe that this would be the appropriate place to formulate it. To do so would require selective evaluation of the evidence presented by others. Our judgment would not necessarily correspond with those of our authors whom we invited to contribute. Moreover, we might well interpret their evidence differently than they have, but they would have no opportunity to respond. They are our guests in this text. As their hosts, we do not think it seemly to use our editorial advantage to have the last word.

Richard F. Curlee
William H. Perkins
Editors

Characteristics of
stuttering and stutterers

Chapter 1

Epidemiology of Stuttering
Gavin Andrews

This chapter is concerned with some aspects of the epidemiology of stuttering, particularly prevalence, onset, development, and recovery. Epidemiology is a field of inquiry that deals with rates of disease among populations and the extent to which these rates are affected by variables such as age, sex, marital status, or social class. There are at least three reasons why epidemiology is important: first, because it may produce information which contributes to the understanding of the cause or remedy of a disorder. In a famous example, John Snow, in 1848, noted that high rates of cholera were occurring in a particular area of London. Further study showed that the people affected used water from the Broad Street pump, while those living in the same area, but not using the pump water, were not affected. He had the pump dismantled, and the epidemic ended. Thus, his epidemiological investigation led to a possible cause as well as a remedy. Second, information about the frequency of a disorder can be helpful in planning health care services for that disorder. Third, epidemiological data can be valuable in counseling patients and families about the natural course their disorder is likely to take in the absence of treatment.

The frequency of a disease can be expressed in two ways, prevalence and incidence. The *prevalence* of a disease is the number of cases that exist within a population at a given time, divided by the total number in the population. *Treated prevalence* is the number of cases in treatment divided by the total number of persons in the population. This number is sometimes quoted; but clearly, as not all persons suffering from a disease come for treatment, this index is usually less than the true prevalence. *Incidence* refers to the number of new cases arising in a population during a given time period, usually over a year, although life time risks, the risk of ever developing a disease, are also important.

The relationship between prevalence and incidence is mediated by the *duration* of illness in question. For instance, the common cold has a very high yearly incidence, for most people develop one cold per year.

Because the duration of each cold is usually short, the prevalence, or the number of people with a cold at any given time, is quite low. Conversely, the yearly risk of developing childhood autism is low, but because the duration of the disorder is long, the prevalence at any one time is always higher than the yearly incidence.

Because prevalence depends on both incidence and duration, a change in the prevalence of a disorder may be due either to a change in incidence or to a change in average duration, or to both. Often changes in prevalence can be attributed to a change in a characteristic or circumstance of the population which indirectly affects incidence or duration. For example, the dismantling of the Broad Street pump lowered the incidence or occurrence of new cases, thereby reducing the prevalence. Conversely, effective treatment of a disease such as tuberculosis should reduce duration and lower its prevalence even if the incidence remains constant. Checking to see if the prevalence of a disorder is falling is the best method of testing whether a new treatment being applied to a population is effective. After randomized controlled trials and multicenter field trials have been conducted, this is usually the final and conclusive step in proving a treatment to be effective. If there are effective treatments for stuttering, we should measure the prevalence of stuttering in a high school system, institute an energetic treatment program in the schools, and then see if the prevalence of stuttering has declined in those schools.

THE THOUSAND FAMILY STUDY

The ideal way of establishing incidence, prevalence, duration, and, hence, the natural history of a disorder is to take a series of individuals and follow them throughout the entire period of their lives during which the disorder can be expected to develop or remit. In the case of stutterers, this can largely be achieved by taking a cohort of children and following them from their first birthday until they are grown. There is one small prospective study that did approach this ideal.

In 1947 in England, the University of Durham and the health services of the city of Newcastle-upon-Tyne combined to study the speech development of all children born in the city during the months of May and June. The study began with 1,142 babies, but through death and migration the numbers declined, so that there were only 967 children available for study one year later, 847 five years later, and 763 fifteen years later. Dr. Muriel Morley organized the study of speech development of these children. Under her direction, all of the families were seen regularly by health visitors, who reported on the child's acquisition of speech and her/his progress toward intelligibility, and on the presence of any defects or abnormalities. At regular intervals, speech therapists saw all the children in whom defective speech development or stuttering had been reported, as well as seeing a 1-in-10 sample of the total group. Of the 944 children included in the survey, 37 were reported by Dr. Morley as having, between the ages of 2 and 7 years, some form of interference in their fluency, "usually described as stammering or hesitating." In 16 of these children the episode was mild and transient, but in the remaining 21 children the difficulty was more persistent, lasting for 6 months or more. Compared with the other children in the survey, these 37 were late in acquiring words, phrases, and intelligible speech. There was also a significant trend for these children to come from lower socioeconomic groups (Morley, 1957).

In 1963, as part of my doctoral thesis, Mary Harris and I searched the records for all children noted to have had a period of stuttering. We found an additional six children whose stutter had begun after Dr. Morley's analysis, but in each case the stuttering had lasted less than a year. In all, therefore, 43 children had been noted to stutter and 9 were noted to still be stuttering when last seen during their 16th year. A schematized diagram of the age of onset and age of recovery is presented as Figure 1-1. This is redrawn from the original source (Andrews, Note 1) and differs in two small ways from that published in Andrews, Harris, Garside and Kay (1964): Cases 1, 2, and 3 are now shown as beginning after their second birthday and Case 42 at Age 6. The order of the cases is unchanged from the original account, although I have deleted the three arbitrary divisions, developmental, benign, and persistent stuttering, into which I had divided the data at that time. When these children were compared to those children in the survey who never stuttered, there were significant associations between stuttering and late onset of speech, articulation disorder, below average intelligence, and an adverse social environment, exactly the same findings as were revealed in our retrospective survey of 9- to 11-year-old school children conducted in the same city at that time (Andrews et al., 1964).

One important issue is whether Cases 1–16, who showed less than a 6-month period of "developmental stuttering, " should be included as stutterers. At that time, as any doctoral student should be, I was unwilling to commit myself. In retrospect, I think they should have been classified as stutterers. First, the diagnoses were made by trained health visitors and were usually verified by speech pathologists as having interference in their fluency, "usually described as stammering or hesitating. " One cannot be certain how diagnostic criteria may have altered over the 15 years, but in 1963, when we began the reanalysis, stuttering was defined by us, in collaboration with Dr. Morley, as an interruption in the normal rhythm of speech in which the stutterer "knows precisely what he wishes to say, but at the time is unable to say it easily because of an involuntary

FIGURE 1-1. The age of onset and duration of stuttering in the 43 children identified as stutterers in a birth-to-15 years prospective population survey.

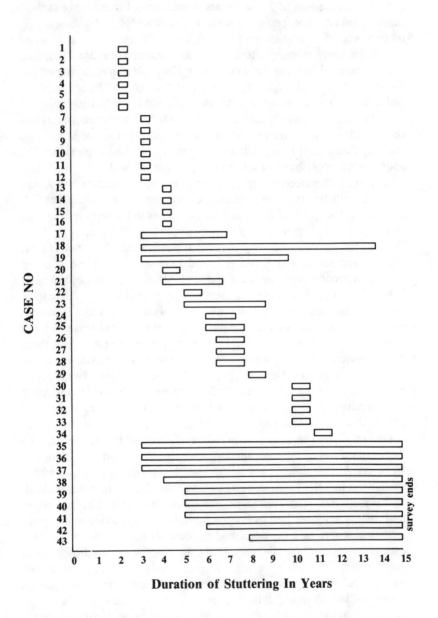

repetition, prolongation or cessation of sound" (Andrews et al., 1964). The health visitors and speech pathologists must have been hearing a great deal of normal nonfluencies in the 900 three-year-olds, but obviously something deviant made them identify these 16 children as stuttering, albeit transiently and mildly. Perkins (1983) has recently discussed this point in detail, highlighting the importance of the involuntary loss of control aspect of the moment of stuttering. Another reason for considering these 16 cases to be stutterers is that, although I divided them into a separate group because of their short duration, I failed to demonstrate the importance of this grouping by showing that they differed from the other stutterers in characteristics such as intelligence, speech development, or social background, characteristics which differentiated the stutterers from the remainder of the children.

If we consider all 43 children to have been stutterers, the following data emerge when Figure 1-1 is analyzed.

Incidence. The risk of beginning to stutter for these children was 12/900 or 1.3% between the 3rd and 4th birthday; 5/847 or 0.6% Age 5, 2/800 or 0.25% while Age 8 and zero from Age 12 and thereafter. The cumulative age of onset curves show that 50% of the risk of ever stuttering was passed between 3 and 4 years old and 75% between 5 and 6 years. The lifetime expectancy of ever stuttering (at least before age 15) was 43/875, based on the median number in the study, or 4.9%.

Prevalence. The proportion of 3-year-old children actually stuttering was 1.3%, of 5-year-olds 1.5%, of 8-year-olds 1.6%, and of 15-year-olds 1.2%.

Duration. As this study ended before the children were 16 we cannot know the precise situation in regard to duration of those still stuttering at that time. In these data, the average child stuttered for less than a year and only one quarter stuttered for longer than 7 years.

Remission. On the basis of the survey data, 34 of the 43 (79%) children stopped stuttering before the age of 16. I would expect that some further remission would be likely in subsequent years. Some of the children who did recover had speech therapy, but so did the children whose stutter persisted, so it is not possible to be certain that any of the remissions were induced by treatment. Nevertheless, given the treatment techniques presently available, if one is forced to select only some children for active treatment, then clearly, preference should be given to those who have stuttered for longer than 1 year, for then only 6/15 or 40% would be expected to recover, while after stuttering for 5 years only 2/11 or 18% would be expected to remit in the absence of effective treatment.

CONCORDANCE WITH OTHER STUDIES

In recent years these issues have been reviewed in three publications (Andrews, Craig, Feyer, Hoddinott, Howie, & Neilson, 1983; Bloodstein, 1981; Van Riper, 1982). The references cited in these publications should be consulted by those interested in the primary sources.

Incidence. There are no other studies that allow calculation of the incidence of new cases at each age, but a number of studies have sought to determine the lifetime incidence. Bloodstein (1981) cites seven studies of populations over the age of 12 who have been asked if they used to, or do presently, stutter. Two studies of high school students returned values of 3.7 and 5.8%. Three studies of university students found values that ranged from 0.93 to 5.5%, and two studies of adults reported values of 4.8 and 5.0%. None of the groups was representative of the general population in terms of age or sex, but the median figure from these studies is in accord with the 1,000-family estimate of the risk of ever stuttering being just less than 5%. It is not a rare condition.

The average stutterer appears to begin to stutter without any obvious cause. It is useful to call this idiopathic stuttering and contrast it to acquired stuttering. Acquired stuttering can begin after brain damage in a previously fluent speaker of any age. The clinical picture can be similar to idiopathic stuttering, although either an age of onset after puberty or history of cerebral insult makes diagnosis relatively simple. Some children probably acquire stuttering because of brain injury at birth, but as it is difficult to be certain in an individual child, such cases may be confused with cases of idiopathic stuttering.

Idiopathic stuttering begins in childhood. To get information about the frequency of onset at various ages, it is necessary either to study a group of children prospectively until an age when the risk of new cases is small, or alternatively, to study a group of older children retrospectively and ascertain the age at which stuttering began. We have used both strategies. The 1,000-family prospective study age of onset data are displayed in Figure 1-2 together with that from a retrospective study of 9- to 11-year-old stutterers in a city school system (Andrews et al., 1964). In the prospective study, onset ranged from 2 to 11 years, 50% beginning before 4 years of age and 75% before 6 years. In the retrospective school survey, onset was reported to have ranged from 2 to 9 years, with 50% beginning before 4 years and 75% by 6 years. Both Bloodstein (1981) and Van Riper (1982) cite studies of mixed age populations (i.e., kindergarten through ninth grade) or clinic populations. Because of selection factors and the presence of young children who may later stutter, neither the percentage of risk passed at each age nor the age of median risk can be calculated. There is need for further

FIGURE 1-2. The age of first beginning to stutter (a) in children detected in a birth-to-15 years prospective population survey and (b) in a school survey of 9- to 11-year-old children whose families were questioned at that time about the onset of the stuttering in Newcastle, England.

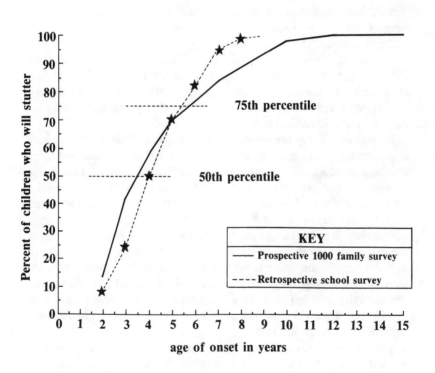

Age of Onset of Stuttering
in Newcastle, England

retrospective studies of the age of onset of a population sample of stutterers obtained from a junior high school system. On the basis of data presently available, half the risk of ever stuttering is passed by Age 4, three quarters by Age 6, and virtually all by Age 12.

Prevalence. There are no studies of the prevalence of stuttering in unselected adult populations. However, there are many accounts of the prevalence of stuttering in school children using both interview and questionnaire methods. Bloodstein (1981) lists 13 studies of U.S. school children and Van Riper (1982) lists two additional studies. The prevalence rates vary widely from 0.30 to 2.12 but 8 of the 15 studies reported prevalence rates between 0.7 and 1.0 with the median prevalence being 0.8%, the value reported by the National Speech and Hearing Survey.

Bloodstein (1981) lists 18 studies of non-U.S. school children and Van Riper (1982) mentions an additional 7 studies. The 25 prevalence figures range from 0.55 to 1.9, and 13 of the studies gave values clustering between 0.9 and 1.3, the median of the 25 values being 1.1%. From inspection of the above figures it seems likely that the foreign surveys did find significantly more stutterers than did the U.S. surveys. The prevalence rates appear to be relatively constant through the elementary school years, then may decline slowly thereafter, presumably because of continuing remission and lack of new cases.

Factors which vary the prevalence of stuttering. This topic is usually discussed from the opposite viewpoint, that is, what attributes are more common in people who stutter (see Andrews et al., 1983). That list is relatively well known, but three conditions affect prevalence considerably. Three times as many boys as girls stutter, and this disproportion increases with age so that the prevalence in elementary school boys is four times higher than in girls. Being a first-degree relative of a stutterer increases the prevalence about threefold, depending on the sex of the stutterer and the sex of the relative, with male relatives of female stutterers showing the highest risk. The prevalence is increased threefold among the mentally retarded, a finding consistent with the observation that a sample of stutterers score half a standard deviation less on intelligence tests than do nonstutterers.

The prevalence differences noted in family history have been used to argue that genetic factors are a major cause of stuttering. The sex difference and intelligence deficit may not be causative factors, but may be evidence of factors that inhibit recovery and, hence, as most recovery occurs in the preschool years, become more obvious among school age stutterers.

Duration. There appear to be no other studies of the duration of stuttering in unselected samples of stutterers. Information about recovery from stuttering would give some clues about its usual duration, especially if recovery occurs in the absence of significant therapy. Recovery as a consequence of therapy is becoming more frequent, but that is not the issue under consideration here. Bloodstein (1981) lists eight studies in which the likelihood of remission was estimated. Van Riper (1982) lists an additional four studies. Remission rates varied from 18 to 80%, the median value being 60%. All these studies are retrospective and could be flawed by problems of selection and by accuracy of recall.

Another way of estimating the likelihood of recovery is to divide the prevalence of stuttering at Age 16 years, say 1%, by the cumulative likelihood of ever having stuttered by that time, say 4.9%, which yields 0.20. The proportion recovering is, therefore, $1 - 0.20$ or .8 or 80%.

A better method of estimating the likelihood of recovery is to identify a group of children who are stuttering and then review them a number of years later to discover how many still stutter. The 1,000-family study did this and 79% were found to have recovered before reaching 16 years of age. There are five other studies (see Andrews et al., 1983) that followed selected groups of children for varying periods of time. When their recovery rates were compared to recovery rates for age-matched children selected from the 1,000-family study, a similar picture emerged. For example, if a study followed children from age 4.2, when they were all stuttering, until they were 6.8 years and found that 54% had recovered, we selected the 13 cases from Figure 1-1 who were stuttering at 4.2 years and asked what proportion had recovered by 6.8 years to find that seven, or 53%, had recovered. On this basis, when comparing the 1,000-family survey with the other five studies, we concluded that the 79% recovery rate by Age 16 was a reasonable estimate.

DEVELOPMENT OF THE SEVERE SYNDROME

Bloodstein (1981), referring to his 1960 review of 418 case histories of persistent stutterers, suggested that it was possible to describe four phases which could act as reference points on the continuum of development from mild to severe stuttering. Obviously, many stutterers remain mildly afflicted all their lives, while a few young stutterers show severe symptoms soon after onset. In my view, the dominant features of the phases in the child who will become severe are as follows: Phase 1 is seen typically in the preschool and kindergarten child. Stuttering is episodic, repetitions predominate, especially at the beginning of a sentence or phrase, and the child is often unconcerned. In Phase 2, the disorder has become chronic, the child considers himself a stutterer, but still seems little concerned, and stuttering is worse when the child is excited or talking fast. The initial repetitions are now often joined by prolongations and tension. In Phase 3, prolongations and cessations of sound now occur frequently. Associated face and body movements now appear. Word fears begin and word avoidance is common, but situation avoidance is rare. Phase 4 is the fully developed pattern seen in adolescents or adults. Tense repetitions, prolongations, and cessations of sound are associated with movements of face or body. Word and situation fears and avoidance are common. The stutterer is constantly preoccupied with his speech problem.

Van Riper (1982) is unhappy with this continuum of development of severity and describes instead a number of tracks along which stutterers can develop. The most common path—Track 1—seems quite consistent with the original Bloodstein data. However, Track 2, which he suggests occurs in children with concurrent language and articulation problems, does appear to be different in that such children begin late and seldom become severe or develop the complicated Phase 3 or 4 symptoms.

In our school survey (Andrews et al., 1964) repetitions were by far the most commonly remembered initial symptom and remained the dominant symptom in the milder cases. The presence of prolongations or cessations of sound were clearly associated with severity, and as predicted by Bloodstein, situation fears were rare among these 10-year-olds. Most of the mild stutterers had had a reasonable period of fluent speech before the onset of stuttering, whereas the one-third who were severe stutterers tended to show an early onset with evidence of articulation problems, a finding contrary to Van Riper's Track 2 concept. Indeed, in the paper by Andrews et al. (1983) we report that despite our ability to apportion the 80 stutterers in the school survey to Van Riper's tracks, we were unable to demonstrate that track membership had any predictive validity with regard to the other variables measured in that survey.

At present I consider idiopathic stuttering to be a homogeneous syndrome in which some children show only repetitions, the symptoms of others vary considerably, and a few, particularly those who have been stuttering for some years, show the full complex of speech symptoms, associated body movements, word and situation avoidances, and a preoccupation with their fate as a stutterer. When this occurs, their education is imperiled and their employability impaired.

CLINICAL IMPLICATIONS

First let us summarize the epidemiological data that we have unearthed and then ask, what are the implications as to cause or for treatment, what are the implications for planning the delivery of speech pathology services, and what are the implications for patient counseling.

Stuttering is a condition which will, at some time, affect about 5% of children. It is particularly common in relatives of stutterers. Most children begin to stutter before they are of school age and virtually none, unless they become brain damaged, begin after puberty. In the majority of cases the stutter will last for less than 1 year and will seldom become a cause for concern; it will persist in only 1% of children. Even so, in many of these persistent stutterers, the stutter will be relatively mild and will not handicap or cause educational or vocational disadvantages. Nevertheless, the life adjustment of about 3 in 1,000 children will be seriously affected by their stuttering.

These epidemiological data have the following implications:

- As the risk of stuttering within families occurs in a way that is not compatible with familial or cultural transmission, it is probable that the condition is controlled by genetic factors.

- If the majority of preschool stutterers is likely to recover within a year, then treatment of most very young stutterers is not likely to be cost effective, and speech-language pathologists should give first priority to treating children whose stutter is persisting. Because the chance of remission is so high, no study claiming to benefit preschool stutterers should be accepted unless it is a randomized controlled trial of treatment compared against a placebo regime.

- If parents of young stutterers are concerned about their child's speech they should be counseled about coping with the child's difficulties and reminded that 60% of children who have stuttered for less than 1 year can be expected to recover without active treatment.

- If only 1% of children become persistent stutterers, and most of these remain mild and do not ask for treatment, then a school speech pathology service should ensure that energetic and effective treatment is offered first to the 3 children in 1,000 who will have a severe and persistent stutter.

- Because of the backlog of untreated cases, clinics that treat adult stutterers should find no difficulty in attracting clients even if only 1 in 1,000 adults want help.

- Information on the natural history of stuttering is of value in counseling parents and stutterers, and for the most part the news will be better than they expected.

- Information on family risks is important, especially for women who stutter, for one in three of their sons is likely to develop stuttering. It is vital to train these women so that, in turn, they can better help their children master fluent speech.

NOTE

[1] Andrews, J. G. *The syndrome of stuttering.* MD thesis, University of Otago, New Zealand, 1964.

REFERENCES

Andrews, G., Craig, A., Feyer, A-M., Hoddinott, S., Howie, P., & Neilson, M. Stuttering: A review of research findings and theories circa 1982. *Journal of Speech and Hearing Disorders,* 1983, *48,* 226–246.

Andrews, G., Harris, M., Garside, R., & Kay, D. The syndrome of stuttering. *Clinics in Developmental Medicine,* 1964, *17,* 1–191.

Bloodstein, O. *A handbook on stuttering.* Chicago, IL: National Easter Seal Society, 1981.

Morley, M. E. *The development and disorders of speech in childhood.* London: Livingstone, 1957.

Perkins, W. Commentary on Andrews et al., Stuttering: A review of research findings and theories circa 1982. *Journal of Speech and Hearing Disorders,* 1983, *48,* 246–249.

Van Riper, C. *The nature of stuttering.* Englewood Cliffs, NJ: Prentice-Hall, 1982.

Chapter 2

Identification of Stuttering and Stutterers

Martin A. Young

Stuttering instances are frequently referred to as perceptual events. This is a condensed way of expressing complex and often controversial ideas. Because all events in nature are one-time unique occurrences, every classification system is arbitrary, including those that observers employ to classify fluency departures as stuttering or normal disfluency and speakers as stutterers or nonstutterers. The uniqueness of all phenomena is not necessarily contrary to the scientist's goal of explaining events through subsumption under general laws. It is taken on faith that certain events are sufficiently similar so that scientific explanation is feasible, for if this were not true then explanation and prediction would be impossible.

There is no test within science which can determine once and for all whether a fluency departure is a stuttering instance or a nonstuttering disfluency. This is true because "stuttering" and "disfluency" are labels used by observers to classify fluency departures, each unique and absolutely distinct from every other one. Moreover, the label *stuttering* generally implies abnormality or undesirability, and this may be more a property of the observer's cognitive status than any particular fluency departure. Fluency departures are not inherently defective or objectionable distinct from an observer's belief that such is the case.

Having said that all fluency departures are unique, that all classification systems are arbitrary, and that stuttering is a component of an observer's cognitive structure, that is, a perceptual event, is not to imply that stuttering exists only in the minds of observers. First, all phenomena studied by science share the features just described. Second, the problem of stuttering does indeed exist insofar as there is any world that exists apart from our mental states. The difficulty here is that perceptible behavioral events are identified and classified only with some effort and often with considerable disagreement, as might be expected when human observers are deployed as detection and measurement devices with nonmetric, multidimensional, intermittent phenomena of relatively brief duration.

The primary task of a science of stuttering is to describe the conditions under which stuttering occurs and to discover the relevant laws of nature which, given the aforementioned antecedent conditions, logically necessitate the occurrence of stuttering. This is a fancy way of verbalizing how science would explain stuttering. Because stuttering is, in large part, a perceptual event, an important component of the scientific study of stuttering is the examination of the situational and cognitive contexts in which these perceptual events (observer judgments) occur. This focus, the subject matter of the chapter, is stated as follows: What are the conditions under which observers detect fluency departures and classify them as instances of stuttering? A closely related but distinct question also considered is: What are the conditions under which observers classify speakers as stutterers?

Table 2-1 lists the research studies to be discussed, organized by type of judgment and by research strategy. As research findings reveal, stuttering and stutterer judgments are clearly distinct for some observers. The two major research strategies, experimental and descriptive, approach problems in different ways and permit different kinds of conclusions. In the experimental method, variables whose effects are studied are under the direct control of the researcher, every attempt being made to exclude or make identical the effects of extraneous or unwanted variables. In the descriptive research strategy, however, investigators do not control variables. Instead, relationships among variables are sought. The experimental strategy is generally more able than the descriptive method to reveal causal connections between variables. In order to gain the needed control, however, investigators must usually conduct experimental studies in laboratory settings with artificially constructed variables. This is thought to limit the potential for generalization. On the other hand, although the descriptive method may examine phenomena in more natural settings, correlations between variables, even of a high magnitude, are not prudently interpreted as representing causal links. Both strategies are appropriate and useful for describing conditions under which fluency departures and speakers are classified as stuttering or stutterers as long as investigators and readers recognize the strengths and limitations of each method.

EXPERIMENTAL STUDIES—JUDGMENTS OF STUTTERING

Disfluency characteristics. In an early, widely cited study by Boehmler (1958), a large number of brief speech samples containing a single

TABLE 2-1. Studies of stuttering and stutterer judgments.

	Stuttering Judgments	Stutterer Judgments

Experimental Research: Conditions Manipulated	Disfluency Characteristics
	  Boehmler, 1958
	  Huffman & Perkins, 1974
	  Hegde & Hartman, 1979a
	  Hegde & Hartman, 1979b
	  Curran & Hood, 1977a
	  Berlin, 1960
	Instructions
	  Williams & Kent, 1958
	  MacDonald & Martin, 1973
	  Curlee, 1981
	  Bar, 1967
	  Sander, 1965
	  Curran & Hood, 1977b
	  Martin & Haroldson, 1981
	Observation Mode
	  Williams et al., 1963
	  Coyle & Mallard, 1979
	  O'Keefe & Kroll, 1980
		Disfluency Characteristics
		  Sander, 1963
		  Huffman & Perkins, 1974
		Instructions
		  Bloodstein & Smith, 1954
		  Sander, 1965
		Observation Mode
		  Wingate, 1977

Descriptive Research: Conditions Observed	Group Membership
	  Tuthill, 1946
	Cognitive Status
	  Sander, 1968
	Attitude
	  Emerick, 1960
		Group Membership
		  Bloodstein et al., 1952
		  Mysak, 1959
		Cognitive Status
		  Sander, 1968
		Fluent Speech
		  Wendahl & Cole, 1961
		  Young, 1964
		  Few & Lingwall, 1972
		Post-treatment Speech
		  Ingham & Packman, 1978
		  Runyan & Adams, 1978
		  Runyan & Adams, 1979
		  Runyan et al., 1982
		  Prosek & Runyan, 1982

disfluency instance had been obtained from stutterers and nonstutterers. After they were rated for severity, samples were discarded for which poor agreement was shown, leaving 300 samples from stutterers and 300 from nonstutterers. Three groups of observers listened to all the samples and noted which samples contained an example of stuttering and which were examples of nonstuttering nonfluencies. These instructions, of course, were likely to convey to the observers that not all instances of disfluency are instances of stuttering, and to the trained observer, at least, that some of the speakers were stutterers. Samples were labeled "stuttering" more often if they were produced by stutterers and were rated as severe. Boehmler's more interesting and widely cited findings were derived from his after-the-fact analysis of the relationship between disfluency types and frequency of stuttering judgments. Sound-syllable instances of disfluency were more likely to be labeled as stuttering while revisions were more likely to be classified as nonstuttering disfluencies. Further analysis showed that the stutterers generated samples of greater severity and also produced more instances of sound-syllable repetitions. Boehmler then showed that the average severity rating for the sound-syllable repetitions was essentially the same as the average rating for all the rest of the samples and concluded that type of disfluency was probably the major factor in eliciting judgments of stuttering instances.

Subsequent investigators refined Boehmler's research strategy in two ways. First, greater control over variables was obtained by having speakers simulate disfluencies. Second, the effects of another variable, frequency of disfluency, were also explored. Huffman and Perkins (1974) considered the effects of three variables on judgments of stuttering. One adult male simulated sound repetitions, prolongations, or hesitations 1, 3, or 5 times in a 50-word passage in an "easy" or "strained" manner. The samples conveyed all possible combinations of these three variables. Observers were asked to judge each passage for "whether or not the speaker stuttered. " What variation there was ranged from 24 (out of a possible 40) judgments of stuttering for one easy hesitation to 39 (of 40) judgments of stuttering for five strained repetitions. With this small range, not many of the differences were significant and what emerged was essentially a pattern. Sound repetitions elicited more stuttering judgments than prolongations and hesitations, and more frequent disfluency instances per sample generated more stuttering judgments than fewer instances.

Frequency of disfluency was also considered in two studies by Hegde and Hartman (1979a, 1979b). They focused on two disfluency types, interjections and word repetitions, which in previous investigations observers tended to label as instances of nonstuttering disfluencies. Hegde and Hartman wished to determine if more frequent instances of these disfluency types would shift observer judgments from disfluent to stuttered. In the first study, a nonstuttering speaker read a passage six times, simulating various frequencies of interjections, and untrained observers judged each sample as fluent, disfluent, or stuttered. The results showed that with increasing frequency of interjections, judgments of fluent decreased and judgments of disfluent and stuttered increased. In Hegde and Hartman's second study, identical procedures were employed except that frequency of word repetitions was varied. The same general pattern of labeling emerged as in the first study. Fluent judgments decreased and disfluent/stuttered judgments increased as the frequency of word repetitions increased. But there were differences in labeling as a function of the two disfluency types. Observers, it would seem, much more readily applied the label stuttering rather than disfluent to word repetitions than to interjections as the frequency of these fluency departures increased. The results of Hegde and Hartman's studies also suggested that considerable disagreement prevailed among observers as to whether samples containing interjections or word repetitions should be labeled as disfluent or stuttered. At all but the lowest frequencies, there were sizable proportions of observers who employed either label for the same stimulus, and at the 5% frequency level, some observers showed even greater disagreement with each other by applying fluent and stuttered to the same samples.

The effects of disfluency type and frequency were explored less directly in other studies, but with essentially the same results. Curran and Hood (1977a) had nonstuttering boys simulate disfluency types, one type per short sentence, and including fluent utterances, constructed a test tape of samples considered to include the most representative examples of each disfluency type. The observers were parents of stutterers, parents of nonstutterers, school teachers, and clinicians. The samples containing double unit part-word and word repetitions were more likely to be labeled as stuttering than as normal disfluencies.

In an earlier study, Berlin (1960) constructed passages which differed in the frequency level of a variety of disfluency types. These samples were generated by third-grade children (nonstutterers) who simulated the disfluency types and frequencies. The observers were parents of stutterers, children with other speech problems, and children without speech problems. The passage was played to the observers twice. On the first occasion, observers responded to the question: If this were your 2- to 5-year-old child, would you be concerned, and if so, why? During the second playing of the samples, the question was: If this were your 2- to 5-year-old child, would you say that he stuttered? The second question elicited more judgments of stuttering than the first, and the proportion of parents in all three groups using the label of stuttering in answer to both questions increased directly as a function of increased frequency of disfluency.

Instructions.   Another group of studies focused on the cognitive status of observers as determined by instructions. In several studies, observers have been asked to detect fluency departures and label them as either stuttering or normal disfluency. The goal of these studies has been to learn to what degree observers are consistent in their identifications, as well as to study the effects of the order of instructions on the level of marking. In an often cited study by Williams and Kent (1958), a nonstuttering speaker simulated different types of fluency departures in a 900-word speech. Untrained observers, provided with transcripts of the speech and told that the speaker stuttered, marked words and spaces between words three times. Half of the observers were instructed to mark all stuttered interruptions, then all interruptions, and then all normal interruptions. The other half of the observers made their judgments in the reverse order. Although the results showed observers marked more of what they were instructed to mark first, this bias occurred only for word and phrase repetitions and interjections. Single- and multiple-unit syllable repetitions and prolongations were identified more often as stuttered than as normal interruptions, no matter what the order of instructions, and revisions were more likely to be judged as normal interruptions, independent of order of instructions.

The effect of order of instruction on consistency of stuttering and disfluency judgments was also examined by MacDonald and Martin (1973). Stuttering speakers each contributed brief videotaped samples of spontaneous speech. The observers were given transcripts on which words and spaces between words were separated by diagonal lines, and were instructed to mark either instances of stuttering or disfluencies. The investigators made it very clear through the instructions and by example that a word or space could be marked as an instance of stuttering, as a disfluency, or as *both* at the same time. Unfortunately, the judgments on each trial were not independent, since the same transcript was used for both trials. While the overall trend was for observers to mark more of what they were instructed to mark first, the only significant difference between the groups was that the group who marked stuttering first marked more items as stuttering (only) than the group who marked disfluencies first. A large proportion of the items marked by both groups was unambiguous, that is, not marked as both stuttering and disfluent. Item-by-item agreement, however, was quite low for both stuttering and disfluency judgments. In MacDonald and Martin's terminology, an ambiguous application of the terms stuttering and disfluency existed when a unit or item was identified as both. Low unit-by-unit agreement, however, implies that many items were marked by one or only a few observers, so their general conclusion of minimal ambiguity may reflect, in part, only poor observer agreement.

In Curlee's replication of the MacDonald and Martin study (Curlee, 1981), observers marked words and spaces between words as stuttered or disfluent on separate transcripts to increase independence of judgments. In addition, Curlee studied the effect on labeling (a) of defining stuttering for the observers as compared to no definition, (b) of the order with which stuttering/disfluency judgments were made, and (c) of observer–group differences—undergraduate–trained as compared to graduate–trained. None of these variables revealed statistically significant differences in mean frequency of judgments of stuttering or disfluency. In addition, inter- and intraobserver unit-by-unit agreement for all conditions for the judgments of both stuttering and disfluency was uniformly quite low. Contrary to MacDonald and Martin's findings, Curlee reported that a majority of the marked items were marked as instances of both stuttering and disfluency.

The effects of differing instructions on the detection and classification of fluency departures was the subject matter of four additional studies. Bar (1967) had observers estimate the percentage of stuttering in a 154-word passage read by a single severe stutterer under two instructions: Listen to the content of the speech or listen to the manner of speaking. The difference between the mean estimates was not significant. In a somewhat more elaborate study, Sander (1965) randomly assigned untrained observers, mothers in a supermarket, to one of three prelistening instructions. Each heard only one sample, a 6-year-old boy simulating instances of single-unit syllable repetition in a 100-word speech. In the recall condition, the observers were asked to listen to what the child was saying. In the control condition, they were merely asked to listen, while in the stuttering condition the observers were asked to pay close attention to the way the child was talking. Sander asked the observers if they felt the child was stuttering. For the 40 observers in each condition, the number of stuttering judgments were 16, 21, and 29 for the recall, control and stuttering conditions, respectively, supporting Sander's belief in the bias created by the perceptual set to hear speech errors, presumably determined by the prelistening conditions.

Curran and Hood (1977b) attempted to influence the cognitive status of observers through three sets of instructions dealing with the presumed status of the speakers. A test tape was prepared by having nonstuttering boys simulate a variety of disfluency types. Observers were randomly divided among three instruction conditions, differing with respect to the presumed status of the speakers: (a) Children may or may not be stutterers, (b) children are being seen for stuttering therapy, and (c) children have successfully completed stuttering therapy. The three sets of instructions did not generate different severity categorizations of the samples.

Most studies report low unit-by-unit inter- and intraobserver agreement for the identification of stuttering instances. Some writers (Wingate, 1977; Adams, 1976) have suggested that observer agreement would improve if they were asked to mark experimenter-defined specific behaviors rather than use idiosyncratic criteria for stuttering instances. To test this assumption, Martin and Haroldson (1981) played brief samples of the spontaneous speech of stutterers to untrained observers. A no-definition group was told to underline words using their own individual definition of stuttering, while the definition group also underlined stuttered words but was provided with a behavioral definition of stuttering. A small but statistically significant difference in average words marked as stuttering instances favored the stuttering-defined condition. With respect to unit-by-unit agreement, two different measures of interobserver agreement revealed, first, low agreement for both conditions, and second, statistically significant lower agreement for the stuttering-defined condition. Repeating the study with the same observers, Martin and Haroldson reported low intraobserver agreement for both conditions, and, not unexpectedly, statistically significant lower self-agreement for the stuttering-defined condition. These results are slightly discrepant from those of Young (1975). Young had observers mark stuttering instances on transcripts, supplying the observers with a behavioral definition of stuttering. Young found unit-by-unit interobserver agreement indexes of the same general magnitude as Martin and Haroldson, although contrary to their results, Young found more stuttering instances marked under the stuttering undefined condition.

Observation mode. Because some behaviors associated with the problem of stuttering are visible but not audible, investigators have suggested that detection of stuttering instances should be made under conditions in which observers can view as well as listen to the speaker. To test this assumption, Williams, Wark, and Minifie (1963) filmed the spontaneous speech of stutterers. The test film was shown to observers in three observation modes: audio alone, visual alone, and audiovisual combined. Analysis of the average number of stuttering instances tallied under each condition revealed essentially identical mean tallies for the audio alone and the audiovisual conditions, with a lower mean tally for the visual alone condition.

Good agreement among observers for marking total instances of stuttering is not uncommon in most studies. Unit-by-unit agreement is another matter. Coyle and Mallard (1979) played videotaped samples of the reading of stutterers to observers with audio alone and audiovisual combined. Average indexes for unit-by-unit interobserver agreement were of the same low magnitude as found in earlier studies and were essentially identical for both observation modes.

Another observation mode whose effects were examined was time expansion, in which the rate of speech was slowed down electronically without changing the pitch. O'Keefe and Kroll (1980) had a nonstutterer generate samples with simulated stuttering in order to control for total words, total stuttering instances, and total number of disfluencies of various types. Trained observers analyzed the samples under two observation modes: normal and with the rate of speech slowed 67%. A comparison of the effects of normal and time-expanded modes showed no difference in average total stuttering instances. It is a provocative finding that when we know exactly how much stuttering there was, because instances were simulated, a significant number of observers regularly identified more stuttering instances and more instances of specific disfluency types than were actually recorded.

EXPERIMENTAL STUDIES—JUDGMENT OF STUTTERER

Disfluency characteristics. Sander (1963) prepared a test tape on which a nonstuttering adult recorded samples differing with respect to frequency of syllable repetition and severity, that is, single- or double-unit repetitions. Each sample was evaluated by a different group of untrained observers, eliminating the need for prelistening instructions. Three questions were asked after each observer listened individually to a sample: (a) Describe the speech you just heard; (b) did you consider his speech defective? and (c) would you classify him as a stutterer? Plots of stutterer judgments as a function of repetition instances showed increasing stutterer judgments with increasing instances, and double-unit repetitions elicited about two times as many stutterer judgments as single-unit repetitions. For the higher frequency levels of both single- and double-unit repetitions, the majority of observers were willing to classify the speaker as a stutterer.

Replicating and elaborating Sander's study, Huffman and Perkins (1974) also asked observers whether a speaker was a stutterer in response to samples on which a speaker simulated three disfluency types, three disfluency frequencies, and two manners of production. Not unexpectedly, repetitions generated more stutterer responses than prolongations and hesitations, while the higher disfluency frequencies also elicited more stutterer judgments. There was a somewhat smaller number of stutterer than stuttering judgments, and from an analysis of individual judgments the authors note that there were a number of observers who classified samples as stuttering but not stutterer.

Instructions to observers. Theories of stuttering have often included attempts to explain the sex ratio. One such approach postulates that boys, although less fluent than girls, are subjected to unrealistically high standards of performance in our society, especially in speech fluency. To test this proposition, Bloodstein and Smith (1954) attempted to influence observers to believe that some speakers were boys and some girls and then examined the frequency with which the speakers were classified as stutterers. The results showed no difference in frequency of stutterer judgments as a function of presumed sex status, and male observers made significantly more stutterer judgments than the female observers.

As a portion of a study already described (Sander, 1965), mothers had been randomly assigned to one of three prelistening conditions. In addition to asking the mothers if they felt the child was stuttering, Sander also asked if they felt the child was a stutterer. There were more than twice as many stutterer judgments for the stuttering condition as for the recall condition, and in all three conditions, there were more stuttering than stutterer judgments.

Observation mode. Wingate (1977) had trained observers make stutterer/nonstutterer judgments under three observation modes: (a) lexical—a transcription containing all the complete words spoken; (b) complete—a transcription which included all words, word segments, sounds, and dashes to indicate silent intervals; and (c) audio—a tape recording. The speakers were stutterers and nonstutterers who generated spontaneous speech in response to a picture. Very few observers were uncertain of their judgments and were, as a group, largely accurate in their labeling. The average number of correct identifications under the lexical, complete and audio conditions was, respectively, 21.1, 25.4, and 27.5 (out of 32).

DESCRIPTIVE STUDIES—JUDGMENT OF STUTTERING

Tuthill's study (1946) is usually cited as the earliest to examine the perceptual aspects of the problem of stuttering. The speaking and reading of stutterers and nonstutterers constituted the sample for evaluation. In the first of three studies, stutterers, trained observers, and untrained observers were asked to follow a transcript and mark the places (sounds) where stuttering occurred. The observers were not told the identification of the speakers. In the second study, the observers were "experts, " janitors, and mothers carrying out essentially the same marking procedures. In the third study, a sound motion picture was made of stutterers and nonstutterers speaking extemporaneously, and observers were asked to push a button to indicate occurrences of stuttering. Tuthill's first study showed a wide variation in the frequency of marking for all three observer groups, with untrained observers marking considerably fewer instances of stuttering than the other two groups. All three groups demonstrated about the same average low magnitude of unit-by-unit intraobserver agreement. In the second study, unit-by-unit interobserver agreement indexes were of the same general magnitude for the three groups, but "experts" marked more instances of stuttering than mothers, who marked more than janitors. In the third study, the addition of visual information for the observers did not change the number of stuttering instances marked or the indexes of agreement.

Sander (1968) studied the degree to which mothers' stuttering/stutterer judgments were associated with their reported attributions and action tendencies. Mothers listened to a sample of a mildly stuttering boy while looking at a photo of a child and his mother. The observers were then asked labeling and attribution questions. The responses to the labeling question divided the observers into three labeling categories: not stuttering/not stutterer, stuttering/not stutterer, and stuttering/stutterer. Membership in the labeling groups was significantly related to some attributions and action tendencies.

As we have seen, a specific fluency departure can be labeled as an instance of stuttering, or an observer can note the location of stuttering instances, whether the speaker stuttered, whether the sample represented stuttering, or, as in the last study in this group, can merely tally the number of stuttering instances. Emerick (1960) asked elementary school teachers to listen to a short recording of a stutterer's reading and count instances of stuttering. The tallies ranged from 8 to 87. In addition to categorizing each observer as above or below the group's median number of tallied stuttering instances, Emerick also categorized each observer into one of three levels of attitude toward stuttering, and into a sophisticated group (one or more courses in speech pathology) or an unsophisticated group. Although the relationships between pairs of these categorical variables were all significant, the associations were small in magnitude. Coursework in speech pathology was positively associated with a better attitude toward stuttering and a higher tally of stuttering instances. A better attitude toward stuttering was positively related to a higher frequency count of stuttering instances.

DESCRIPTIVE STUDIES—JUDGMENT OF STUTTERER

An often cited study by Bloodstein, Jaeger, and Tureen (1952) was designed to be a partial test of one element of the diagnosogenic theory of the onset of stuttering: the presumed extrareadiness of parents of stutterers to make judgments of stutterer. The observers in this study were parents of stutterers and nonstutterers who listened to samples of young stutterers and nonstutterers and then noted if the child was a stutterer or a normal speaker. The results showed that parents of stutterers made significantly more judgments of stutterer, on the average, than the parents of nonstutterers. Since this was a correlational study between group membership (parents of stutterers and nonstutterers) and number of stutterer judgments, it is appropriate to note that group membership accounted for only 19% of the variation in the number of stutterer judgments.

A concern with possible sex differences in fluency standards led Mysak (1959) to examine the relationship between teenage observers' sex status and number of stutterer judgments. Nonstuttering children generated brief samples of spontaneous speech. The observers were girls and two groups of boys whose average ages were 13.7, 13.8, and 15.6 years, respectively. The difference in average number of stutterer judgments between the younger males and females was small but significant (5%), but only 6% of the variation of number of stutterer judgments was explained by knowledge of the observer's sex status.

In a study already discussed (Sander, 1968), mothers were classified in three judgment groups (stuttering/stutterer, stuttering/nonstutterer and nonstuttering/nonstutterer) on the basis of their response to a single sample. The relation between membership in these three groups and certain attributions and action tendencies was examined. Contrasting the stuttering/stutterer group to the other two groups, the mothers who used the stutterer label more frequently assented to the attributions of "perceives difficulty" and "emotional disturbance. " They were also more likely to "express alarm" and "seek help, " but not more likely to "correct at home. "

That stuttering instances in the speech flow, so-called moments of stuttering, are embedded in essentially normal speech has been an important theoretical and therapeutic belief. Some writers, notably Williams (1957), have called attention to behaviors stutterers perform prior to moments of stuttering, and as a response to this suggestion, Wendahl and Cole (1961) decided to determine to what degree observers could differentiate between stutterers and nonstutterers on the basis of samples from which "overt behavioral units ordinarily considered to represent moments of stuttering had been. . .deleted. " In their study, stutterers were matched on the basis of reading ability with nonstutterers. Disfluencies were edited out and replaced by pauses. For each matched nonstutterer, the same edited sentences were available, creating a test tape of sentence pairs. Untrained observers were given the option of labeling each sentence pair as nonstutterer/nonstutterer, stutterer/stutterer, stutterer/nonstutterer or nonstutterer/stutterer. In every case, the stutterer in each speaker pair received more stutterer judgments than the matched nonstutterer. Indeed, ranking the 16 speakers on the basis of total number of stutterer judgments produced only a single misclassification, one nonstutterer.

Young (1964) replicated Wendahl and Cole's study, using their test tape, because their tape had all samples from each speaker pair in consecutive order, ruling out any assumption of independent judgments. In this replication, therefore, trained observers made the same kind of judgment as in the earlier study but did so only after listening to all sentences from each speaker pair. Young reasoned that because one speaker gets more stutterer judgments than another speaker does not mean that the first speaker is correctly identified as a stutterer. The majority of observers may consider both speakers to be nonstutterers, as was true for many of Wendahl and Cole's samples. Using this mode of analysis, Young's results showed that only two stutterers were correctly identified, and one nonstutterer was incorrectly labeled better than chance as a stutterer. Two stutterers were labeled as nonstutterers along with six nonstutterers. The rest of the speakers fell in the uncertainty range where the observers' judgments did not sufficiently deviate from chance or guessing.

These two conflicting modes of analysis are reflected again in a study by Few and Lingwall (1972). Samples of spontaneous speech were obtained from stutterers and nonstutterers. The experimenters selected a brief speech segment from each speaker which was judged to be fluent. Observers were told that some speakers were stutterers and some were nonstutterers and were asked to check which were which. They made about three times as many nonstutterer as stutterer judgments, and for only one stutterer did the number of stutterer judgments exceed chance. Yet a different analytical model would reach alternate conclusions. Assuming that each observer's judgments were independent of one another, we can categorize all the judgments in a 2-by-2 contingency table of actual and judged categories. The small ($r\phi$ = .15) but significant correlation (1%) portrayed by this contingency table indicates that the observers gave more stutterer judgments to stutterers and nonstutterer judgments to nonstutterers than would be expected by chance. Although Few and Lingwall's results are usually cited as evidence contrary to the hypothesis that observers can identify stutterers on the basis of their fluent speech, the interpretation presented here does reach the opposite conclusion.

The remainder of the descriptive studies dealing with the judgment of stutterer focus on whether observers can differentiate between stutterers and nonstutterers on the basis of the stutterers' fluent post-treatment speech. The emphasis on post-treatment speech performance comes about because there are many therapies which employ modified rate or rhythm or prolonged speech to achieve speech from which stuttering instances are absent. Clinical researchers are interested in discovering to what degree such fluent speech is perceived by observers as being normal.

Ingham and Packman (1978) obtained samples from stutterers who had completed prolonged speech and rate control therapy and were judged by clinicians to be "stutter-free." Samples from nonstutterers were matched to those of the stutterers. Observers made a variety of judgments after listening to each sample, including a decision as to which speakers were stutterers and which were normal. The nonstutterers received more judgments of normal than the stutterers, but not a single stutterer was correctly identified beyond chance (5%). The reader is again faced with deciding what interpretation is to be placed on the finding that a stutterer may accrue more stutterer judgments than a nonstutterer, but the majority of observers consider both to be normal speakers, or cannot identify the stutterers correctly better than chance.

Identification of stutterers from their post-treatment speech was examined by Runyan and colleagues in four related studies (Runyan & Adams, 1978, 1979; Runyan, Hames, & Prosek, 1982; Prosek & Runyan, 1982). The stimulus tape was constructed from samples sent by proponents of various therapy strategies of their "successfully treated" stutterers. From these samples, and from those of nonstutterers, the experimenters deleted all overt stuttering, long pauses, and other likely clues to the speakers' classification. In their first study (Runyan & Adams, 1978), observers were told that each speaker pair contained one stutterer who had completed therapy and whose speech was free of disfluencies. The stutterers were identified at greater than chance levels, and the correct identification rate was related to reported initial (pretreatment) severity. In the next study (Runyan & Adams, 1979), the procedure was repeated with untrained observers, and the judgments of stutterer were evaluated separately for each of the therapy type groups. In five of the seven therapy type groups, stutterers received more stutterer judgments than would be expected by chance.

Using the same samples as in the previous two studies, Runyan et al. (1982) compared single- and paired-stimulus methods of identifying stutterers from their fluent post-treatment speech. Observers who served in both listening tasks were asked which member of each pair was a stutterer or whether the samples were produced by stutterers or normal speakers. For the paired-stimulus method, the overall correct rate was 68.1%. For the single-stimulus method, using the same analytic model as was suggested in Few and Lingwall's study, the correlation between the actual and judged classification was $r\emptyset = .26$ (1%). As in the earlier study of Few and Lingwall, a small but significant relationship indicated that observers generated more stutterer judgments for stutterers than for nonstutterers than would be expected by chance.

Prosek and Runyan (1982) treated correct identification of stutterers from their fluent post-treatment speech as a continuous variable and related it to four dimensions that observers might employ to make their classifications: (a) number of syllables per second; (b) number of pauses 100 msec or longer; (c) average pause duration; and (d) average duration of stressed vowels. The variables of syllable rate and number of pauses accounted for 71% of the variation in percent correct identification scores, and the addition of the other two independent variables did not significantly increase the predictive potential. Syllable rate alone explained 65% of the variation.

SUMMARY

A variety of factors can be identified which influence observers' detection and identification of stuttering instances and classification of speakers as stutterers. Disfluency type, frequency, and severity are among the important determinants of whether instances of fluency departures and passages containing fluency departures are more likely to be labeled as instances of stuttering or as stuttered. This applies whether fluency departures are spoken by stutterers, are simulated by nonstutterers to represent stuttering, or are normal disfluencies performed by nonstutterers. Sound, syllable, and part-word repetitions, and to a lesser extent prolongations, are those disfluency types which observers are likely to classify as stuttering instances, or when appearing in extended samples, as representing stuttering. Extended passages containing other disfluency types, especially interjections and word repetitions, may also be classified as stuttering if these occur with sufficient frequency. In addition, severity of individual instances, often represented by repetitions within single disfluency units, contributes to stuttering judgments in a like manner. Type, frequency, and severity of disfluency influence observers' classification of speakers as stutterers in essentially the same way. Untrained observers, however, make a clear distinction between stuttering and stutterers, using the former classification more frequently than the latter label, and believe that an individual can stutter without also being a stutterer. The cognitive status of observers is influenced by prelistening instructions. Observers are more likely to detect stuttering instances and identify speakers as stutterers if their attention is directed toward making these judgments by prelistening instructions than if they are asked first to identify nonstuttered or normal fluency departures or if their attention is directed toward the content of the speaker's talk. Some disfluency types, such as word and phrase repetitions and interjections, are particularly susceptible to such biasing influences. Agreement among observers for identifying stuttering instances, or for consistently differentiating stuttering instances from normal disfluencies, is very low. The same pattern of poor agreement holds for individual observers on repeated trials. Measures of inter- and intraobserver agreement do not increase in magnitude when observers are presented with behavioral definitions of stuttering, with visual as well as auditory information, or when the rate of speech has been electronically slowed. Moreover, these different observation modes do not increase the frequency with which stuttering instances are detected, although this finding may not apply to individual stutterers.

Observers show wide differences in their frequency counts of stuttering instances and in the frequency with which speakers are classified as stutterers. Some of these variations are associated with membership in groups, such as being a trained rather than an untrained observer, a parent of a stutterer rather than a nonstutterer, or a male rather than a female. Group membership is not related to measures of inter- and intraobserver agreement. Some observers can correctly identify some stutterers on the basis of speech from which disfluencies have been edited out or on the basis of presumed fluent post-treatment speech. Correct identifications are associated with rate and pause pattern differences between stutterers and nonstutterers.

The ultimate detection and measurement instrument for stuttering and stutterers is a human observer, as it should be, since "stuttering" and "stutterers" represent human judgments. All other tools of measurement, both acoustical and physiological, eventually must be validated against the judgments of human observers. Because observers are influenced by a variety of extraneous factors and inescapable biases, progress in understanding the problem of stuttering necessarily depends upon our skillful use of observers to generate the data which our research endeavors require.

REFERENCES

Adams, M.R. Some common problems in the design and conduct of experiments in stuttering. *Journal of Speech and Hearing Disorders*, 1976, *41*, 3-9.

Bar, A. Effects of listening instructions on attention to manner and content of stutterers' speech. *Journal of Speech and Hearing Research*, 1967, *10*, 87–92.

Berlin, C.I. Parents' diagnoses of stuttering. *Journal of Speech and Hearing Research*, 1960, *3*, 372–379.

Bloodstein, O., Jaeger, W., & Tureen, J. A study of the diagnosis of stuttering by parents of stutterers and nonstutterers. *Journal of Speech and Hearing Disorders*, 1952, *17*, 308–315.

Bloodstein, O., & Smith, S.M. A study of the diagnosis of stuttering with special reference to the sex ratio. *Journal of Speech and Hearing Disorders*, 1954, *19*, 459–466.

Boehmler, R.M. Listener responses to non-fluencies. *Journal of Speech and Hearing Research*, 1958, *1*, 132–141.

Coyle, M.M., & Mallard, A.R. Word-by-word analysis of observer agreement utilizing audio and audiovisual techniques. *Journal of Fluency Disorders*, 1979, *4*, 23–28.

Curlee, R.F. Observer agreement on disfluency and stuttering. *Journal of Speech and Hearing Research*, 1981, *24*, 595–600.

Curran, M.F., & Hood, S.B. Listener ratings of severity for specific disfluency types in children. *Journal of Fluency Disorders*, 1977, *2*, 87–97. (a)

Curran, M.F., & Hood, S.B. The effect of instructional bias on listener ratings of specific disfluency types in children. *Journal of Fluency Disorders*, 1977, *2*, 99–107. (b)

Emerick, L.L. Extensional definition and attitude toward stuttering. *Journal of Speech and Hearing Research*, 1960, *3*, 181–186.

Few, L.R., & Lingwall, J.B. A further analysis of fluency within stuttered speech. *Journal of Speech and Hearing Research*, 1972, *15*, 356–363.

Hegde, M.N., & Hartman, D.E. Factors affecting judgments of fluency: I. Interjections. *Journal of Fluency Disorders*, 1979, *4*, 1–11. (a)

Hegde, M.N., & Hartman, D.E. Factors affecting judgments of fluency: II. Word repetitions. *Journal of Fluency Disorders*, 1979, *4*, 13–22. (b)

Huffman, E.S., & Perkins, W.H. Dysfluency characteristics identified by listeners as "stuttering" and "stutterer. " *Journal of Communication Disorders*, 1974, *7*, 89–96.

Ingham, R.J., & Packman, A.C. Perceptual assessment of normalcy of speech following stuttering therapy. *Journal of Speech and Hearing Research*, 1978, *21*, 63–73.

Johnson, W. Measurements of oral reading and speaking rate and disfluency of adult male and female stutterers and nonstutterers. *Journal of Speech and Hearing Disorders*, Monograph Supplement 7, 1961, 1–20.

MacDonald, J.D., & Martin, R.R. Stuttering and disfluency as two reliable and unambiguous response classes. *Journal of Speech and Hearing Research*, 1973, *16*, 691–699.

Martin, R.R., & Haroldson, S.K. Stuttering identification: Standard definition and moment of stuttering. *Journal of Speech and Hearing Research*, 1981, *24*, 59–63.

Mysak, E.D. Diagnoses of stuttering as made by adolescent boys and girls. *Journal of Speech and Hearing Disorders*, 1959, *24*, 29–33.

O'Keefe, B.M., & Kroll, R.M. Clinician's molar and molecular stuttering analyses of expanded and nonexpanded speech. *Journal of Fluency Disorders*, 1980, *5*, 43–54.

Prosek, R.A., & Runyan, C.M. Temporal characteristics related to the discrimination of stutterers' and nonstutterers' speech samples. *Journal of Speech and Hearing Research*, 1982, *25*, 29–33.

Runyan, C.M., & Adams, M.R. Perceptual study of the speech of 'successfully therapeutized' stutterers. *Journal of Fluency Disorders*, 1978, *3*, 25–39.

Runyan, C.M., & Adams, M.R. Unsophisticated judges' perceptual evaluation of 'successfully treated' stutterers. *Journal of Fluency Disorders*, 1979, *4*, 29–38.

Runyan, C.M., Hames, P.E., & Prosek, R.A. A perceptual comparison between paired stimulus and single stimulus methods of presentation of the fluent utterances of stutterers. *Journal of Fluency Disorders*, 1982, *7*, 71–77.

Sander, E.K. Frequency of syllable repetition and 'stutterer' judgments. *Journal of Speech and Hearing Disorders*, 1963, *28*, 19–30.

Sander, E.K. Comments on investigating listener reaction to speech disfluency. *Journal of Speech and Hearing Disorders*, 1965, *30*, 159–165.

Sander, E.K. Interrelations among the responses of mothers to a child's disfluencies. *Speech Monographs*, 1968, *35*, 187–195.

Tuthill, C.E. A quantitative study of extensional meaning with special reference to stuttering. *Speech Monographs*, 1946, *13*, 81–98.

Wendahl, R.W., & Cole, J. Identification of stuttering during relatively fluent speech. *Journal of Speech and Hearing Research*, 1961, *3*, 281–286.

Williams, D.E. A point of view about 'stuttering'. *Journal of Speech and Hearing Disorders*, 1957, *22*, 390–397.

Williams, D.E., & Kent, L.R. Listener evaluations of speech interruptions. *Journal of Speech and Hearing Research*, 1958, *1*, 124–131.

Williams, D.E., Wark, M., & Minifie, F.D. Ratings of stuttering by audio, visual, and audiovisual cues. *Journal of Speech and Hearing Research*, 1963, *6*, 91–100.

Wingate, M.E. Criteria for stuttering. *Journal of Speech and Hearing Research*, 1977, *20*, 596–607.

Young, M.A. Identification of stutterers from recorded samples of their 'fluent' speech. *Journal of Speech and Hearing Research*, 1964, *7*, 302–303.

Young, M.A. Observer agreement for marking moments of stuttering. *Journal of Speech and Hearing Research*, 1975, *18*, 530–540.

Chapter 3

Stuttering Secondary to Nervous System Damage

John C. Rosenbek

Stutter-like speech disruption subsequent to nervous system damage, which Canter (1971) called neurogenic stuttering, is in speech pathology's penumbra. This chapter's content will neither shift the light so as to better illuminate the topic nor define and describe the disorder (assuming it is only one disorder) so as to move it closer to the light. Instead this chapter's purposes are much less grand. They are to (1) summarize and evaluate what is known about neurogenic stuttering in adults so that clinicians will not start when they catch a glimpse of it in their next patient's symptomatology, (2) compare neurogenic stuttering to developmental stuttering, and (3) help light the way for systematic research so that subsequent reviews can begin more confidently.

PROBLEMS OF DEFINITION

Neurogenic stuttering has not been specifically defined. Helm, Butler, and Benson (1978) begin their discussion of "acquired stuttering" by quoting Espir and Rose's (1970) definition of stammering.[1] "Stammering is a deviation of speech which attracts attention or affects adversely the speaker or listener because of an interruption in the normal rhythm of speech by involuntary repetition, prolongation or arrest of sounds" (p. 122). And it was evidence of such interruptions of rhythm that they used as their criterion for selecting brain-damaged stutterers for study. Rosenbek, Messert, Collins, and Wertz (1978) based their subject selection and analysis of "cortical stuttering" on Wingate's (1964) definition which highlights a variety of kernel, accessory, and associated features of stuttering and of the stutterer. Many other authors have either ignored definitions altogether or have been content with some unadorned statement about sound, syllable, and word repetitions subsequent to brain damage.

That we have had to borrow definitions from developmental stuttering creates problems for clinicians and researchers. Foremost among these is that patients labeled as neurogenic stutterers may share only a few, perhaps insignificant, characteristics—sound and syllable repetitions, for example—and be dissimilar in many significant ways. Another problem is that some patients so labeled may merely be trying to self-correct motor or linguistic errors. A third problem is that we may be ignoring the presence of distinct subgroups of neurogenic stutterers. Patients with stuttering secondary to subcortical damage may be different from stutterers with cortical damage, for example.

Despite such problems, probably the majority of clinicians working with brain-damaged men and women have seen the condition in some percentage—perhaps small—of their patients. Some of these clinicians have published their observations so that a modest literature on neurogenic stuttering is available. The rest of this chapter is a summary and evaluation of that work.

CHARACTERISTICS OF NEUROGENIC STUTTERING

Canter (1971) appears to have developed the most complete list of neurogenic stuttering's characteristics. He says (1) disfluencies such as repetitions occur on final syllables as well as on initial ones, (2) phonemes on which stuttering occurs include /s/, /l/, and /h/ and are different from the phonemes that attract traditional stuttering, (3) disfluency is not related systematically to "grammatical function," (4) there may be an inverse relationship of propositionality and disfluency (5) neurogenic stuttering does not show the adaptation effect, and (6) accessory or secondary features are not present. Unfortunately, his observations are not supported by data, but like other seminal efforts they have spurred others to collect data.

Rosenbek et al. (1978) studied the spontaneous and imitative speech of seven patients selected as neurogenic stutterers because "repetitions appeared in their speech subsequent to brain damage" (p. 82). These authors counted the number of sound–syllable, monosyllabic word, polysyllabic word, and phrase repetitions and the number of audible prolongations. They did not count silent repetitions or prolongations, even though Wingate (1964) considers these to be among developmental stuttering's "kernel features." They did note the location of sound–syllable repetitions, whether in word-initial, medial, or final position and the presence of what Wingate (1964) calls accessory features, such as grimacing. Sound–syllable repetitions were the most frequent type of disfluency for six of these seven patients. The one exception had more monosyllabic word repetitions than sound–syllable repetitions. While the majority of repetitions occurred in the initial position, six of the seven repeated medial sounds or syllables as well. This characteristic was especially prominent for the more severely involved speakers. No word-final, sound–syllable repetitions were noted. Five of the seven exhibited some accessory features such as grimacing. Three patients were more disfluent in spontaneous speech; two were more disfluent on imitative tasks; and two showed similar difficulty on both kinds of tasks. Canter's hypotheses about loci of stuttering and absence of "secondary features" were not confirmed.

Caplan (1972) studied five persons who had "predominately expressive" aphasia and who manifested "some degree of non-fluency in their speech" (p. 54), according to their clinicians. As a way of classifying their disfluencies, Caplan used Johnson's (1961) categories: interjections; part-word, word, and phrase repetitions; revisions; incomplete phrases; broken words; and prolonged sounds. To elicit speech for evaluation, he used a spontaneous speech task, a propositional speech sample, and an adaptation measure.

He found more disfluencies on "function" words such as prepositions than on "lexical" words such as nouns and verbs. This observation lends support to Canter's (1971) hypothesis about the relationship of grammaticality and locus of disfluency. Certainly the more lexical items were not more frequently stuttered, as is the case with developmental stutterers. Other of Canter's hypotheses are not supported. Caplan found no systematic "phonetic factor" because each patient seemed to be idiosyncratic. Neither did he find a trend in the data on stuttering and propositionality, nor could Rosenbek et al. (1978). The data on adaptation are equivocal. Caplan's five neurogenic stutterers adapted in one condition and got worse in another. Given the Rosenbek et al. and Caplan data, the most that can be said is that Canter may be correct for some neurogenic stutterers but not for the population as a whole.

TYPES OF NEUROGENIC STUTTERING

Neurogenic stuttering, like headache and body type, may not come in a single form. Canter (1971) has identified three general types: dysarthric, dyspraxic, and dysnomic and provides several subtypes of dysarthric stuttering.

Dysarthric stuttering

Dysarthria refers to a group of motor speech disorders (Darley, Aronson, & Brown, 1975) resulting from damage to the central or peripheral nervous systems. A number of conditions such as Parkinson's disease, stroke, multiple sclerosis, myasthenia gravis, or too much sour mash whiskey can affect the nervous system and cause a dysarthria. Dysarthric people sound different from each other depending on what portions of their nervous systems have been affected. This observation has led researchers to adopt the term "dysarthrias" rather than "dysarthria. "

Canter has apparently identified several subtypes of neurogenic, dysarthric stutterers. The dysarthria associated with Parkinson's disease is called hypokinetic dysarthria. According to Canter, the hypokinetic dysarthric's speech may be characterized by one of three stuttering patterns: (1) "frequent prolongations with a consequent disruption of the flow of speech," which he equates with "articulatory freezing" (p. 140); (2) "rapid syllable, word, and phrase repetitions" (p. 141), which he further describes as being "effortless"; and (3) "long silent blocks" associated with "a transient inability to initiate any kind of motor activity" (p. 141). Damage to the cerebellum can result in what is usually called an ataxic dysarthria, and the ataxic speaker may also stutter. Canter calls that stuttering "perhaps the most severe and dramatic of the varieties of dysarthric stuttering" (p. 141). Symptomatic of this condition are "violent prolongations" (presumably Parkinson speakers have tamer prolongations) resulting from their "inability to properly gauge the speed and force of movements leading to articulatory contacts (dysmetria)" (p. 141). He also mentions, as typical of this group, accelerating repetitions that may end in silent or audible prolongations "due to a paroxysmal spasm of the vocal tract musculature triggered by the increased muscle tension" (p. 141).

Apraxic stuttering

Apraxia of speech, like the dysarthrias, is a motor speech disorder; but, unlike them, it results from impairment to the highest level of motor control. It is usually described as a deficit of motor programming, and experienced clinicians can distinguish apraxic speech from dysarthric speech. Canter (1971) suggests the stuttering that accompanies apraxia of speech and the dysarthrias can be distinguished as well. According to Canter, "apraxic stuttering tends to occur as the individual re-approaches the initial sound of a word in his attempt to 'zero in' on the correct sound" (p. 141). Also, "the apraxic stutterer sometimes experiences silent speech blocks because of his impairment in voluntarily triggering the motor speech mechanism" (p. 141). As previously noted, it is probably inappropriate to label as stuttering those sound repetitions and prolongations that are reflections of the speaker's attempt to correct articulation or movement errors. This is not to say, however, that apraxic speakers do not have stuttering repetitions and prolongations. We have seen several who had multiple repetitions of the correct initial sound or syllable. That the repetition was on a correct sound suggests that the speaker was not trying to self-correct. These repetitions, like prolongations of a correct sound, may result from their "impairment in voluntarily triggering the motor speech mechanism" (p. 141) and may properly be called neurogenic stuttering.

Others have also noted the appearance of stuttering in the symptomatology of apraxia of speech (cf. Johns & Darley, 1970; Trost, 1971). Johns and Darley observed, for example, that speakers with apraxia of speech do a "creditable job of miming secondary stutterers" (p. 50). Trost (1971) said, "the prolongation and repetition behaviors in apraxic adults showed noteworthy similarities with those behaviors observed in ostensibly non-organic stutterers" (p. 8). Schuell, Jenkins, and Jiménez-Pabón (1964) observed that every speaker with apraxia (they called it sensorimotor involvement) passes through a period of stuttering during recovery. And some authors are so convinced of the co-occurrence of speech apraxia and stuttering that they argue that stuttering is an apraxia (Shtremel, 1963).

Dysnomic stuttering

Dysnomia refers to difficulty in recalling words. It results typically from damage to the left or dominant hemisphere and is part of the more general syndrome of aphasia in which reading, writing, understanding, and even gesturing are impaired. Canter (1971) offers this description of dysnomic stuttering: "Sometimes these word lapses are marked by pauses and articulatory gropings. In other cases, the patient repeats the preceding word or phrase, or fills in the impending silence with prosodic grunts or interjections" (p. 142).

Numerous other authors have described stuttering among the symptoms of aphasia (Schiller, 1947; Arend, Handzel, & Weiss, 1962; Farmer, 1975). That Arend, Handzel, and Weiss describe one of their case's speech deficit as "spluttering" does not diminish their observation that stuttering can coexist with aphasia following dominant (usually left) hemisphere damage. Farmer tried to measure the stuttering associated with aphasia, and hers is a welcome addition to the literature because, prior to her research, most reports had been primarily anecdotal rather than experimental. She studied "stuttering repetitions" in the speech of a group of nonaphasic, brain-damaged adults and in three patients with Wernicke's aphasia, two with conduction aphasia, four with Broca's aphasia, and three with anomic aphasia. The Wernicke's aphasic people had the most disfluencies, the conductions were next, the Broca's were third, and the anomics were fourth. Statistically, however, the only significant differences were between the Wernicke's and Broca's aphasics and between the Wernicke's and anomic aphasics. Farmer concludes that "lesions to the left hemisphere resulting in inefficient language performance may reflect temporal disorganization in the form of stuttering repetitions" (p. 395).

Eventually, the profession may decide not to call such symptoms of language deficit "stuttering. " In my opinion the decision, if it comes, will be a wise one. Stuttering is not the manifestation of a language deficit, although it may certainly accompany one. Nor is a language deficit a necessary prerequisite to neurogenic stuttering. Stuttering also appears in the absence of any language deficit. Helm, Butler, and Canter (1980) make this last point best. They say, "little support was found for either the notion that acquired stuttering results from the emotional strain created by aphasia or that acquired stuttering is invariably an inherent part of some aphasic syndrome" (p. 271).

Canter's paper (1971) is quoted widely. Its major contribution may be that it identifies the problem with the neurogenic stuttering literature—too many kinds of disfluency have been called by one name: stuttering. This may explain why it is difficult to make sense of the rest of the literature to be reviewed which does not appear to present a unified picture of either neurogenic stuttering or the neurogenic stutterer. But do not despair; that the literature does not make sense does not mean it is nonsense. Much less is known for sure in most fields including science and medicine—those bastions of truth—than many lay people think. Speech pathology merely joins its better known brethren in ignorance. Besides, some patterns seem to be emerging.

WHAT NEUROGENIC STUTTERING IS NOT

The definitions and descriptions of neurogenic stuttering are sufficient to separate it from another pattern of abnormal repetition secondary to brain damage—palilalia. As described by Critchley (1927), palilalia is characterized by word and phrase repetitions, which get faster and faster and progressively more unintelligible. Kent and LaPointe (1982) confirmed the repetitions but not the progressive rate or increasing unintelligibility. LaPointe and Horner (1981) reported an exhaustive (to complete, not to read) study of one palilalic speaker. Word and phrase repetitions accounted for 88% of all his palilalic repetitions. Syllable repetitions accounted for only 1.4%. This pattern contrasts sharply with that of six of the seven neurogenic stutterers described by Rosenbek et al. (1978) for whom sound–syllable repetitions were the most frequent type of repetition. Probably palilalia is distinct from neurogenic stuttering, not only in the type of repetitions but also in the underlying mechanism that produces it and in the site of the lesion or damage that causes it. But we cannot yet be sure, especially about mechanism and site. What we can be sure of is that the clinician who hears a patient say, "I was born in Grand Island, in Grand Island, in Grand Island, " recognizes immediately that the pattern is different from "I w-w-w-w-wa-was born in Grand Island. "

And as noted in an earlier section (but important enough to warrant repetition), neurogenic stuttering also is not the result merely of a speaker's attempt to self-correct. The patient who says, "My name is b-p-b-uh-deb" is different from the one who says, "My name is de-de-de-de-deb. " Many speakers with brain damage, especially involving the left or language hemisphere, make errors in articulation, word selection, or word ordering, which they may or may not try to repair. If they try to fix their mistakes, they will be disfluent; but they are not necessarily neurogenic stutterers. Neurogenic stuttering is the repetition, primarily, of correct sounds and syllables although a neurogenic stutterer may both self-correct and "stutter" as he talks. Whether neurogenic stutterers, like developmental ones, change the vowel in stuttered syllables to (Λ) has not been reported. My impression is that they do.

CONDITIONS WITH WHICH NEUROGENIC STUTTERING IS ASSOCIATED

Stroke

Neurogenic stuttering has been associated with several conditions that cause nervous system disfunction. Foremost among these is stroke, but the relationship between stroke and stuttering remains to be clarified. Rosenbek et al. (1978) hypothesized that less severe strokes were more likely to be associated with stuttering than were more severe ones, but this possibility demands considerably more research. Such research is especially crucial because of the Helm et al. (1980) statement that multiple strokes, if they involve only one side of the brain, are necessary to cause stuttering. They say, "in no case did the stuttering occur with the first stroke" (p. 273). They also say that "with bilateral brain damage resulting from vascular disease . . . the onset of stuttering may be abrupt" (p. 274). Both the timing of stuttering onset and the severity of the stroke with which it is associated warrant further study for the insights that such relationships might provide about why those with a damaged brain stutter.

Tumors and penetrating missile wounds

Tumors can also be associated with stuttering, as can a variety of traumatic injuries, including penetrating missile wounds (as when someone is shot in the head; Schiller, 1947). Adding to the argument that both tumors and penetrating missiles can cause stuttering are reports of remission of stuttering symptoms after removal of tumor (Shtremel, 1963) and after removal of shrapnel (Luchsinger & Arnold, 1965). In contrast to the onset of stuttering following cerebral vascular accident, stuttering following such trauma may be slow to evolve, perhaps in conjunction with the increasing complexity of a coexisting seizure disorder (Helm et al. 1980). Its timing with a tumor has not been reported, probably because it is difficult to know how long a tumor has been growing before it is discovered.

Closed-head injury

Helm et al. (1980) appear to have made the most careful observations of patients who begin stuttering following closed-head injury. They say the distinctive features of this group are (1) bilateral involvement, (2) loss of consciousness, (3) development of a seizure disorder, and (4) emerging stuttering as the seizure disorder becomes "more complex" (p. 273). They present an extensive review of the course and symptoms for a 54-year-old male who, 18 years prior to their evaluation, had suffered a closed-head injury and loss of consciousness. Four years after the trauma, the patient developed focal seizures in the left arm. He gradually developed a "generalized seizure disorder. " With one of the seizures (presumably generalized), he had a severe cardiorespiratory collapse. After a period of coma he awoke but was speechless. When speech returned, he "stammered. " He continued to speak with "phoneme and occasional whole-word repetition" (pp. 273–274) 14 years later. They seem less impressed with the seizure disorder per se than with the possibility that "the evolutionary aspect of the stuttering may be attributed to a 'daughter focus', which slowly arises in the opposite hemisphere, thus creating bilateral brain dysfunction" (p. 274).

Other conditions

Other conditions have also been associated with neurogenic stuttering. Canter (1971) reports stuttering in parkinsonism, especially in postencephalitic parkinsonism. Rosenbek, McNeil, Lemme, Prescott, and Alfrey (1975) report stuttering as the earliest symptom in a patient with dialysis dementia. Dialysis dementia sometimes occurs in patients who have been undergoing dialysis for from 2 to 8 years. This syndrome, which can now be cured, appeared to begin with stuttering and inevitably ended in death. Stuttering has also been associated with dementia or acquired intellectual impairment (Quinn & Andrews, 1977).

COURSE OF THE SYMPTOMS

Clinicians encountering neurogenic stuttering for the first time are especially interested in its course. They want to know, for example, the likelihood that it will resolve spontaneously. Helm et al. (1978) make the strongest statement about prognosis that I could find in the literature. They say that stuttering associated with bilateral brain damage persists, while that associated with unilateral brain damage does not. Other researchers have added observations that help complete the picture. Schiller (1947) reports parallel improvement in stuttering and coexisting aphasia. Based on these data, one might assume that once an aphasic stutterer's prognosis for recovery from aphasia has been established, the course of the stuttering symptoms can also be predicted. This is such a neat formula, it is unfortunate that data in support of it are inconsistent. Andrews, Quinn, and Sorby (1972), for example, report one case whose aphasia improved substantially but whose severe stuttering persisted. Of the three aphasic stutterers in the Rosenbek et al. (1978) group of seven, one showed improvement of aphasia and of stuttering; one showed improvement of aphasia and persistence of stuttering; one showed persistence of both; four of the patients did not have aphasia. Even if the data on the parallel courses of aphasia and stuttering remission were compelling, the prognosticator would still have to cope with predicting the course of symptoms in cases of stuttering unaccompanied by aphasia. Initial severity does not seem to be a predictor. The two most severe of the Rosenbek et al. (1978) patients had the most complete recovery. Nor have any specific symptoms been associated with recovery. My own experience suggests that bilateral brain damage and stuttering's persistence after 2 or 3 months are bad prognostic signs unless stuttering coexists with another speech–language deficit that is responding to treatment.

WHY NEUROGENIC STUTTERING OCCURS

Opinions abound as to why neurogenic stuttering occurs. Some have been tested; other have not. No single opinion prevails, but one has attracted more interest than the rest. This is the opinion that neurogenic stuttering results from a lack of cerebral dominance. Presumably, lack of clear-cut dominance leads to competition between the brain's left and right hemispheres with disastrous results for behavior such as speech. This and other opinions are reviewed in this section.

Lack of cerebral dominance

In its simplest form this theory, which was formulated initially to explain developmental stutterers, holds that the stutterer's brain is abnormal because one hemisphere does not clearly dominate the other in motor speech control. Such lack of dominance causes the two hemispheres to compete, with the result that signals about movement sent to the speech mechanism are abnormal and the speaker stutters. Orton (1928), on whose early work most of this hypothesis rests, said it this way: "Confusion in choice of antitropic engrams . . . also might result in failure of accurate synthesis of the reflex patterns which enter the speech act" (p. 1051-1052). Antitropic means existing in both the left and right hemispheres. Failure in synthesis is manifest in stuttering. See Moore (chap. 4 in this volume) for a different interpretation of the data on cerebral dominance and stuttering.

In more recent years, the theory got considerable support from a now famous study by Jones (1966), who reported the evaluation and surgical management of four patients who had presumably been stuttering since childhood. All four came to Jones's attention when they developed neurological symptoms as adults. One was discovered to have a tumor in the left hemisphere; each of the other three suffered from a subarachnoid hemorrhage caused by the rupturing of a weakened artery wall (aneurysm). Jones is confident that the neurological conditions could not have been responsible for the stuttering. All four had surgically treatable conditions, and prior to and after surgery Jones completed intracarotid amytal testing, called the Wada test (Wada & Rasmussen, 1960). In Wada testing a substance is injected, first into one and then into the other carotid arteries. The substance travels to the cortical hemisphere on the side of the injection and any ability which is served by that hemisphere is interrupted for several minutes. This method is useful for determining hemispheric dominance for speech and language. The tests were interpreted as showing bilateral speech representation in all four patients. Following surgery to remove the tumor (one case) or to repair the aneurysms (three cases), Wada testing was repeated. All four cases were reported to have clear hemispheric dominance and stuttering was absent. This study should not be used as evidence that surgery is the treatment of choice for neurogenic stutterers. It was seized on by many, however, as proof of the lack of dominance hypothesis.

Unfortunately, Andrews et al. (1972) and Luessenhop, Boggs, La Borwit, and Walle (1973) could not replicate Jones's finding. Andrews et al. studied three developmental stutterers and one neurogenic stutterer. They found clear-cut cerebral dominance in their three developmental stutterers. The fourth subject, a brain-damaged adult whose stuttering developed 2 years after severe head trauma, was apparently a severe neurogenic stutterer but was not aphasic, although it is not clear how his language was evaluated. Wada testing demonstrated that this right-handed man had bilateral motor speech representation. The authors' conclusion was, "it would appear that in the absence of an adventitial neurological lesion, typical stutterers have no general tendency to show bilateral speech centers as revealed by the intracarotid sodium amylobarbitone test" (p. 417). In a later report, Quinn and Andrews (1977) say of the patient whose stuttering developed after brain damage that the findings "suggested a post-traumatic inter-hemispheric redistribution of language function which may represent a process of division rather than of reduplication" (p. 700). Luessenhop et al. (1973) failed to demonstrate bilateral speech representation in three young adults who had begun stuttering as children. They say, "mixed dominance for speech, as indicated by Wada testing, is not uniformly present in adult stutterers, irrespective of handedness. This finding does not exclude, however, the possibility of ambilaterality of other less obvious speech mechanisms not readily definable by Wada testing" (p. 1192).

The failure of other researchers to replicate Jones's findings with developmental stutterers has not dissuaded researchers from using hemispheric competition as an explanation for stuttering that appears unequivocally to have resulted from brain damage. For example, Rosenfield (1972) reported the case of a 53-year-old right-handed female who "had a vascular headache associated with stuttering" (p. 991). After reviewing the case he says "an insult to a nonstutterer's dominant hemisphere can facilitate competition between the two hemispheres" (p. 991), resulting in stuttering. Donnan (1979) reviewed two cases of neurogenic stuttering and posited "sudden left cortical damage may have resulted in . . . an ambivalence of cerebral dominance in a previously left hemisphere dominant person" (p. 45). Rosenbek et al. (1978), after reviewing seven cases of neurogenic stuttering, include among their hypotheses about why stuttering develops, a slightly modified version of the competition hypothesis. They say, "perhaps stuttering can profitably be viewed as but one more example of loss of equilibrium in a bilaterally innervated system—the speech system" (p. 93).

That Helm et al. (1978) say neurogenic stuttering seems to result only from multiple, focal lesions in one hemisphere or from involvement of both hemispheres may or may not detract from the hemispheric competition hypothesis. Their report of persisting stuttering in patients with lesions in both hemispheres does not seem to support the hypothesis, but they did not report the size or location of lesions in all cases so the hypothesis may be able to accommodate their data. The presence of stuttering after both unilateral and bilateral nonhemispheric lesions would seem to be a greater threat to the theory. That so few brain-damaged people develop stuttering, however, is the greatest threat of all.

Other hypotheses

A variety of other hypotheses have been formulated to explain stuttering's presence after brain damage. None is any better at explaining why some and not others, but several of them are interesting despite this weakness. Schiller (1947) anticipated Eisenson's (1958) perseveration hypothesis as an explanation of the stuttering in one group of brain-damaged soldiers. Trost (1971), Shtremel (1963), and Canter (1971) all developed the hypothesis that stuttering results from an apraxia of the speech musculature. Canter (1971) posited that a variety of movement disorders, such as difficulty initiating movement and incoordination, may explain stuttering in some dysarthric speakers. And several authors (cf. Luchsinger & Arnold, 1965) have posited that stuttering results as a reaction to the presence of another communication deficit, usually aphasia, or as a reaction to brain-damage itself (Rosenbek et al., 1978).

CHARACTERISTICS OF NEUROGENIC STUTTERERS

The search for a profile of neurogenic stuttering has been shadowed by the search for a profile of the neurogenic stutterer. A profile is emerging. Neurogenic stutterers must, first of all, have suffered some kind of nervous system damage such as stroke, trauma, infection, or tumor. Their stuttering must be subsequent to that damage and not be accountable for in any other way. Other characteristics of neurogenic stutterers have been proposed by Canter (1971) and Helm et al. (1980). Canter says the stutterer is not anxious about his stuttering. If this is true, it is probably most likely to be true early after onset. We have heard several chronic patients complain about their stuttering. Helm et al. (1980) catalog five "neuropsychological behaviors" of neurogenic stutterers: (1) difficulty drawing and copying three dimensional figures, (2) difficulty copying block designs, (3) difficulty with sequential hand positions, (4) difficulty with singing, and (5) difficulty tapping out rhythms. Future research will determine which if any of these five characteristics combine with stuttering, and perhaps other abnormalities, to form a distinct syndrome.

LOCALIZING SIGNIFICANCE OF NEUROGENIC STUTTERING

Various kinds of speech and language deficits can be used to help localize where damage has occurred to the nervous system. Neurogenic stuttering, however, may not be one such deficit. It has occurred following damage to the low and high brainstem, to the basal ganglia, cerebellum, left and right cortical hemispheres, and to the white matter (tracts) of the frontal lobes of both the right and left hemispheres (Ludlow, Rosenberg, Dillon, & Buck, 1982). Stuttering has also been reported after frontal, parietal, and temporal lobe lesions within the left hemisphere. About the only sites within the nervous system which have not been associated with stuttering are the occipital lobes of the brain, which are devoted primarily to vision and the cranial nerves once they leave the brainstem.

This is not a cause for melancholy. A variety of other symptoms such as anomia, or word retrieval impairment, are seldom useful in helping health care professionals localize lesions. But there is another reason not to despair. Subsequent research will make more sense out of the ruck of symptoms presently grouped together as "neurogenic stuttering. " With increased understanding may come knowledge about what cortical and subcortical areas are important to fluency and—if damaged—to disfluency.

TREATING NEUROGENIC STUTTERING

Only a handful of treatment reports have been published, but this is all right. Treatment can profitably await considerable knowledge about a condition, so that once initiated it is intelligent and appropriate. When treatments spring up in an environment of ignorance, they may be easily abused. The few discussions of treatment are prudent. They seem meant to focus the harsh light of investigation rather than deflect it.

Medication

Baratz and Mesulam (1981) describe the use of anticonvulsants to treat the acquired stuttering of one 42-year-old female whose stuttering began following trauma. The patient was right-handed. A computerized tomography (CT) scan, which permits cross-sectional viewing of the brain and other organs, showed a left frontal subdural hematoma and multiple lesions in the right hemisphere. In other words, this lady had damage to both cortical hemispheres. Her speech was apparently evaluated during her hospitalization for control of seizures. How long she had been stuttering is not reported, but she had been having seizures since the accident. The speech pathologist concluded that the patient had an anomic aphasia with normal auditory and reading comprehension. Spontaneous speech was characterized by "frequent hesitations, prolongations, repetitions, and blocks on initial sounds of words" (p. 132). Facial grimaces accompanied her stuttering. She was fluent when reading aloud.

The seizures were treated with 300 mg of phenytoin and 90 mg of phenobarbital daily. According to the authors, "within one week there was a marked decrease in seizure activity. Right-sided body sensations and stuttering were diminished" (p. 132). The type of seizure is not identified, but after a time, the seizures and stuttering returned. Medications were changed to daily doses of 200 mg of phenytoin and 800 mg of carbamazepine. Stuttering was apparently reduced and "spoken and written word-finding abilities were improved" (p. 132).

Surgery

Donnan (1979) reports on a 65-year-old right-handed female whose stuttering appears to have been treated by left carotid endarterectomy. This surgical procedure removes matter clogging an artery. In November 1976, this patient suffered transient sensory impairment in her right arm with no other symptoms. In January of 1977, she again developed sensory loss accompanied by weakness and clumsiness, which lasted for several days. "Concurrently, sudden, severe, and persistent stuttering commenced" (p. 44). In February 1977, after an episode of transient blindness in one eye, the patient was again admitted to the hospital. At that time her stuttering was described as "rapid easy repetition of the initial sound syllable of every other word" (p. 44). Dysnomia or word-finding difficulty was also noted; grimacing was not. Carotid angiography, a method for determining the amount of occlusion in carotid arteries, revealed "tight left internal carotid stenosis and mild right internal carotid stenosis with some mild atheromatous ulceration" (p. 44). In other words, neither carotid was completely open and healthy. A left carotid endarterectomy to reduce stenosis was done, and "upon recovering from anaesthesia the patient was found to be completely free from stutter" (p. 44). A postoperative angiogram showed "uninterrupted left carotid blood flow" (p. 44). The patient was still fluent 2 months after surgery.

Donnan's second case was a 60-year-old, right-handed female who, in February 1978, suffered a sudden onset of weakness in her right arm and leg and "complete expressive aphasia" (p. 44). Her weakness improved over the next 2 days, but she "was unable to speak until the third day when her husband noted a marked stutter" (p. 44). In March 1978, she was again admitted with transient, right-sided weakness and exacerbation of stuttering. She was described as having "repetition of initial phonemes" and a slight word-finding deficit. Her carotid angiogram was normal. Her stuttering is reported to have decreased during her hospitalization and after discharge from the hospital.

Donnan bases his speculations about the cause of neurogenic stuttering and its amelioration following surgery primarily on the first case. He says, "sudden left cortical damage may have resulted in an element of dysphasia and perhaps an ambivalence of cerebral dominance in a previously left hemisphere dominant person . . . sudden remission after endarterectomy may have been due to sudden increase in cerebral blood flow to the left hemisphere improving speech function and reversing the state of incomplete cerebral dominance" (p. 45).

Donnan's data are not sufficiently compelling to make surgeons recommend endarterectomy for treatment of neurogenic stuttering, but combined with Jones's (1966) findings mentioned earlier during discussion of the hemispheric competition hypothesis, the data are compelling enough to alert other researchers to the possible palliative effects on neurogenic stuttering of surgery performed for other reasons, such as improvement of blood flow to the brain.

Behavioral management

Canter (1971) says, "Our therapy experience with adults with neurogenic stuttering has been very encouraging" (p. 143). Mine has not, but one case reported earlier (Rosenbek, Messert, Collins, & Wertz, 1978) warrants mention.

That patient was a 53-year-old right-handed male who began stuttering approximately 24 hours following a stroke involving the right parietal lobe. Treatment began 24 hours later, and he was fluent 96 hours after treatment began. Treatment included equal portions of counseling to reassure the patient that he could regain his fluency, and instruction to speak effortlessly and at approximately 50 words per minute by increasing both his articulation time and his pause time. The speech he chose was an effortless, stereotyped drawl with prolonged vowels and consonants and reasonably long pauses between most words.

COMPARISON TO DEVELOPMENTAL STUTTERING

Canter highlighted a number of features that he thought distinguished neurogenic from traditional stutterers. As Rosenbek et al. (1978) observed, however, "a clinical impression, developed over the years, was that a set of symptoms reminiscent of traditional, developmental stuttering was prominent in the speech of some proportion of brain-damaged patients" (p. 94). They went on to point out that the presence of a high proportion of sound, syllable, and monosyllabic word repetitions, especially in word-initial position, is typical of both neurogenic and developmental stutterers. Among the other similarities they report are mild accessory features such as grimacing, especially when neurogenic stuttering is severe.

Caplan, in his study of five aphasic speakers, was primarily concerned with determining whether their disfluencies resembled traditional stuttering. He says first that the amount of disfluency for three of his five subjects was great enough to justify calling them stutterers. He adds that for no subject was the distribution of disfluencies like that of traditional stutterers, however. He concludes: "It appears that the non-fluencies shown by the subjects in this experiment are similar to the non-fluencies exhibited by normal speakers, and not those considered to be the distinguishing features of stuttering" (p. 59).

He subsequently had three judges " 'comment on' the speech samples . . . in terms of what the judges believed the speech problems of the subjects were" (p. 58). It appears that the judges thought the speech sounded stuttered. This led him to conclude: "It appears that there are other more subtle attributes of the disfluencies that contribute to the diagnosis of stuttering" (p. 59). He also says, "symptoms that have been regarded as peculiar to dysphasia (anomia, incomplete sentences, sequencing difficulties) can be reinterpreted and viewed within the framework of stuttering behaviour" (p. 59).

The similarity of neurogenic and traditional stuttering may eventually be demonstrated. Probably the two conditions will not be identical, however. Disfluencies beginning after a long period of normal speech-language use may well be different from disfluencies beginning in childhood, if for no other reason than that the adult may react differently to their appearance. The data will eventually tell us.

Some opinions and guidelines

I think stuttering following nervous system damage is an identifiable entity that ought to be included in speech pathology's nosology. Disfluencies such as repeated words, broken words, revisions, and inappropriate pauses can and do accompany any speech-language disorder. In my view, however, these disfluencies are not neurogenic stuttering. They are symptomatic of efforts to say the right word, or phrase, or sound. It has been my experience that neurogenic stuttering consists primarily of involuntary repetition primarily of correct sounds and syllables any place in a word. These sound-syllable repetitions may be accompanied by prolongations and by word and phrase repetitions, but they are more numerous than such accompanying abnormalities.

Speech, like gait and other behavior, has only a limited number of ways to go wrong. It seems likely, therefore, that researchers will continue to find neurogenic stuttering after lesions to a variety of cortical and subcortical (e.g., basal ganglia and cerebellum) regions, especially those serving sensory-motor speech performance. Slight differences in symptoms may be discernible, however, and may depend on whether damage is to cortical or subcortical areas and on accompanying emotional, linguistic, and cognitive deficits.

The unanswered question is why some persons stutter and others do not. The literature survey reported in this paper found no common threads. The closest thing to a unifying observation is that many neurogenic stutterers have relatively mild, transient neurogenic deficits following stroke. The exception are those stutterers who suffer closed-head injury, often with accompanying seizures. Perhaps a clue lies in the quick appearance of stuttering after stroke but its delayed appearance after closed-head injury. And while we are searching for answers we can trust, we probably would do well to avoid embracing that old standby—stuttering can have several causes, it depends on the individual. It may well have nothing to do with the individual. Sometime we will know.

For now, clinical researchers should be careful to describe their patient's disfluencies in excruciating detail. The profession might be well served by declaring a moratorium on the use of neurogenic stuttering, or even neurogenic disfluency, as labels. Neurogenic stuttering is too specific and implies that we know more about the condition than we do. Neurogenic disfluency is too general; the majority of speech-language impaired speakers are disfluent. We need as much light as possible if we are ever going to see what we are treating. I am confident that subsequent research will provide that light if we prevent labels from coming between researchers and patients.

NOTE

[1]Espir and Rose consider stammering and stuttering to be synonymous.

REFERENCES

Andrews, G., Quinn, P.T., & Sorby, W.A. Stuttering: An investigation into cerebral dominance for speech. *Journal of Neurology, Neurosurgery, and Psychiatry,* 1972, *35,* 414–418.

Arend, R., Handzel, L., & Weiss, B. Dysphatic stuttering. *Folia Phoniatrica,* 1962, *14,* 55–66.

Baratz, R., & Mesulam, M.M. Adult-onset stuttering treated with anti-convulsants. *Archives of Neurology,* 1981, *38,* 132.

Canter, G.J. Observations on neurogenic stuttering: A contribution to differential diagnosis. *British Journal of Disorders of Communication,* 1971, *6,* 139–143.

Caplan, L. An investigation of some aspects of stuttering-like speech in adult dysphasic subjects. *Journal of the South African Speech and Hearing Association,* 1972, *19,* 52–66.

Critchley, M. On palilalia. *Journal of Neurological Psychopathology,* 1927, *8,* 23–31.

Darley, F.L., Aronson, A.E., & Brown, J.R. *Motor Speech Disorders.* Philadelphia: Saunders, 1975.

Donnan, G.A. Stuttering as a manifestation of stroke. *The Medical Journal of Australia,* 1979, *1,* 44–45.

Eisenson, J. A perseverative theory of stuttering. In J. Eisenson (Ed.), *Stuttering: A symposium.* New York: Harper & Row, 1958. 223–271.

Espir, M.L.E., & Rose, F.C. *The basic neurology of speech.* Oxford: Blackwell, 1970.

Farmer, A. Stuttering repetitions in aphasic and nonaphasic brain damaged adults. *Cortex,* 1975, *11,* 391–396.

Helm, N.A., Butler, R.B., & Benson, D.F. Acquired stuttering. *Neurology,* 1978, *28,* 1159–1165.

Helm, N.A., Butler, R.B., & Canter, G.J. Neurogenic acquired stuttering. *Journal of Fluency Disorders,* 1980, *5,* 269–279.

Johns, D.F., & Darley, F.L. Phonemic variability in apraxia of speech. *Journal of Speech and Hearing Research,* 1970, 556–583.

Johnson, W. *The onset of stuttering.* Minneapolis: University of Minnesota Press, 1961.

Jones, R.K. Observations on stammering after localized cerebral injury. *Journal of Neurology, Neurosurgery, and Psychiatry,* 1966, *29,* 192–195.

Kent, R., & LaPointe, L.L. Acoustic properties of pathologic reiterative utterances: A case study of palilalia. *Journal of Speech and Hearing Research,* 1982, *25,* 95–99.

LaPointe, L.L., & Horner, J. Palilalia: A descriptive study of pathological reiterative utterances. *Journal of Speech and Hearing Disorders,* 1981, *46,* 34–38.

Luchsinger, R., & Arnold, G.E. *Voice-Speech-Language.* Belmont, CA: Wadsworth, 1965.

Ludlow, C.L., Rosenberg, J., Dillon, D., & Buck, D. *Persistent speech dysprosody following penetrating head injury.* Paper presented at the American Speech–Language–Hearing Association Convention, Toronto, Canada, 1982.

Luessenhop, A.J., Boggs, J.S., La Borwit, L.J., & Walle, E.L. Cerebral dominance in stutterers determined by Wada Testing. *Neurology,* 1973, *23,* 1190–1192.

Orton, S.T. A physiological theory of reading disability and stuttering in children. *New England Journal of Medicine,* 1928, *199,* 1046–1053.

Quinn, P.T., & Andrews, G. Neurological stuttering: A clinical entity. *Journal of Neurology, Neurosurgery, and Psychiatry,* 1977, *40,* 699–701.

Rosenbek, J., McNeil, M.R., Lemme, M.L., Prescott, T.E., & Alfrey, A.C. Speech and language findings in a chronic hemodialysis patient: A case report. *Journal of Speech and Hearing Disorders,* 1975, *40,* 245–252.

Rosenbek, J., Messert, B., Collins, M., & Wertz, R. Stuttering following brain damage. *Brain and Language,* 1978, *6,* 82–96.

Rosenfield, D.B. Stuttering and cerebral ischemia. *New England Journal of Medicine,* 1972, *287,* 991.

Schiller, F. Aphasia studied in patients with missile wounds. *Journal of Neurology, Neurosurgery, and Psychiatry,* 1947, *10,* 183–197.

Schuell, H., Jenkins, J.J., & Jiménez-Pabón, E. *Aphasia in adults.* New York: Harper & Row, 1964.

Shtremel, A.K. Stuttering in left parietal lobe syndrome. *Zhurnal Nevropatologii i Psikhiatrii imeni S.S. Korsakova,* 1963, *63,* 828–832.

Trost, J.E. *Apraxic dysfluency in patients with Broca's aphasia.* Paper presented at the American Speech and Hearing Association Convention, Chicago, 1971.

Wada, J., & Rasmussen, T. Intracarotid injection of sodium amytal for the lateralization of cerebral speech dominance. Experimental and clinical observations. *Journal of Neurosurgery,* 1960, *17,* 266–282.

Wingate, M.E. A standard definition of stuttering. *Journal of Speech and Hearing Disorders,* 1964, *29,* 484–489.

Chapter 4

Central Nervous System Characteristics of Stutterers

Walter H. Moore, Jr.

The central nervous system (CNS) characteristics of stutterers can best be examined in terms of information processing strategies of the cerebral hemispheres. In seeking to understand CNS characteristics, we observe behavioral events and relate them to known or theorized CNS functions. Interpretations of such observations have ranged from viewing them as evidence of CNS dysfunctions to evidence supporting a difference in information processing strategies. This chapter views stuttering as the outcome of a manipulable process, rather than as a static disorder resulting from CNS dysfunction which can be compensated for but not remediated.

In this chapter we review procedures used in studying hemispheric processing, review variables that affect processing strategies, review the processing literature for stutterers, and critically examine the conclusions of such literature.

METHODS FOR THE INVESTIGATION OF HEMISPHERIC PROCESSING

Dichotic listening

Dichotic listening is probably the most familiar method of investigating hemispheric processing. It has been widely used for several years (i.e., Kimura, 1961a, 1961b). Typically, two auditory stimuli of equal intensity and onset times are delivered to different ears. Following presentation of single pairs of stimuli or several sets of pairs, listeners are asked to indicate, by recall or recognition, what they heard. The examiner records the number of responses associated with left and right ear presentations and determines an "ear preference score." Typically, within stimulus and task constraints, normal subjects obtain a right ear preference score for verbal material (particularly nonsense syllables).

Such findings are thought to reflect more direct neural pathways from the right ear to the "language" processing areas in the left hemisphere, since left ear stimuli travel to the right hemisphere before being relayed to the left for processing. This relay process produces a time lag for left ear stimuli or a possible degradation of the signal which results in a right ear advantage (Kimura, 1961a, Rosenzweig, 1951).

A major limitation of the dichotic listening method is the duration of the stimuli used for presentation. Often, nonsense consonant–vowel (CV) syllables beginning with stop-plosives have been used because of the ease in aligning syllable pairs. However, such stimuli do not reflect the semantic and syntactic components of language and represent, at best, a phonologic component only.

Tachistoscopic visual methods

Analogous to dichotic listening is the tachistoscopic visual method in which stimuli are presented to the left and/or right visual half fields. Typically, vertically arrayed information is presented to visual half fields, either monocularly or binocularly, for brief durations (under 100 msec). Pathways from the right half field project directly to the left hemisphere and from the left half field to the right hemisphere, and a right visual half field preference is often obtained for verbal information, with left visual half field preference for nonverbal information (Hines, 1972; McKeever & Huling, 1971; Moore, 1976). Presentations of verbal information to the right visual field have a temporal advantage over those presented to the left field, since information from the right field can travel directly to language processing areas of the left hemisphere, while stimuli presented to the left field go first to the right hemisphere before being shunted to the left for processing.

This method, too, has several limitations. Because information can be presented only for short durations, to control for eye movement, only short stimulus arrays can be used. Most investigations have used letters, digits, syllables or, at best, short words with information presented vertically. As in dichotic listening studies, many linguistic variables cannot be examined due to these important limitations. Luminous conditions must also be carefully controlled, requiring sophisticated equipment to present and time the stimulus parameters.

Scalp recorded averaged evoked responses

Averaged evoked responses (AER) are a neuroelectrical measure of cortical activity in an area of the cortex. Surface scalp electrodes are placed over a cortical area, and changes in electrical potential (relative voltage) are recorded referenced to a ground. Recordings are time-locked to stimulus presentations. Changes in cortical electrical activity are averaged over trials and are displayed as consistent voltage changes, since random activity tends to cancel when averaged (Gruber & Segalowitz, 1977; Seitz, Weber, Jacobson, & Morehouse, 1980).

One advantage to AER is that it allows for observation of a specific cortical response over cortical areas, which may be pertinent to localization of hemispheric function. It can also be used to study relative activation latencies of different cortical areas (Brown, Marsh, & Smith, 1973, 1976; Kutas & Donchin, 1979; Molfese, 1980; Molfese, Freeman, & Palermo, 1975; Neville, 1980; Thatcher, 1977).

Typically, stimuli are restricted to under 1 sec in duration, with rapid rise and fall times, and must be replicable over numerous trials with computer averaging. Such equipment requirements restrict the method to individuals with sophisticated laboratory equipment and skills.

Hemispheric alpha asymmetries

Numerous investigations (Galin & Ornstein, 1972; Haynes & Moore, 1981a, 1981b; McKee, Humphrey, & McAdam, 1973; Moore & Haynes, 1980a, 1980b; Morgan, McDonald, & MacDonald, 1971; Robbins & McAdam, 1974) have shown increased suppression of alpha brain wave frequency (8–13 Hz) over the hemisphere primarily processing specific kinds of information under specific task conditions. Moore and Haynes (Moore and Haynes, 1980a, 1980b; Haynes & Moore, 1981a, 1981b; Moore, 1979) have found that asymmetries are affected by such variables as gender of the subject, task to be performed, stimuli, and the interactions of these variables. One advantage of this procedure is that it can be used to study hemispheric processing over time using a variety of stimuli, including more natural units of language (phrases, sentences, connected discourse).

The fact that scalp electrodes are used in this method means that results reflect activity of many small zones of cortical surface beneath the electrodes (Cooper, Osselton, & Shaw, 1974). Consequently, a small, discrete area cannot be said to be responsible for the electrical activity observed. The method also requires sophisticated equipment for recording and measuring electroencephalographic (EEG) activity.

Cortical blood flow (CBF)

Cortical blood flow methods are based upon the observation that the flow of blood through various tissues of the body changes as a direct result of metabolism and activity of the tissues (Lassen, Ingvar, &

Skinhøj, 1978). Thus, if one hemisphere or region is more or less active than another, we should expect to find differences in regional cerebral circulation.

Recently a noninvasive xenon-133 inhalation method has been developed, in which a patient inhales xenon for approximately 1 minute followed by 10 minutes of normal air breathing (Risberg, 1980). Detectors are placed at selected locations on the scalp, and the level of radioactivity is monitored via computer analysis. Changes in localized blood flow are indicative of metabolic changes and, consequently, neuronal activity of various sites of the brain. (Interested readers can refer to a special issue of *Brain and Language, 9* (1), 1980, devoted to noninvasive blood flow studies and methods.)

The xenon-133 inhalation method is noninvasive, and numerous detectors permit observation of regional blood flow within and between hemispheres. While this method has clear advantages over some of the techniques already described, it, too, has limitations.

According to Wood (1980), EEG has much greater temporal resolution than does the CBF technique, which requires a minimum of 2 to 3 minutes of repetitive behavioral activation. Changes in cortical/cognitive activity that take place during the long interval required for CBF recording cannot be seen. However, the degree of spatial resolution obtained with CBF methods is not possible with typical EEG methods. CBF also requires experience, sophisticated equipment, and highly specialized training on the part of the user. Wood's point that cerebral blood flow methods supplement and do not replace other measurement methods and procedures is well taken.

Temporary anesthetization of the cerebral hemispheres

Anesthetization of the cerebral hemispheres is another method used to determine hemispheric "lateralization" for language. The method, which was developed by Wada (1949), requires a general anesthetic (for example, sodium amytal) to be injected into the left or right carotid artery. With injection into the left carotid, the left hemisphere is temporarily anesthetized, while injection into the right carotid results in a temporary anesthetization of the right hemisphere. Anesthetization lasts for a period of 2 to 3 minutes. In most subjects temporary loss of language/speech is seen when the left carotid artery is injected, an indication that the left hemisphere is importantly involved in language functions.

While this procedure has been used to infer hemispheric "language dominance, " it is more often than not a test of "speech dominance. " Most studies with this method have used motor speech tasks. Perhaps the greatest limitation of the procedure is that it gives only a gross indication of interhemispheric activation. The method, of course, is invasive and does place the patient at risk; therefore, its use is restricted to trained medical personnel, primarily neurosurgeons and neurologists.

ASYMMETRIES OF THE CEREBRAL HEMISPHERES: MORPHOLOGICAL AND COGNITIVE DIFFERENCES

There is overwhelming evidence of morphological asymmetries of the cerebral hemispheres, which may be reflected in cognitive/behavioral strategies of each hemisphere.

Morphological asymmetries

Morphological asymmetries of the upper surface of the left and right temporal lobes have been reported by numerous independent investigators (Geschwind, 1979; Geschwind & Levitsky, 1968; Hochberg & LeMay, 1975; LeMay & Culebras, 1972; Ratcliff, Dila, Taylor, & Milner, 1980; Wada, 1969; Wada, Clarke, & Hamm, 1975; Witelson & Pallie, 1973). The planum temporale, which extends from Heschl's gyrus on the superior temporal gyrus posteriorly to the Sylvian fossa, has been found to be from one-third to seven times larger in the left hemispheres of normal right-handed subjects (Geschwind & Levitsky, 1968). Additionally, McRae, Branch, and Milner (1968) reported that the left occipital horn of the lateral ventricle is larger and broader than the right, suggesting that there may be more white matter in the posterior portion of the right hemisphere than in the left.

The left hemisphere, with a larger planum temporale, may be better equipped to process brief sounds (less than 100 msec), to analyze constituent parts of auditory stimuli, and to sequence information temporally (Tallal & Newcomb, 1978; Thatcher, 1980; Zaidel, 1979, 1978, 1976). The right hemisphere, with greater tissue mass in the posterior occipital lobe, is better suited to process visual information, to scan the auditory and visual environment, and to process steady state information or information associated with high visual imagery (Day, 1977, 1979; Tallal & Piercy, 1974).

Work begun by Ojemann, Fedio, and Van Buren (1968) and Fedio and Van Buren (1975) has shown the left and right pulvinars (thalamic nuclei) to be importantly involved in information processing. Fedio and Van Buren observed that the right pulvinar was involved in processing visual stimuli, and the left pulvinar with processing verbal/auditory stimuli.

These findings support the hypothesis that language is not lateralized to the left hemisphere; what are lateralized are certain processing strategies or mental operations, which process the verbal/acoustic parameters of linguistic stimuli. According to Thatcher (1980) "the combination of an enhanced neural mass devoted to associative and cognitive functions, plus an hemispheric specialization of the processing of speech-related sounds . . . is at the root of man's distinctive and elaborate linguistic capabilities" (p. 254).

Cognitive/behavioral asymmetries

The literature does not support an absolute dichotomy of left-linguistic, right–nonlinguistic processing, and it is probably more correct to conceive of the right hemisphere as a holistic–gestalt, time-independent processor and the left hemisphere as an analytic–segmental, time-dependent processor (Gordon, 1979; Segalowitz & Gruber, 1977; Whitaker & Whitaker, 1975, 1976, 1977). Both the nature of the stimuli and the way in which a subject approaches a given task is associated with activation of the cerebral hemispheres. For example, Willis, Wheatley, and Mitchell (1979) have shown that spatial stimuli, under analytic task demands, is processed left hemispherically, while Gates and Bradshaw (1977) found trained musicians process music more left hemispherically than nonmusicians.

Zaidel (1979) has suggested that speech is the most lateralized linguistic function, usually to the left hemisphere, while language comprehension is the least lateralized, being present in various degrees in both hemispheres. Shankweiler and Studdert-Kennedy (1975) also suggest that language lateralization is a continuum, not a dichotomy.

If the nature of right hemispheric processing is qualitatively distinct from left hemispheric processing, then one might reasonably expect the comprehension strategies and lexicons of the two hemispheres to be different. Zaidel (1979) has reported that the right hemisphere may comprehend spoken words by performing an acoustic pattern match with stored exemplars, rather than performing a phonetic analysis as does the left hemisphere. The lexicon of the right hemisphere, compared to the left, has been described as connotative, associative, and imagined rather than precise, denotative, and phonologic (Bradshaw, 1980).

Variables which affect right and left hemispheric processing. If each hemisphere uses different strategies for processing information, then it should not be surprising to find that each hemisphere is more or less activated by different task, stimulus, and subject variables. For example, the left hemisphere, which operates in a segmental mode, is more efficient at processing phonologic information, while the right nonsegmental hemisphere is better at processing semantic information. Numerous studies have explored how different variables are likely to activate the

TABLE 4-1. Variables affecting hemispheric activation.

Authors	Method	Variable	Results
Zaidel (1979)	Dichotic/Tachistoscopic	Phonological component in nonsense syllables.	The greater the phonological component the greater the left hemispheric activation.
Day (1977, 1979)	Tachistoscopic	High ("house") and low ("hypothesis") imagery nouns, verbs, and adjectives.	High imagery nouns and adjectives in left and right hemispheres. Low imagery nouns, adjectives, and all verbs in left hemisphere.
Springer and Gazzaniga (1975)	Dichotic	CV nonsense syllables and concrete words.	Split-brain subjects had a right ear preference for CV nonsense syllable, but could verbally report some of the concrete words presented to their left ears.
Tallal and Newcombe (1978)	Responding to sounds of varying duration.	Duration of auditory stimuli.	Left hemisphere damaged subjects were impaired in their ability to respond to sounds of brief duration.
Heeschen and Jürgens (1978)	Dichotic	Pragmatic–semantic and syntactic components.	Left hemisphere is responsive to syntactic structuredness, both left and right responsive to semantic–pragmatic structuredness.
Dennis (1980a, 1980b)	Metalinguistic judgments of left and right hemidecorticates.	Reversible and nonreversible passive sentences and negatives.	Theme and focus relations of the passive sentence are available to the left hemisphere but not the right. Both hemispheres encode the same sentence in different ways.
Faber-Clark and Moore (1983)	Alpha suppression	Recall and recognition of word lists.	Greater left hemisphere suppression with recall; greater right hemisphere suppression with recognition.

(Cont'd)

TABLE 4-1. Variables affecting hemispheric activation. (Cont'd)

Authors	Method	Variable	Results
Moore and Haynes (1980a)	Alpha suppression	Activity–passivity of subject task in males and females.	No difference in sexes for passive listening; active tasks found greater lateralization in females and less in males.
Faber-Clark and Moore (1983)	Alpha suppression	Subjects strategy for recalling and recognizing words.	"Visualizers" have greater right hemisphere suppression; "verbalizers" have greater left hemisphere suppression.
Satz et al. (1975) (Porter & Berlin, 1975)	Dichotic	Ear preference of children.	No ear preference in children below age 9 suggesting development of lateralization (different dichotic tests may assess different levels of language processing).
Willis et al. (1979)	Alpha suppression	Spatial and verbal–analytic tasks.	Hemispheric processing is a function of task demands and not just perceptual requirements.
Niederbahl and Springer (1979)	Tachistoscopic	Cognitive strategies	Strategy affects hemispheric asymmetry.

cerebral hemispheres. Table 4-1 provides a summary of variables that affect left and right hemispheric processing.

It is apparent from Table 4-1 that numerous variables interact to influence the activation of left and/or right hemispheric processing strategies. A nondiscerning view of hemispheric processing could give one an impression of inconsistency across studies. Yet, when they are analyzed in terms of variables known to influence hemispheric activation, considerable consistency among them emerges. With this in mind, we now turn to studies that have investigated the hemispheric processing of stuttering individuals.

HEMISPHERIC PROCESSING OF STUTTERING INDIVIDUALS

CNS investigations suggested that stutterers lack cerebral dominance for speech (Orton, 1927; Travis, 1931). Travis (1931) hypothesized that stuttering results from the asynchronous arrival of nerve impulses in the bilaterally paired jaw muscles. In 1934 Travis presented electromyographic (EMG) data recorded from the left and right masseter muscles of 24 adult stutterers and nonstutterers. He reported that action potentials from normal subjects were "practically identical, " while those from stuttering subjects were "strikingly different. " Other EMG investigations (Morley, 1935; Steer, 1937; Strother, 1935) seemed to support Travis's findings, and it was believed that competition between the cerebral hemispheres during motor speech behavior resulted in out-of-phase arrival of action potentials that disrupted speech.

While some early data were interpreted as suggesting a lack of cerebral dominance for stutterers (Lindsley, 1940; Freestone, 1942), other data were also being gathered, which suggested that stutterers demonstrate right hemispheric dominance for language. For example, an investigation reported by Douglass (1943), and replicated by Knott and Tjossen (1943), found that stutterers as a group have less percent time alpha in their right occipital areas compared to their left occipital areas during silence, while nonstutterers evidenced just the opposite.

While momentum gathered for a "cerebral dominance" explanation of stuttering during the 1930s and 1940s, it all but stopped during the 1950s and early 1960s. One of the important investigations that contributed to a rethinking of the role of cerebral dominance in stuttering was published by Williams in 1955. Williams failed to find significant differences in bilateral amplitude or timing of action potentials between the two sides of the jaw. Differences that were found between the two groups were attributed to the excessive muscular tension and different patterns of jaw movements accompanying stuttering. Thus, EMG differences were viewed as a consequence of stuttering rather than its cause. Additionally, EEG studies which sought to find *neuronal dysfunction*, rather than hemispheric differences (Fox, 1966), deemphasized hemispheric asymmetry differences between stutterers and nonstutterers during language processing.

For the remainder of this section, investigations grouped by specific methodologies will be discussed. One advantage of this approach is that we can better compare procedures relative to variables known to affect hemispheric processing.

Wada technique. Using the Wada technique, with intracarotid injection of sodium amytal, Jones (1966) found bilateral motor speech control in four stutterers prior to neurological surgery. Following surgery speech was no longer controlled bilaterally, and all four stutterers were reported to have normal speech. While these results seemed to provide powerful evidence for implicating cerebral dominance as a causal factor in stuttering, there were several variables that may have accounted for bilateral speech control. Three of the four subjects were left-handed, all had neurological lesions, and all had undergone a neurological surgical procedure. Subsequent investigations by Andrews, Quinn, and Sorby (1972) and Luessenhop, Boggs, LaBorwit, and Walle (1973) using the Wada technique and controlling for some of the confounding variables in the Jones study have failed to replicate the earlier observation of bilateral motor speech control in stutterers.

Investigations using the Wada technique are difficult to interpret for several reasons: handedness was different; neurological integrity was heterogeneous; onset of stuttering was not always controlled; age of subjects varied; a number of potentially important observations were not always adequately explained. For these and other reasons, categorical statements of the contributions of cerebral dominance or processing to stuttering cannot be made.

Dichotic listening. Dichotic listening methods have generated the largest number of investigations exploring hemispheric processing in stutterers. Unfortunately, this also is one of the more confusing and seemingly inconsistent areas of information. However, when investigations are viewed relative to methodological commonalities (i.e., words vs. nonsense syllable, recall vs. recognition, etc.), confusion and inconsistency give way to predictable findings.

Studies employing meaningful linguistic stimuli have usually reported a significantly larger proportion of stutterers with a left ear preference (Curry & Gregory, 1969; Davenport, 1979; Perrin & Eisenson, 1970; Quinn, 1972; Sommers, Brady, & Moore, 1975). Perrin and Eisenson found a left ear preference for words but no ear preference for nonsense syllables for their stutterers. Their investigation highlighted the importance of the nature of the auditory stimuli used when exploring dichotic ear preferences of stutterers. Davenport reported that severe stutterers failed to show a strong right ear preference, while least severe stutterers' performance was similar to a nonstuttering group. These investigations illustrate the importance of controlling both stimulus and subject variables when conducting and interpreting dichotic research with stutterers.

Dichotic investigations, using nonsense syllables, have not reported findings similar to those using meaningful stimuli (Brady & Berson, 1975; Cerf & Prins, 1974; Dorman & Porter, 1975; Liebetrau & Daly, 1981; Pinsky & McAdam, 1980; Rosenfield & Goodglass, 1980; Sussman & MacNeilage, 1975). However, in many investigations, a larger number of stutterers than nonstutterers were shown to have either a left ear preference or no ear preference under dichotic stimulation (Brady & Berson, 1975; Liebetrau & Daly, 1981; Rosenfield & Goodglass, 1980; Strong, 1978).

If the right hemisphere is less capable of processing nonsense syllables than the left (Zaidel, 1979), we should not expect stutterers to process nonsense syllables differently from nonstutterers or to process them less efficiently if their primary mode of processing such stimuli is right hemispheric. Support for such a hypothesis is found in the results of dichotic listening studies by Rosenfield and Goodglass (1980) and Pinsky and McAdam (1980). Rosenfield and Goodglass found that stutterers were inferior to nonstuttering controls in all comparisons of reporting CV nonsense syllables and interpreted these findings as evidence of a phoneme perception "deficiency. " Since a larger proportion of stutterers in their study obtained left ear preference scores, the reported deficiency could reflect the right hemisphere's reduced capacity to process phonological information. Pinsky and McAdam's data revealed apparent differences between stutterers and nonstutterers for correctly pointing to nonsense syllables, and an analysis of variance confirmed that their stutterers correctly pointed to significantly fewer nonsense syllables than did nonstutterers.

When dichotic studies are controlled for the nature of stimuli used, consistent trends emerge: Meaningful linguistic stimuli evoke right hemisphere processing in stutterers and larger numbers of stutterers show either a left ear or no preference for nonsense syllables which they also process less efficiently than most nonstutterers.

Tachistoscopic visual procedures. All investigations with stutterers using this method (Hand & Haynes, 1983; Moore, 1976; Plakosh, 1978) have used meaningful linguistic stimuli (Hand & Haynes used both meaningful stimuli and nonmeaningful stimuli in a linguistic decision task). Moore reported a significantly larger proportion of stutterers had a left field (right hemisphere) preference than did nonstutterers. Similarly, Plakosh found no visual field differences for stutterers and concluded that stutterers were more dependent on visuospatial aspects of visually presented linguistic stimuli than were normals.

Hand and Haynes, measuring manual and voice reaction time responses to tachistoscopically presented words, showed stutterers' reaction times to be slower for stimuli presented to the right visual field. Furthermore, stutterers' vocal reaction time was significantly slower than their manual reaction time, and both of these reaction times were significantly slower than those of nonstutterers.

Electrophysiological methods. In a series of investigations conducted by Moore and his associates (McFarland & Moore, 1982; Moore, Craven, & Faber, 1982; Moore & Haynes, 1980a; Moore & Lang, 1977; Moore & Lorendo, 1980) alpha was surpressed over the right posterior temporal–parietal areas in stutterers. Stutterers have also been found to recall and recognize fewer numbers of words than nonstutterers in these studies (Moore & Lorendo; Moore, Craven, & Faber) and by another investigator (Daly, 1981). These findings may reflect the right hemisphere's shorter span for verbal short-term memory (Zaidel, 1979). Moore and Haynes (1980a) found that comprehension of connected verbal discourse was unaffected in male stutterers who also demonstrated reduced right hemispheric alpha, a finding which could also reflect the right hemisphere's superiority in processing semantic aspects of language.

After analyzing the alpha hemispheric asymmetries of male stutterers, Moore and Haynes (1980a) suggested:

> Stuttering may emerge when both hemispheric processing of incoming information and motor programming of segmental linguistic units is in the right hemisphere (a non-segmental processor). These processing differences may be related to an inability, under certain circumstances, to handle the segmentation aspects of language. This may suggest the importance of linguistic segmentation as it relates to motor programming in some stutterers. (p. 244).

Boberg, Yeudall, Schopflocher, and Bo-Lassen (1983) gathered hemispheric alpha asymmetry data from anterior and posterior brain sites pre- and post-treatment. Prior to treatment, stutterers showed less alpha over the right posterior frontal region for verbal tasks, while after treatment there was less alpha over the left posterior frontal region. These findings suggest that alpha ratios over frontal motor areas may implicate motor programming aspects of stuttering and that increased fluency accompanying treatment shifts alpha suppression from the right to the left hemisphere.

McFarland and Moore (1982), using a double reversal single subject experimental biofeedback design, demonstrated a reduction of laryngeal electromyographic (EMG) activity with a corresponding decrease in disfluency. Alpha hemispheric asymmetries were also recorded pre- and post-treatment sessions. Results revealed right hemispheric alpha suppression during baseline (relatively high frequency of stuttering) with a gradual and consistent suppression of left hemispheric alpha as fluency increased. The importance of these later observations is that following treatment that increases fluency, stutterers apparently show a shift to more segmental, left hemispheric processing strategies.

Pinsky and McAdam (1980), when treating their data as categorical, did not support the contention that hemispheric alpha asymmetry patterns differ between stutterers and nonstutterers. Left and right hemisphere alpha ratios were collapsed over five tasks for the left hemisphere and four tasks for the right hemisphere. These ratios were not analyzed statistically but any change, no matter how small, between collapsed means was taken as evidence for reliable differences between tasks. The grouping of tasks *a priori* as left or right hemispheric also does not allow for observing differences between tasks that might differentiate the two groups. Consequently, it is difficult to assess the differences, if any, between the stutterers and nonstutterers from the data presented in this investigation.

Averaged evoked responses (AER) have been used by Ponsford, Brown, Marsh, and Travis (1975) to investigate hemispheric differences between stutterers and nonstutterers. Potentials were evoked with meaningful words embedded in phrases. Results indicated that normals' responses were most different in the left hemisphere. Stutterers showed a reversal of this trend, with greater differences in the right hemisphere and greater variance among subjects.

Zimmerman and Knott (1974) used the contingent negative variation (CNV) method (a specialized form of AER) to investigate hemisphere differences in stutterers and nonstutterers. Two control conditions with nonverbal stimuli (tones) requiring a nonverbal response were compared with two experimental conditions in which meaningful linguistic stimuli (words) were used. In one experimental condition subjects indicated whether or not they thought they would stutter on the word presented by pushing one of two keys marked "yes" and "no. " In the second experimental condition, subjects were instructed to speak each word upon signal. Results revealed differences between groups for frontal electrodes placed over Broca's area on the left and its contralateral homologue on the right. Zimmerman and Knott stated:

When processing verbal stimuli stutterers appear to show more variable interhemispheric relationships and do not show a shift that is consistently larger
in the left hemisphere than in the right. (p. 604)

Pinsky and McAdam presented data using the CNV method for
average evoked responses. In their study nonlinguistic stimuli were used
(1000-Hz tone) under two response conditions. One condition required
subjects to press a button with each thumb simultaneously when a tone
stopped. For the second condition subjects uttered the same fluent word
each trial at the termination of the tone, in constrast to the Zimmerman and Knott study in which subjects were required to utter each word
presented whether fluent or not. Pinsky and McAdam concluded that
their results provided insufficient evidence to support hemispheric
asymmetries between stutterers and nonstutterers with their CNV
method.

In the two AER investigations that used meaningful linguistic stimuli,
stutterers were found to show greater right hemispheric activation during
such tasks. In a third study, which used nonverbal stimuli and the
repetition of a single fluent word, it was concluded that there were no
differences between groups. Differences in behavioral tasks between
studies may well account for the disparate conclusions reached. For
example, saying fluent words may activate different processing strategies
in stutterers than saying disfluent words (see below).

Other methods. The only investigation to study cortical blood flow
with stutterers was conducted by Wood, Stumps, Sheldon, and Proctor
(1980). Using noninvasive measurement of regional cerebral circulation,
as described by Stump and Williams (1980), two stutterers were subjected
to cerebral blood flow measurements while reading aloud. During one
condition they read aloud while under the influence of haloperidol,
which resulted in improved fluency, and under a second condition
without medication. Wood et al. reported that both stutterers showed
higher cortical blood flow in Broca's area on the right compared to the
left hemisphere *during stuttering*. With regard to posterior areas, greater
cerebral blood flow was found in Wernicke's area in the left compared
to the right hemisphere during stuttering. Interestingly, when subjects
were fluent, greater flow was observed in the left hemisphere compared
to the right. These results provide further support of the relationship
between stuttered speech and hemispheric processing reported by Boberg
et al. (1983) and McFarland and Moore (1982), whose investigations
found a shift in alpha suppression from right to left hemisphere
accompanied improvement in fluency.

The last investigation to be discussed in this section implicates the
importance of subcortical structures in stuttering. In the section on

morphological asymmetries of the brain, we noted the importance of the left and right pulvinars (thalamic nuclei) in language processing. The pulvinars are association nuclei and have inputs from all primary sensory pathways. Work conducted by Ojemann and his colleagues (Fedio & Van Buren, 1975; Ojemann, 1975; Ojemann et al., 1968) suggests that the left pulvinar/thalamus may direct attention to linguistic stimuli in the external environment. The right pulvinar seems more involved with directing attention to visual–spatial stimuli. Brown (1975) has also suggested that anterior and posterior cortical connections from the pulvinar may allow for simultaneous activation of these areas for both motor and perceptual aspects of language. If stuttering is a behavioral manifestation of a central disorder, then we might also hypothesize subcortical deviations that relate to cortical findings.

Support for the above speculation can be found in an investigation by Hall and Jerger (1978). Using a battery of clinical auditory tests, they found depressed performance for their stutterers on three measures— the acoustic reflex amplitude function, synthetic identification with ipsilateral competing messages, and staggered spondaic word test. While stressing the subtlety of their findings, they concluded that stutterers presented evidence of a central auditory deficiency and that patterns of test results suggested a disorder at the brainstem level.

Hall and Jerger's results may reflect a central linguistic difference in stutterers which manifests itself as a "central auditory deficiency" due to the nature of the auditory stimuli used in their test battery. One potentially important suggestion from their data is a possible link between subcortical and cortical structures, which may include the pulvinars, that results in a central linguistic dysfunction among stutterers.

CONCLUSIONS

There is compelling evidence of asymmetries in both cognitive capacities and morphological structures of the cerebral hemispheres. Enhanced neural mass in the left planum temporale, together with the specific alerting response to auditory–verbal stimuli provided by the left pulvinar, may make the left hemisphere uniquely suited for processing time-dependent, segmental, auditory stimuli. The greater tissue mass in the posterior portion of the right hemisphere and the importance of the right pulvinar for directing visual–spatial information to the right hemisphere, may specialize it for time-independent, nonsegmental information. There are also a variety of task, stimulus, and subject variables that influence hemispheric activation. Also, the right hemisphere is capable of processing linguistic information, but differently from the left hemisphere. It is less capable of performing phonetic analyses but better suited to performing auditory and visual pattern matching with stored exemplars. Consequently, the right hemisphere is able to process high imagery, meaningful linguistic information that is embedded in nontransformed versus transformed sentences. We should not view hemispheric processing as left–linguistic, right–nonlinguistic, but should consider stimulus and task variables as variables which differentially evoke hemispheric activation.

Investigations with stutterers that have used meaningful linguistic stimuli with dichotic, tachistoscopic, hemispheric alpha asymmetries, averaged evoked response, contingent negative variation, and blood flow methods have *all* reported right hemispheric activation for perceptual and motor processing.

While not predicting right hemispheric processing of nonsense syllables, which depend on phonological aspects of language, many investigations of dichotic listening with nonsense syllables reported subgroups of stutterers with left ear preferences for such stimuli. Perhaps of greater importance are results from two dichotic studies that found stutterers to be inferior to nonstutterers in reporting nonsense syllables, which may reflect a "phoneme deficiency" disorder. It was suggested that these findings may be related to stutterers' greater dependency on right hemispheric processing and a reflection of the right hemisphere's decreased capacity to process phonologic information.

Several investigations have addressed the CNS mechanism of fluent and disfluent speech in stutterers. Two clinical investigations have shown a shift in hemispheric activation in stutterers from the right to the left hemisphere as fluency increases from clinical intervention. One blood flow study found higher left frontal hemispheric flow during fluent speech and greater right frontal flow during stuttered speech.

There is considerable evidence for right hemispheric processing of meaningful linguistic stimuli in stutterers. One can hypothesize that tasks and stimuli requiring time-dependent, segmental processing will be more defective than those requiring time-independent, nonsegmental strategies in stutterers. A review of those variables associated with stutterers' language lends support to such a hypothesis.

Research has shown that stuttering frequency increases: on the same words of initial segments of long sentences compared to short sentences (Tornick & Bloodstein, 1976); on low-frequency words compared to high-frequency words (Palin & Peterson, 1982; Ronson, 1976; Schlesinger, Melkman, & Levy, 1966); from base structure sentences to transformations (Bloodstein & Gantwerk, 1967; Hannah & Gardner, 1968; Palin & Peterson, 1982; Ronson, 1976; Soderberg, 1967); at clause boundaries compared to internal (nonboundary) positions of clauses

(Wall, Starkweather & Cairns, 1981); and when voicing adjustments are required (see Molfese, 1978a, 1978b for a discussion of voicing and hemispheric processing; Adams & Reis, 1971, 1974; Wall, Starkweather, & Harris, 1981). Observations of the occurrence of disfluencies in stutterers' language reveal greater fluency breakdowns associated with linguistic variables that are not typically processed by the right hemisphere.

The above observations may have clinical and assessment implications for the management of disfluent verbal behavior. One might predict that the greater the severity of stuttering, the greater a stutterer's dependency on right hemispheric processing. The research reviewed supports this prediction and suggests that we evaluate not only stutterers' verbal behaviors, but also their primary modes of hemispheric information processing.

From a clinical management perspective, the data suggest that disfluent verbal behavior may result from hemispheric processing differences. These processing differences may be related to an inability, under certain circumstances, to handle the segmentation aspects of language. Clinical investigations in these areas have only just begun. The future looks bright for understanding the process of which stuttered verbal behavior is the outcome—a long neglected area of inquiry.

REFERENCES

Adams, M. R., & Reis, R. The influence of the onset of phonation on the frequency of stuttering. *Journal of Speech and Hearing Research,* 1971, *14,* 639–644.

Adams, M. R., & Reis, R. Influence of the onset of phonation on the frequency of stuttering: A replication and re-evaluation. *Journal of Speech and Hearing Research,* 1974, *17,* 752–754.

Andrews, G., Quinn, P. T., & Sorby, W. A. Stuttering: An investigation into cerebral dominance of speech. *Journal of Neurology, Neurosurgery, and Psychiatry,* 1972, *25,* 414–418.

Bloodstein, O. *A handbook of stuttering.* Chicago: The National Easter Seal Society, 1981.

Bloodstein, O., & Gantwerk, B. F. Grammatical function in relation to stuttering in young children. *Journal of Speech and Hearing Research,* 1967, *10,* 786–789.

Boberg, E., Yeudall, L., Schopflocher, D., & Bo-Lassen, P. The effects of an intensive behavioral program on the distribution of EEG alpha power in stutterers during the processing of verbal and visuospatial information. *Journal of Fluency Disorders,* 1983, *8,* 245–263.

Bradshaw, J. L. Right-hemisphere language: Familial and nonfamilial sinistrals, cognitive defects and writing hand position in sinistrals and concrete-abstract, imageable-nonimageable dimensions in word recognition. A review of interrelated issues. *Brain and Language,* 1980, *10,* 172–188.

Brady, J. P., & Berson, J. Stuttering, dichotic listening, and cerebral dominance. *Archives of General Psychiatry,* 1975, *32,* 1449–1459.

Brown, J. W. On the neural organization of language: Thalamic and cortical relationships. *Brain and Language,* 1975, *2,* 18–30.

Brown, W. S., Marsh, J. T., & Smith, J. C. Evoked potential waveform differences produced by the perception of different meanings of an ambiguous phrase. *Electroencephalography and Clinical Neurophysiology,* 1976, *41,* 113-123.

Brown, W. S., Marsh, J. T., & Smith, J. C. Contextual meaning effects on speech evoked potentials. *Behavioral Biology,* 1973, *9,* 755-761.

Cerf, A., & Prins, D. *Stutterers' ear preference for dichotic syllables.* Paper presented to the American Speech and Hearing Association Convention, Las Vegas, 1974.

Cooper, R., Osselton, J. W., & Shaw, J. C. *EEG Technology.* London: Butterworth, 1974.

Curry, F., & Gregory, H. The performance of stutterers on dichotic listening tasks thought to reflect cerebral dominance. *Journal of Speech and Hearing Research,* 1969, *12,* 73-82.

Daly, D. *An investigation of immediate auditory memory skills in "functional" stutterers.* Paper presented at the Annual Meeting of the International Neuropsychological Society, Atlanta, 1981.

Davenport, R. W. Dichotic listening in four severity levels of stuttering. Paper presented at the Annual Convention of the American Speech and Hearing Association, Atlanta, 1979.

Day, J. Right-hemisphere language processing in normal right-handers. *Journal of Experimental Psychology: Human Perception and Performance,* 1977, *13,* 518-528.

Day, J. Visual half-field word recognition as a function of syntactic class and imageability. *Neuropsychologia,* 1979, *17,* 515-519.

Dennis, M. Capacity and strategy for syntactic comprehension after left or right hemidecortication. *Brain and Language,* 1980, *10,* 287-317.(a)

Dennis, M. Language acquisition in a single hemisphere: Semantic organization. In D. Caplan (Ed.), *Biological studies of mental processes.* Cambridge, MIT Press, 1980.(b)

Dorman, M. F., & Porter, R. J., Jr. Hemispheric lateralization for speech perception in stutterers. *Cortex,* 1975, *11,* 181-185.

Douglass, L. C. A study of bilaterally recorded electroencephalograms of adult stutterers. *Journal of Experimental Psychology,* 1943, *32,* 247-265.

Faber-Clark, M., & Moore, W. H., Jr. Sex, task, and strategy effects in hemispheric alpha asymmetries for the recall and recognition of arousal words: Results from perceptual and motor tasks. *Brain and Cognition,* 1983, *2,* 233-250.

Fedio, P., & Van Buren, J. M. Memory and perceptual deficits during electrical stimulation in the left and right thalamus and parietal subcortex. *Brain and Language,* 1975, *2,* 78-100.

Fox, D. R. Electroencephalographic analysis during stuttering and nonstuttering. *Journal of Speech and Hearing Research,* 1966, *9,* 488-497.

Freestone, N. W. A brainwave interpretation of stuttering. *Quarterly Journal of Speech,* 1942, *28,* 466-470.

Galin, D., & Ornstein, R. Lateral specialization of cognitive mode: An EEG study. *Psychophysiology,* 1972, *9,* 412-418.

Gates, A., & Bradshaw, J. The role of the cerebral hemispheres in music. *Brain and Language,* 1977, *9,* 403-431.

Geschwind, N. Anatomical foundation of language and dominance. In C. L. Ludlow & M. E. Doran-Quine (Eds.), *The neurological bases of language disorders in children: Methods and directions for research.* Bethesda: NIH Publication 79-440, 145-153, 1979.

Geschwind, N., & Levitsky, W. Left-right asymmetries in temporal speech regions. *Science,* 1968, *161,* 186-187.

Gordon, W. H. Left hemisphere dominance of rhythmic elements in dichotically-presented melodies. *Cortex,* 1979, *15,* 58–70.

Gruber, F., & Segalowitz, S. Some issues and methods in the neuropsychology of language. In S. Segalowitz & F. Gruber (Eds.), *Language development and neurological theory.* New York: Academic Press, 1977.

Hall, J. W., & Jerger, J. Central auditory function in stutterers. *Journal of Speech and Hearing Research,* 1978, *21,* 324–337.

Hand, C. R., & Haynes, W. O. Linguistic processing and reaction time differences in stutterers and nonstutterers. *Journal of Speech and Hearing Research,* 1983, *26,* 181–185.

Hannah, E. P., & Gardner, J. G. A note on syntactic relationships in nonfluency. *Journal of Speech and Hearing Research,* 1968, *11,* 853–860.

Haynes, W. O., & Moore, W. H., Jr. Sentence imagery and recall: An electroencephalographic evaluation of hemispheric processing in males and females. *Cortex,* 1981, *17,* 49–62.(a)

Haynes, W. O., & Moore, W. H., Jr. Recognition and recall: An electroencephalographic investigation of hemispheric alpha asymmetries for males and females on perceptual and retrieval tasks. *Perceptual and Motor Skills,* 1981, *53,* 283–290.(b)

Heeschen, C., & Júrgens, R. Pragmatic-semantic and syntactic factors influencing ear differences in dichotic listening. *Cortex,* 1978, *14,* 17–24.

Hines, D. Bilateral tachistoscopic recognition of verbal and non-verbal stimuli. *Cortex,* 1972, *7,* 313–322.

Hochberg, F. H., & LeMay, M. Arteriographic correlates of handedness. *Neurology,* 1975, *25,* 218–222.

Jones, R. K. Observations on stammering after localized cerebral injury. *Journal of Neurology, Neurosurgery and Psychiatry,* 1966, *29,* 192–195.

Kimura, D. Cerebral dominance and the perception of verbal stimuli. *Canadian Journal of Psychology,* 1961, *15,* 166–177.(a)

Kimura, D. Some effects of temporal lobe damage in auditory perception. *Canadian Journal of Psychology,* 1961, *14,* 156–165.(b)

Knott, J. R., & Tjossen, T. D. Bilateral encephalograms from normal speakers and stutterers. *Journal of Experimental Psychology,* 1943, *32,* 357–362.

Kutas, M., & Donchin, E. Variations in the latency of P300 as a function of variations in semantic categorization. In D. Otto (Ed.), *New perspectives in event-related potential (EPR) research.* Washington, D. C.: U.S. Government Printing Office, 1979.

Lassen, N. A., Ingvar, D. H., & Skinhøj, E. Brain function and blood flow. *Scientific American,* 1978, *239,* 62–71.

LeMay, M., & Culebras, A. Human brain—Morphological differences in the hemispheres demonstrable by carotid arteriography. *New England Journal of Medicine,* 1972, *287,* 168–170.

Liebetrau, R. M., & Daly, D. A. Auditory processing and perceptual abilities of "organic" and "functional" stutterers. *Journal of Fluency Disorders,* 1981, *6,* 219–231.

Lindsley, D. Bilateral differences in brain potentials from the two hemispheres in relation to laterality and stuttering. *Journal of Experimental Psychology,* 1940, *26,* 211–225.

Luessenhop, A. J., Boggs, J. S., LaBorwit, L. J., & Walle, E. L. Cerebral dominance in stutterers determined by Wada testing. *Neurology,* 1973, *23,* 1190–1192.

McFarland, D. H. II, & Moore, W. H., Jr. *Alpha hemispheric asymmetries during an electromyographic biofeedback procedure for stuttering.* Paper presented to the Annual Convention of the American Speech-Language-Hearing Association, Toronto, 1982.

McKee, G., Humphrey, B., & McAdam, D. Scaled lateralizations of alpha activity during linguistic and musical tasks. *Psychophysiology*, 1973, *10*, 441-443.

McKeever, W. F., & Huling, M. D. Lateral dominance in tachistoscopic word recognition as a function of hemisphere stimulation and interhemispheric transfer time. *Neuropsychologia*, 1971, *9*, 291-299.

McRae, D. L., Branch, C. L., & Milner, B. The occipital horns and cerebral dominance. *Neurology*, 1968, *18*, 95-98.

Molfese, D. L. Hemispheric specialization for temporal information: Implications for the perception of voicing cures during speech perception. *Brain and Language*, 1980, *11*, 285-299.

Molfese, D. L. Electrophysiological correlates of categorical speech perception in adults. *Brain and Language*, 1978, *5*, 25-35.

Molfese, D. L. Left and right hemisphere involvement in speech perception: Electrophysiological correlates. *Perception and Psychophysics*, 1978, *23*, 237-243. (b)

Molfese, D. L., Freeman, R. B., Jr., & Palermo, D. S. The ontogeny of brain lateralization for speech and nonspeech stimuli. *Brain and Language*, 1975, *2*, 356-368.

Moore, W. H., Jr. Alpha hemispheric asymmetry of males and females on verbal and nonverbal tasks: Some preliminary results. *Cortex*, 1979, *15*, 321-326.

Moore, W. H., Jr. Bilateral tachistoscopic word perception of stutterers and normal subjects. *Brain and Language*, 1976, *3*, 434-442.

Moore, W. H., Jr., Craven, D. C., & Faber, M. Hemispheric alpha asymmetries of words with positive, negative, and neutral arousal values preceding tasks of recall and recognition: Electrophysiological and behavioral results from stuttering males and nonstuttering males and females. *Brain and Language*, 1982, *17*, 211-224.

Moore, W. H., Jr., & Haynes, W. O. Alpha hemispheric asymmetry and stuttering: Some support for a segmentation dysfunction hypothesis. *Journal of Speech and Hearing Research*, 1980, *23*, 229-247.(a)

Moore, W. H., Jr., & Haynes, W. O. A study of alpha hemispheric asymmetries and their relationship to verbal and nonverbal abilities in males and females. *Brain and Language*, 1980, *9*, 338-349.(b)

Moore, W. H., Jr., & Lang, M. K. Alpha asymmetry over the right and left hemispheres of stutterers and control subjects preceding massed oral readings: A preliminary investigation. *Perceptual and Motor Skills*, 1977, *44*, 223-230.

Moore, W. H., Jr., & Lorendo, L. Alpha hemispheric asymmetries of stuttering and nonstuttering subjects for words of high and low imagery. *Journal of Fluency Disorders*, 1980, *5*, 11-26.

Moore, W. H., Jr., & Weidner, W. E. Bilateral tachistoscopic word perception in aphasic and normal subjects. *Perceptual and Motor Skills*, 1974, *38*, 1003-1011.

Morgan, A. H., McDonald, P. J., & MacDonald, H. Differences in bilateral alpha activity as a function of experimental task with a note on lateral eye movements and hypnotizability. *Neuropsychologia*, 1971, *9*, 459-469.

Morley, A. J. An analysis of the associative and predisposing factors in the symptomatology of stuttering. Unpublished PhD dissertation, State University of Iowa, 1935.

Niederbuhl, J., & Springer, S. P. Task requirements and hemispheric asymmetry for the processing of single letters. *Neuropsychologia*, 1979, *17*, 689-692.

Neville, H. J. Event-related potentials in neuropsychological studies of language. *Brain and Language*, 1980, *11*, 300-318.

Ojemann, G. A. Language and the thalamus: Object naming and recall during and after thalamic stimulation. *Brain and Language*, 1975, *2*, 101-120.

Ojemann, G. A., Fedio, P., & Van Buren, J. M. Anomia from pulvinar and subcortical parietal stimulation. *Brain*, 1968, *91*, 99–116.

Orton, S. T. Studies in stuttering. *Archives of Neurology and Psychiatry*, 1927, *18*, 671–672.

Palin, C., & Peterson, J. M. Word frequency and children's stuttering: The relationship to sentence structure. *Journal of Fluency Disorders*, 1982, *7*, 55–62.

Perrin, K. L., & Eisenson, J. *An examination of ear preference for speech and nonspeech stimuli in a stuttering population.* Paper presented at the Annual Convention of the American Speech and Hearing Association, New York, 1970.

Pinsky, S. D., & McAdam, D. W. Electroencephalographic and dichotic indices of cerebral laterality in stutterers. *Brain and Language*, 1980, *11*, 374–397.

Plakosh, P. *The functional asymmetry of the brain: Hemispheric specialization in stutterers for processing of visually presented linguistic and spatial stimuli.* Unpublished doctoral dissertation, the Palo Alto School of Professional Psychology, 1978.

Ponsford, R., Brown, W., Marsh, J., & Travis, L. Evoked potential correlates of cerebral dominance for speech perception in stutterers and nonstutterers. *Electroencephalography and Clinical Neurophysiology*, 1975, *39*, 434 (abstract).

Porter, R. J., Jr., & Berlin, C. I. On interpreting developmental changes in the dichotic right-ear advantage. *Brain and Language*, 1975, *2*, 186–200.

Quinn, P. T. Stuttering, cerebral dominance and the dichotic word test. *Medical Journal of Australia*, 1972, *2*, 639–643.

Ratcliff, G., Dila, C., Taylor, L., & Milner, B. The morphological asymmetry of the hemispheres and cerebral dominance for speech: A possible relationship. *Brain and Language*, 1980, *11*, 87–98.

Risberg, J. Regional cerebral blood flow measurements by 133Xe-Inhalation: Methodology and applications in neuropsychology and psychiatry. *Brain and Language*, 1980, *9*, 9–34.

Robbins, K. I., & McAdam, D. W. Interhemispheric alpha asymmetry and imagery mode. *Brain and Language*, 1974, *1*, 189–193.

Ronson, I. Word frequency and stuttering: The relationship to sentence structure. *Journal of Speech and Hearing Research*, 1976, *19*, 813–819.

Rosenfield, D. B., & Goodglass, H. Dichotic testing of cerebral dominance in stutterers. *Brain and Language*, 1980, *11*, 170–180.

Rosenzweig, M. R. Representation of the two ears at the auditory cortex. *American Journal of Physiology*, 1951, *167*, 147–158.

Satz, P., Bakker, D., Teunissen, J., Goebel, R., & Van der Vlugt, H. Developmental parameters of the ear asymmetry: A multivariate approach. *Brain and Language*, 1975, *2*, 171–185.

Schlesinger, I. M., Melkman, R., & Levy, R. Word length and frequency as determinants of stuttering. *Psychonomic Science*, 1966, *6*, 255–256.

Segalowitz, S., & Gruber, F. (Eds.) *Language development and neurological theory.* New York: Academic Press, 1977.

Seitz, M. R., Weber, B., Jacobson, J., & Morehouse, R. The use of averaged electroencephalographic response techniques in the study of auditory processing related to speech and language. *Brain and Language*, 1980, *11*, 261–284.

Shankweiler, D., & Studdert-Kennedy, M. A continuum of lateralization for speech perception. *Brain and Language*, 1975, *2*, 212–225.

Soderberg, G. A. Linguistic factors in stuttering. *Journal of Speech and Hearing Research*, 1967, *10*, 801–810.

Sommers, R. K., Brady, W., & Moore, W. H. Dichotic ear preferences of stuttering children and adults. *Perceptual and Motor Skills*, 1975, *41*, 931–938.

Springer, S. P., & Gazzaniga, M. A. Dichotic testing of partial and complete split brain subjects. *Neuropsychologia*, 1975, *13*, 341-346.

Steer, M. Symptomatology of young stutterers. *Journal of Speech Disorders*, 1937, *2*, 3-13.

Strong, J. C. Dichotic speech perception: A comparison between stutterers and nonstutterers. *ASHA*, 1978, *20*, 728 (abstract).

Strother, C. A study of the extent of dyssynergia occurring during stuttering spasm. Unpublished PhD dissertation, State University of Iowa, 1935.

Stump, D. A., & Williams, R. The noninvasive measurement of regional cerebral circulation. *Brain and Language*, 1980, *9*, 35-46.

Sussman, H. M., & MacNeilage, P. F. Hemispheric specialization for speech production and perception in stutterers. *Neuropsychologia*, 1975, *13*, 19-26.

Tallal, P., & Newcomb, F. Impairment of auditory perception and language comprehension in dysphasia. *Brain and Language*, 1978, *5*, 13-24.

Tallal, P., & Piercy, M. Developmental aphasia: Rate of auditory processing and selective impairment of consonant perceptions. *Neuropsychologia*, 1974, *12*, 83-93.

Thatcher, R. W. Neurolinguistics: Theoretical and evolutionary perspectives. *Brain and Language*, 1980, *11*, 235-260.

Thatcher, R. W. Evoked-potential correlates of hemispheric lateralization during semantic information processing. In S. Harnad, R. Doty, L. Goldstein, J. Jaynes, & G. Krauthamer (Eds.), *Lateralization in the nervous system.* New York: Academic Press, 1977.

Tornick, G. B., & Bloodstein, O. Stuttering and sentence length. *Journal of Speech and Hearing Research*, 1976, *19*, 651-654.

Travis, L. E. *Speech pathology.* New York: Appleton-Century-Crofts, 1931.

Travis, L. E. Disassociation of the homologous muscle function in stutterers. *Archives of Neurology and Psychiatry*, 1934, *31*, 127-133.

Wada, J. A. Interhemispheric sharing and shift of cerebral speech function. *Excerta Medica International Congress Series*, 1969, *193*, 296-297.

Wada, J. A new method for the determination of the side of cerebral speech dominance. *Medical Biology*, 1949, *14*, 221-222.

Wada, J. A., Clarke, R., & Hamm, A. Cerebral hemispheric asymmetry in humans. *Archives of Neurology*, 1975, *32*, 239-246.

Wall, M. J., Starkweather, C. W., & Cairns, H. S. Syntactic influences on stuttering in young child stutterers. *Journal of Fluency Disorders*, 1981, *6*, 283-298.

Wall, M. J., Starkweather, C. W., & Harris, K. S. The influence of voicing adjustments in the location of stuttering in the spontaneous speech of young child stutterers. *Journal of Fluency Disorders*, 1981, *6*, 299-310.

Whitaker, H., & Whitaker, H. *Studies in neurolinguistics, 1.* New York: Academic Press, 1975.

Whitaker, H., & Whitaker, H. *Studies in neurolinguistics, 2.* New York: Academic Press, 1976.

Whitaker, H., & Whitaker, H. *Studies in neurolinguistics, 3.* New York: Academic Press, 1977.

Williams, D. E. Masseter muscle action potentials in stuttered and nonstuttered speech. *Journal of Speech and Hearing Disorders*, 1955, *20*, 242-261.

Willis, S. G., Wheatley, G. H., & Mitchell, O. R. Cerebral processing of spatial and verbal-analytic tasks: An EEG study. *Neuropsychologia*, 1979, *17*, 473-484.

Witelson, A., & Pallie, W. Left hemisphere specialization for language in the newborn: Neurological evidence of asymmetry. *Brain*, 1973, *96*, 641-646.

Wood, F. Theoretical methodological, and statistical implications of the inhalation rCBF technique for the study of brain–behavior relationships. *Brain and Language*, 1980, *9*, 1-8.

Wood, F., Stump, D., McKeehan, A., Sheldon, S., & Proctor, J. Patterns of regional cerebral blood flow during attempted reading aloud by stutterers both on and off haloperidol medication: Evidence for inadequate left frontal activation during stuttering. *Brain and Language*, 1980, *9*, 141-144.

Zaidel, E. The split and half brains as models of congenital language disability. In C. L. Ludlow, M. E. Doran-Quine (Eds.), *The neurological bases of language disorders in children: Methods and directions for research.* Bethesda: NIH Publication 79-440, 55-89, 1979.

Zaidel, E. Auditory language comprehension in the right hemisphere following cerebral commissurotomy and hemispherectomy: A comparison with child language and aphasia. In A. Caramazza & E. G. Zuriff (Eds.), *The acquisition and breakdown of language: Parallels and divergencies.* (pp 229-275). Baltimore: Johns Hopkins University Press, 1978.

Zaidel, E. Auditory vocabulary of the right hemisphere following brain bisection or hemidecortication. *Cortex*, 1976, *12*, 191-211.

Zimmerman, G. N., & Knott, J. R. Slow potentials of the brain relation to speech processing in normal speakers and stutterers. *Electroencephalography and Clinical Neurophysiology*, 1974, *37*, 599-607.

Chapter 5

Stuttering and Auditory Function

David B. Rosenfield and James Jerger

Auditory tests have played two important roles in stuttering research: first, as sensitive measures of cerebral dominance for language; second, in the search for abnormalities of the auditory feedback mechanism subserving speech production. In this chapter we review the evidence, both positive and negative, relating stuttering to abnormalities in each of these areas. We then discuss our own conclusions and thoughts about the directions that future research in this area might take.

STUTTERING AND CEREBRAL DOMINANCE
The Orton–Travis thesis

More than 50 years ago, Orton (1928) and Travis (1931) proposed that individuals stutter due to incomplete cerebral lateralization of language. They theorized that many children go through a stage of disfluency because language has not yet lateralized to the appropriate hemisphere. As the child grows older, the language lateralization process becomes more complete and the disfluency disappears. However, a subgroup retain their abnormal bilateral representation and continue to stutter.

As a result of the Orton–Travis thesis, many investigators addressed the prevalence of right- and left-handedness among stutterers, contending that if stuttering were a disorder due to abnormal cerebral laterality, such an abnormality should be reflected in a different matrix of handedness between stutterers and nonstutterers. Due to varying definitions of handedness, and varying methods of ascertaining the presence/absence of stuttering in populations, investigators derived conflicting data and arrived at disparate results. As a result, the Orton–Travis thesis soon lost popularity (Bryngelson, 1935, 1939; Milisen & Johnson, 1936; McAllister, 1937; Daniels, 1940; Spadino, 1941; Meyer, 1945; Despert, 1946).

Jones and the Wada test

The Orton-Travis thesis lay fairly dormant until Jones (1966), a neurosurgeon, had occasion to operate upon four stutterers who had developed cerebral disease necessitating surgical intervention. Aware of the thesis that language might reside in both hemispheres of stutterers, Jones was concerned that his contemplated surgery might render the stutterers aphasic. (That is, would a stutterer undergoing left brain surgery become aphasic if classical areas of speech were surgically compromised? Could the same happen to the right?) In order to obtain this information preoperatively, he performed the Wada test.

The Wada test (Wada & Rasmussen, 1960) consists of an intracarotid injection of sodium amytal, a short-acting barbiturate. Each carotid artery supplies the ipsilateral cerebral hemisphere (although sometimes there is crossover of blood flow). The barbiturate transiently anesthetizes the ipsilateral hemisphere. Patients are transiently hemiplegic on the side contralateral to the injection and are aphasic if the language-dominant hemisphere was exposed to the barbiturate.

Jones noted that all four stutterers became aphasic following amytal injection in either their right or their left carotid artery; this suggested that both hemispheres were contributing significantly to language production. Each patient required surgery on one hemisphere as a result of the underlying cerebral lesion. All four ceased stuttering following surgery. A repeat Wada test elicited aphasia only after injection on the nonoperated side. The patients no longer had bilateral speech representation and they no longer stuttered.

Jones' paper, although exciting, is open to several criticisms. (1) A major obstacle to accepting his findings as having import on the genesis of stuttering is the fact that there are several patients who have bilaterally positive Wada tests but who do not stutter (Milner, Branch, & Rasmussen, 1960). (2) Additionally, there is no statement as to how the presence of stuttering was ascertained. (3) Further, all but one of his four patients were left-handed, thus implying bilateral language representation (Benson & Geschwind, 1977). (4) All but one had a strong family history of left-handedness, also implicating bilateral language representation (Zurif & Bryden, 1969). Why should bilateral speech representation make one stutter as opposed to being hyperfluent, aphasic, mute, or even schizophrenic? Do we know for certain that bilateral language representation causes poor motor regulation of articulation and phonation? Since some people have bilateral language representation and do not stutter, are stutterers "different" on levels other than that of cerebral dominance, even if dominance differences are known to exist?

Several investigators have pursued Wada testing in stutterers (Luessenhop, Boggs, LaBorwit, & Walle, 1973; Andrews, Quinn, & Sorby, 1972). In total, 11 stutterers have had bilateral Wada tests; bilateral speech representation was noted in 5. One of these was an individual who had developed stuttering-like behavior and aphasia following head trauma. This discrepancy may reflect the fact that stuttering is not a homogeneous disturbance.

The Wada test is invasive; it involves intra-arterial puncture with injection of dye. The test carries a risk, not because of the injection of the barbiturate but because of the possible complications associated with the procedure. Although physicians frequently employ this procedure with intracerebral disease, it is not readily employable for research purposes in subjects who do not have brain compromise. There are, however, less invasive techniques that permit analysis of cerebral dominance. One of these is dichotic listening.

Dichotic listening

In the dichotic listening paradigm, different sounds are presented simultaneously to the two ears. The listener must report everything he hears, from both ears. Since the sounds are simultaneous, it is presumed that the listener must alternate attention between the two ears, placing one percept in short-term memory while attending to the other, and vice versa.

When normal adults are tested in the dichotic paradigm, there is a slight advantage for certain sounds delivered to the right ear, and for other sounds delivered to the left ear. Kimura was the first to demonstrate that verbal signals such as words or digits are more accurately reported from the right ear (i.e., left hemisphere) than from the left ear (i.e., right hemisphere) after simultaneous dichotic presentation (Kimura, 1961, 1967). The reverse is true for melodies (Kimura, 1967).

The fact that the dichotic paradigm demonstrates an asymmetry for verbal materials in favor of the hemisphere ordinarily dominant for language suggested, at least to some investigators, that dichotic listening tests might provide a relatively simple test of the Orton–Travis thesis. If stutterers are, indeed, lacking in suitable hemispheric dominance for language, this fact should be readily revealed by a proper dichotic test.

In evaluating this research, it is well to bear in mind that dichotic listening results are influenced by an array of contaminating variables. It is important, for example, to ascertain the handedness of the subjects being tested. Stating that subjects are right- or left-handed is not as meaningful from a laterality standpoint as the administration of a detailed handedness questionnaire (Oldfield, 1971). Another variable is the order in which subjects are instructed to report sounds (i.e., right ear first, left ear first, or either ear first). Most investigators who have controlled this variable have noted that there is a greater index of cerebral laterality when subjects are instructed to report first from the left ear and then from the right ear. When a sound is reported second, it must be held in short-term memory. Perhaps the signal from the right ear (left hemisphere) survives short-term storage better than that from the left ear. Since free report sometimes results in a biased strategy of always first reporting from one ear, it may well be very important to direct the subject to report a particular ear first (Satz, Aschenbach, Pattishall, & Fennell, 1965; Bryden, 1967; Goodglass & Peck, 1972).

Another variable is the stability of the dichotic ear advantage over time. Blumstein, Goodglass, and Tarter (1975), employing a test–retest experiment, contend that 85% of normal right-handed males have a right-ear advantage in dichotic listening and that any such test sample contains 15% misclassified subjects. They observed that as many as 30% may change ear dominance when retested. Thus, consistency between test and retest is an important dimension in studies of cerebral laterality.

Dichotic listening paradigms test a response to a sound input. The test evaluates cerebral laterality in a steady state; it does not evaluate laterality in the dynamic state of speech production. This may be very important in the investigation of stuttering. Suppose, for example, that stutterers have a disturbance in cerebral laterality that causes a compromise in their speech output. This "abnormality" may not be static, that is, it may only appear during speech, or perhaps only at certain times during speech production. There is a challenge to devise a means of investigating laterality as a concomitant of the stuttering act. Interhemispheric competition might exist as a phasic phenomenon. Perhaps one should (ideally) investigate a stutterer at the precise moment of the stuttered disfluency, although this is technically difficult. With these caveats in mind, we turn to a review of dichotic test findings in stutterers.

Dichotic listening in stutterers

Curry and Gregory (1969) used a dichotic listening paradigm with 20 adult stutterers (19 males, 1 female) and 20 appropriate controls. All were stated to be right-handed. The authors employed several dichotic tasks, one of which was the Dichotic Word Test. This test involves the recognition of pairs of consonant–vowel–consonant (CVC) words of high familiarity, presented in groups of 6 pairs with 0.5 sec separating each pair. After each group of 6 word pairs had been presented, the subjects attempted to recall the 12 different words, in any order, and without concern for which words had been presented to any particular ear. The anticipated right ear superiority was significantly less for stutterers than for nonstutterers. Seventy-five percent of the nonstutterers had right ear scores that were higher than their left; this was true for only 45% of the stutterers. Kimura contends that such reversals of ear superiority occur in cases of known reversals of hemispheric dominance, as confirmed by intracarotid amytal test. Finally, the nonstutterers' mean absolute between ears difference score was more than twice that of the stutterers.

Quinn (1972) also investigated dichotic listening in stutterers. His method was similar to that of Curry and Gregory; neither evaluated the order of report. Quinn examined 60 right-handed stutterers (53 males, 7 females) and matched controls. He detected no reliable difference between the two groups. However, he did observe that 12 stutterers had left ear scores that were higher than right ear scores; only two nonstutterers had this "reversal." The author subsequently realized that 5 of these 12 stutterers were left-handed golfers. The remaining 7 were strongly right-handed. Thus, although he initially believed that his sample was right-handed, some were more right-handed than others. Perhaps other discrepancies of handedness existed in other subjects, both in this study and in others.

Dorman and Porter (1975) evaluated 16 right-handed adult stutterers (12 males, 4 females) and compared them to 20 controls (10 males, 10 females). Subjects had to write down responses to synthetically generated consonant–vowel dichotic stimuli. There was no significant difference between stutterers and nonstutterers. Pinsky and McAdam (1980) tested 5 adult stutterers and 5 fluent speakers in a dichotic listening paradigm. All individuals were right-handed except one, who was stated to be "weakly right-handed." The degree of right-handedness was not commented upon. The authors failed to find a significant difference between the stutterers and the nonstutterers.

Slorach and Noehr (1973) examined 15 stutterers, aged 6 to 9 years. They presented dichotic digit pairs and tested not only the free recall of digits but also the performance on instructed order of report from particular ears. The stutterers' scores were similar to those of controls. Gruber and Powell (1974) tested 28 right-handed children using dichotic digit pairs. They failed to find significant interear differences for either stutterers' or controls' free recall reports. At this point, one should note that since 4% of children stutter, whereas only 1% of adults stutter, the mechanism(s) or type(s) of stuttering among children might be different from that among adults.

Rosenfield and Goodglass (1980) queried whether the above studies had failed to take into account a number of variables that might affect results. Children stutterers, for example, might be different from adult stutterers. Perhaps males and females should not be mixed in a stuttering paradigm since the prognosis and prevalence among females is different from that among males. Rigorous handedness questionnaires should be given to stutterers since laterality is an issue, and, therefore, one should be certain that one is testing a homogeneously handed population.

In an effort to control all relevant variables, Rosenfield and Goodglass (1980) evaluated a group of adult male, strongly right-handed, stutterers. They evaluated left cerebral dominance for language using consonant-vowel stimuli, and tested right hemisphere laterality for melodies by testing melody input. Right ear advantages were obtained for consonant–vowel stimuli, and left ear advantages were noted for melodies, without significant differences between the groups of stutterers and controls. However, there was a significantly greater number of stutterers than controls who consistently failed to show the expected ear laterality for either type of material.

In sum, these experiments evaluating dichotic listening performance in stutterers versus nonstutterers have addressed the issue of whether there is a right ear advantage and whether the difference between the groups in the degree of right ear advantage is significant. As pointed out by Moore (1976), stutterers seem to differ from nonstutterers when investigators employ meaningful verbal stimuli. Of the dichotic studies that employ words or digits, rather than meaningless consonant–vowel or other stimuli, most find a difference between stutterers and nonstutterers.

Sussman and MacNeilage (1975) employed a dichotic paradigm and another paradigm, that of pursuit auditory tracking. They reasoned that dichotic listening tested elements of laterality pertaining to speech perception, whereas the tracking paradigm tested speech production. Their experiment involved matching the frequency of a variable tone in one ear to the frequency of an externally varied tone in the other ear. The former tone was altered by a transducer attached to the tongue or jaw. The subject varied the frequency of this tone by appropriately moving the tongue or jaw. Subjects were required to "match" the frequency of this transducer-related tone to the frequency of the externally varied tone. The authors tested right-handed male and female stutterers and nonstutterers for laterality pertaining to speech perception (dichotic listening) and speech production (tracking paradigm). They noted a right-ear advantage for both nonstutterers and stutterers on the dichotic studies; stutterers did not differ from nonstutterers in laterality on the speech perception task. On the tracking paradigm, however, normals had a right ear advantage whereas stutterers did not (i.e., nonstutterers best altered the transducer tone when they heard it in the right ear and had to match it against the externally varied tone in the left, as opposed to having a transducer tone in the left and the externally varied tone in the right). This indicated a left hemisphere "dominance" for nonverbal output. Stutterers failed to demonstrate such laterality for nonverbal output.

Neilson, Quinn, and Neilson (1976) subsequently confirmed the observations of Sussman and MacNeilage in the pursuit auditory tracking for normal speakers, but found no difference between normal speakers and stutterers.

STUTTERING AND AUDITORY FEEDBACK

The notion that stuttering might be due to a defect in the auditory feedback mechanism subserving speech production has a long history in stuttering research. Over 40 years ago, surveys by Harms and Malone (1939) and Backus (1938) noted a low prevalence of stuttering in schools for the deaf. Whether this is a result of a compromised auditory circuit that does not permit stuttering, or the fact the deaf individuals have multiple articulatory disturbances and that their stuttering goes unrecognized, or that this reflects a slowed form of speaking that induces fluency, is not known.

Soon after the delayed auditory feedback (DAF) paradigm was developed, in the early 1950s, several investigators showed that, whereas nonstutterers develop disfluencies under DAF, stutterers show fewer disfluencies. Another research finding strongly implicating the auditory feedback mechanism is the fact that stutterers show increased fluency when external noise masks their own speech (Dewar, Dewar, Austin, & Brash, 1979).

The acoustic reflex

One component of the total auditory monitoring system, the acoustic reflex, has come under particular scrutiny because of its intimate relation to vocalization. The stapedius muscle contracts during vocalization. Borg and Zakrisson (1975) visually and electromyographically evaluated stapedius muscle activity that accompanied vocalization in fluent speakers who had a perforated tympanic membrane. EMG activity in the stapedius muscle accompanied speech, even at low levels of phonation. Stapedius EMG activity occurred before the onset of vocalization in 55% of their cases, and after vocalization in 45% (Borg & Zakrisson, 1975). In the former instance, the time difference between reflex onset and phonation onset was less than 75 msec. The authors concluded that EMG activity in the stapedius muscle is not caused by feedback of the voice signal but, rather, is centrally mediated as a component of the vocalization process.

At this point, we should note that EMG activity necessarily precedes the onset of any consequence of that activity, that is, the laryngeal muscle activity must precede the beginning of the acoustic wave form. Thus, one cannot take the onset of phonation as heralding the point of onset of the laryngeal muscle activity that underlies speech.

McCall and Rabuzzi (1973) offer confirmatory evidence that the activity of the stapedius muscle is a bona fide part of the phonation process. Upon electrical stimulation of the internal laryngeal nerve (similar to the human superior laryngeal nerve) in anesthetized cats, these investigators report concurrent EMG activity in the cricothyroid, tensor tympani, and stapedius muscles. Activation of the cricothyroid, but not the tensor or stapedius muscle, was observed during stimulation of the recurrent laryngeal nerve, the nerve which supplies the majority of laryngeal muscles.

Further evidence for an acoustic–laryngeal link is provided by Jen and Suga's (1976) work on echo-locating bats. When a bat produces a sound, the middle ear muscles contract following onset of laryngeal muscle activity. When the bat hears a sound, the middle ear muscles contract and, following this contraction, laryngeal muscles also contract.

Thus, there is evidence that stapedius muscle activity is involved in the phonatory process. Is it possible, then, that we may find an abnormality of the acoustic reflex in stutterers?

Shearer and Simmons (1965) investigated stapedius muscle activity in stutterers and nonstutterers during ongoing speech. They observed that stapedius muscle activity tended to parallel vocalization in non-stutterers. In stutterers, however, parallelism was less consistent. At times, the onset of stapedius activity seemed to be delayed relative to the onset of vocalization. In general, however, differences between groups were not striking.

Hall and Jerger (1978) compared the acoustic reflex to external sound in stutterers and controls. Reflex threshold was equivalant in the two groups, but reflex amplitude was smaller in the stuttering group. Hannley and Dorman (1982), however, failed to note any differences between the stutterers and nonstutterers.

Phase disparity

Another approach to the question of intrinsic abnormality in the stutterer's auditory monitoring system is to study phase disparities between air- and bone-conducted tones. In 1957, Stromsta exploited the fact that two pure tones, 180 degrees out of phase but equal in frequency and amplitude, will cancel each other out. Stutterers and normal speakers listened to an air-conducted tone introduced to the ear, and to a bone-conducted tone of the same frequency simultaneously introduced at the teeth. Subjects were asked to vary the phase and amplitude of the air-conducted tone until a critical adjustment was achieved at which no sound was audible to them. There was a significant difference between stutterers and nonstutterers in the relative phase angle of the air- and bone-conducted sounds at 2000 Hz. Using a similar method, Stromsta (1972) noted an unusual phase disparity between stutterers' left and right ears. The stutterers adjusted the amplitude and phase of two air-conducted tones, heard at either ear, until they cancelled an identical bone-conducted tone. At the point at which cancellation was achieved, the air-conducted tones of the two ears had a phase disparity at several frequencies that was twice as wide for the stutterers as for the nonstutterers.

If, indeed, stutterers have a brain disturbance such that they lack appropriate auditory feedback of ongoing speech, that same delay might create problems in nonspeech activities that depend upon auditory information for their performance. Stark and Pierce (1970) investigated whether stutterers would produce deviate responses in a simple oral activity such as lip closure under delayed auditory feedback conditions. Stutterers and nonstutterers were trained to reproduce a sequential pattern of lip closures, their lips positioned around an apparatus that generated an audible click with every lip closure. They engaged in these temporal patterns under normal auditory feedback, delayed auditory feedback, and a combination of delayed auditory feedback by air conduction and sensory auditory feedback by bone conduction. The delayed feedback condition caused disturbances in lip closure patterns; there were errors, prolonged lip closures, and prolongations of patterns in both nonstutterers and stutterers. The delayed auditory feedback had the same effect among both the stutterers and nonstutterers. However, the normal, nondelayed, auditory feedback paradigm caused longer lip closures and other errors among stutterers.

Central auditory dysfunction

Is it possible that defects in the auditory feedback mechanism of stutterers may be only part of a more comprehensive disorder of function in their central auditory perceptual mechanism? A number of investigators have attempted to explore this question, using both conventional clinical audiometric measures and testing techniques developed specifically to assess central auditory disorder. In 1959, Rousey, Goetzinger, and Dirks observed that stuttering children perform less well than nonstutterers in localizing sounds in space. Gregory (1964), further pursuing audiometric studies, contended that there was no significant difference between adult stutterers and nonstutterers in tests of sound localization, binaural loudness balance, and understanding of speech distorted by frequency filtering. Other investigators initially supported Gregory's findings (Kamiyama, 1964; Asp, 1968), but in the past 15 to 20 years, more sophisticated tests for central auditory dysfunction have been developed. In this setting, Hall and Jerger (1978) studied stutterers and nonstutterers with a battery of central tests. On most of these, stutterers' responses were normal; in some they were not.

One of the tests employed by Hall and Jerger was the Staggered Spondaic Word Test (SSW). Devised by Katz (1962), this test employs principles similar to dichotic listening. The stimuli are a series of two bisyllabic words, having equal stress on each syllable; the syllables are then overlapped in time. The overlapping syllable provides a dichotic input to the listener, although the syllables are not precisely aligned for simultaneous onset. Thus, the word "upstairs" might be played in the right ear, whereas "downtown" is played in the left ear. The "stairs" and "down" are both heard at approximately the same time. This test is extremely sensitive to temporal lobe dysfunction and recently was included in a battery of tests administered to stutterers by Hawver (1978). The stutterers and nonstutterers significantly differed in their total correct responses to the competing portion of this test. However, the means of the two groups, while satisfying statistical criteria for a significant difference at the .05 level, both fell within the range of normal performance on the test. Hall and Jerger (1978) also noted that stutterers performed less well than nonstutterers on this test.

The Synthetic Sentence Identification Test (SSI), in its contralateral competing message format (CCM), is also a type of dichotic test to assess temporal lobe function. The materials are a set of 10 nonsense sentences, presented in competition with an ongoing conversation. The message and competition are presented to opposite ears. Stutterers and fluent speakers perform in a similar manner on the SSI–CCM (Hall & Jerger, 1978; Toscher & Rupp, 1978).

Another test for central auditory disturbance involves monaural presentation of speech materials through a low-pass filter. Hawver (1978) failed to find any differences between stutterers and nonstutterers on this test.

The SSI can be performed with the competing messages presented to the same ear. In this paradigm, the ipsilateral competing message

(ICM), the test assesses sentence identification as a function of the message-to-competition ratio (MCR) or, more simply, the signal-to-noise ratio. The SSI–ICM test is a sensitive index of brainstem auditory function. Toscher and Rupp (1978) found a difference in the performance of stutterers versus nonstutterers. Their findings were criticized due to the fact that they used a nonstandard competing message for their tests. Further, there was no simultaneous analysis of acoustic reflex or auditory brainstem evoked responses.

Hall and Jerger (1978) employed a standardized version of the SSI and evaluated several other parameters of auditory function. As Toscher and Rupp had noted, these authors also observed that stutterers and fluent speakers differed in performance on the SSI. The mean differences between the two groups were small, and it is possible that such differences resulted from an unusually accurate performance on the part of the normal subjects, rather than from unusually poor performance by the stutterers.

Hannley and Dorman (1982) tested 20 individuals with SSI materials who had completed the fluency training program at the Hollins Communication Research Institute. Their stutterers performed as well as Hall and Jerger's normal listeners, and fell near the mean of normal performance. They contend that Hall and Jerger's normal listeners performed well above normal range and that their stutterers did not have an unusually poor performance. However, as Hannley and Dorman note, one could easily argue that the stutterers whom they tested had completed fluency training and, thus, possibly behaved like normal speakers. It is not known whether fluency training programs alter the manner in which competing messages are processed at the brainstem level. In any event, there is some evidence that stutterers may show a performance deficit on tests designed to assess central auditory function at the brainstem level. The evidence for a temporal lobe disorder is less convincing.

DISCUSSION

What can we conclude about stutterers from auditory measures? Is there any consistent thread of evidence linking stuttering either to failure of cerebral dominance or to a defective auditory feedback system? Our brief review seems laden with contradictory evidence. For every study reporting a positive difference between stutterers and nonstutterers, there seem to be two or three reporting negative results. Should we dismiss sporadic positive findings as an "immaculate perception" of investigators with an axe to grind? Perhaps, but to do so would be to ignore a persistent pattern of findings, based on a variety of measures and techniques, all suggesting abnormality in the central auditory system of some stutterers, especially at the brainstem level. The chain of evidence includes sound localization, stapedius reflex, speech intelligibility under competition, phase disparities between air- and bone-conducted feedback systems, and pursuit tracking by the tongue.

In spite of what seems, at first observation, to be a wealth of negative findings, we are reluctant to abandon the search for the elusive audiomotor link to stuttering. Certainly, part of our motivation is dissatisfaction with the conventional experimental design comparing an experimental group of "stutterers" with a control group of "nonstutterers." The assumption here is that "stutterers" are a homogeneous group, all of whom will either demonstrate, or not demonstrate, the phenomenon under investigation. But there is no reason to believe that all stutterers are the same. Indeed, clinicians constantly remind us of the broad variation and individual differences characterizing the stuttering population. If stutterers differ among themselves on such variables as degree of handedness preference, response to therapy, response to various fluency-evoking maneuvers, and so forth, then is it not also possible that they differ among themselves on response to dichotic listening tests, acoustic reflex measures, and speech intelligibility tests? If such is the case, then important facets of individual performance may be lost in the rote search for group differences.

A second important consideration is that abnormalities in cerebral laterality or in central auditory function may produce deleterious effects on speech production only during the dynamic process of ongoing speech. Such abnormalities may be detected with only indifferent success in the steady state when the subject is merely engaged in passive listening. Abnormality may be maximally manifest only by dynamic measurement during speech production.

These considerations argue for more innovative approaches to experimental design in stuttering research. The conventional two-group design, where the mean for stutterers is compared to the mean for nonstutterers, may need to be replaced by single-subject designs, in which a single stutterer, rather than the group mean, provides the datum of interest, and experimental effects are measured as dynamic modifications to baseline performance.

Certainly, the final answer on stuttering and audition is not yet in. We expect, however, that much of the seemingly contradictory evidence facing us today will be resolved by future research.

ACKNOWLEDGMENT

This work was supported by the Ariel Foundation, the Kitty M. Perkins Foundation, and the M. R. Bauer Foundation.

REFERENCES

Andrews, G., Quinn, P., & Sorby, W. Stuttering: An investigation into cerebral dominance for speech. *Journal of Neurology, Neurosurgery and Psychiatry,* 1972, *35,* 414–418.

Asp, C. W. Time-intensity trade and lateralized location of interaural intensity differences by stutterers and nonstutterers. *Speech Monographs,* 1968, *35,* 316–317.

Backus, O. Incidence of stuttering among the deaf. *Annals of Otology, Rhinology, and Laryngology,* 1938, *47,* 632–635.

Benson, D. F., & Geschwind, N. The aphasias and related disturbances. In A. B. Baker & W. M. Baker (Eds.), *Clinical neurology.* Hagerstown, MD: Harper & Row, 1977.

Blumstein, S., Goodglass, H., & Tarter, V. The reliability of ear advantage in dichotic listening. *Brain and Language,* 1975, *2,* 226–236.

Borg, E., & Zakrisson, J. The activity of the stapedius muscle in man during vocalization. *Acta Otolaryngologica,* 1975, *79,* 325–333.

Bryden, M. P. An evaluation of some models of laterality in dichotic listening. *Acta Otolaryngologica,* 1967, *63,* 595–604.

Bryngelson, B. Sidedness as an etiological factor in stuttering. *Journal of Genetics and Psychology,* 1935, *47,* 204–217.

Bryngelson, B. A study of laterality of stutterers and normal speakers. *Journal of Speech Disorders,* 1939, *4,* 231–236.

Curry, F. K., & Gregory, H. The performance of stutterers on dichotic listening tasks thought to reflect cerebral dominance. *Journal of Speech and Hearing Research,* 1969, *12,* 73–82.

Daniels, E. M. An analysis of the relation between handedness and stuttering with special reference to the Orton-Travis theory of cerebral dominance. *Journal of Speech Disorders,* 1940, *5,* 309–326.

Despert, J. L. Psychosomatic study of fifty stuttering children: I. Social, physical and psychiatric findings. *American Journal of Orthopsychiatry,* 1946, *16,* 100–113.

DeWar, A., Dewar, A. D., Austin, W. T., & Brash, H. M. The long term use of an automatically triggered feedback masking device in the treatment of stammering. *British Journal of Disorders of Communication,* 1979, *14,* 219–230.

Dorman, M. F., & Porter, R. S. Hemispheric lateralization for speech perceptions in stutterers. *Cortex,* 1975, *11,* 181–185.

Goodglass, H., & Peck, E. A. Dichotic ear order effects in Korsakoff and normal subjects. *Neuropsychologia,* 1972, *10,* 211–217.

Gregory, M. Stuttering and auditory central nervous system disorder. *Journal of Speech and Hearing Research,* 1964, *7,* 335–341.

Gruber, L., & Powell, R. L. Responses of stuttering and nonstuttering children to a dichotic listening task. *Perceptual and Motor Skills,* 1974, *38,* 263–264.

Hannley, M., & Dorman, M. Some observations on auditory function and stuttering. *Journal of Fluency Disorders,* 1982, *7,* 93–108.

Hall, J., & Jerger, J. Central auditory function in stutterers. *Journal of Speech and Hearing Research,* 1978, *21,* 324–337.

Harms, M., & Malone, J. The relationship of hearing acuity to stammering. *Journal of Speech Disorders*, 1939, *4*, 363–370.

Hawver, K. *A comparison of the performance of stutterers and nonstutterers on tests of central auditory processing*. Unpublished doctoral dissertation, University of Cincinnatti, 1978.

Jen, P., & Suga, N. Coordinated activities of middle ear and laryngeal muscle in echolocating bats. *Science*, 1976, *191*, 950–952.

Jones, R. K. Observations on stammering after localized cerebral injury. *Journal of Neurology, Neurosurgery, and Psychiatry*, 1966, *29*, 192–195.

Kamiyama, G. A comparative study of stutterers and nonstutterers in respect to critical flicker frequency and sound localization. *Speech Monographs*, 1964, *31*, 291 (abstract).

Katz, J. The use of staggered spondaic words for assessing the integrity of the central auditory system. *Journal of Auditory Research*, 1962, *2*, 327–337.

Kimura, D. Cerebral dominance and the perception of verbal stimuli. *Canadian Journal of Psychology*, 1961, *3*, 166–171.

Kimura, D. Left–right differences in the perception of melodies. *Quarterly Journal of Experimental Psychology*, 1964, *16*, 355–358.

Kimura, D. Functional asymmetry of the brain in dichotic listening. *Cortex*, 1967, *13*, 163–178.

Lussenhop, A. J., Boggs, J. S., LaBorwit, L. J., & Walle, E. L. Cerebral dominance in stutterers determined by Wada testing. *Neurology*, 1973, *23*, 1190–1192.

McAllister, A. H. *Clinical studies in speech therapy*. London: University London Press, 1937.

McCall, G., & Rabuzzi, D. Reflex contraction of middle ear muscles secondary to stimulation of laryngeal nerves. *Journal of Speech and Hearing Research*, 1973, *16*, 56–61.

Meyer, B. C. Psychosomatic aspects of stuttering. *Journal of Nervous and Mental Disease*, 1945, *101*, 127–157.

Milisen, R., & Johnson, W. A comparative study of stutterers, former stutterers and normal speakers whose handedness has been changed. *Archives of Speech*, 1936, *1*, 61–86.

Milner, B., Branch, C., & Rasmussen, T. Evidence for bilateral speech representatives in some non-right-handers. *Transactions of the American Neurological Association*, 1966, *91*, 306–308.

Moore, W. Bilateral tachistoscopic word perception of stutterers and normal subjects. *Brain and Language*, 1976, *3*, 434–442.

Neilson, P., Quinn, P., & Neilson, M. Auditory tracking measures of hemispheric asymmetry in normals and stutterers. *Australian Journal of Human Communication Disorders*, 1976, *4*, 121–126.

Oldfield, R. C. The assessment and analysis of handedness: The Edinburgh inventory. *Neuropsychologia*, 1971, *9*, 97–113.

Orton, S. T. A physiological theory of reading disability and stuttering in children. *New England Journal of Medicine*, 1928, *199*, 1045–1052.

Pinsky, S., & McAdams, D. Electroencephalographic and dichotic indices of cerebral intensity in stutterers. *Brain and Language*, 1980, *11*, 374–397.

Quinn, P. T. Stuttering—Cerebral dominance and dichotic word test. *Medical Journal of Australia*, 1972, *2*, 639–642.

Rousey, C., Goetzinger, C., & Dirks, D. Sound localization ability of normal, stuttering, neurotic, and hemiplegic subjects. *Archives of General Psychiatry*, 1959, *1*, 640–645.

Rosenfield, D. B., & Goodglass, H. Dichotic testing of cerebral dominance in stutterers. *Brain and Language*, 1980, *11*, 170–180.

Satz, P., Aschenbach, K., Pattishall, E., & Fennell, E. Order of report, ear, asymmetry, and handedness in dichotic listening. *Cortex*, 1965, *1*, 377–396.

Shearer, W., & Simmons, F. Middle ear activity during speech in normal speakers and stutterers. *Journal of Speech and Hearing Research*, 1965, *8*, 203–237.

Slorach, N., & Noehr, B. Dichotic listening in stuttering and dyslalic children. *Cortex*, 1973, *9*, 295–300.

Spadino, E. J. *Writing and laterality characteristics of stuttering children.* New York: Columbia University Teachers College, 1941.

Stark, R., & Pierce, B. The effects of delayed auditory feedback on a speech-related task on stutterers. *Journal of Speech and Hearing Research*, 1970, *13*, 245–253.

Stromsta, C. A methodology related to the determinations of the phase angle of bone-conducted speech sound energy of stutterers and nonstutterers. *Speech Monographs*, 1957, *24*, 147–148 (abstract).

Stromsta, C. Interaural phase disparity of stutterers and nonstutterers. *Journal of Speech and Hearing Research*, 1972, *15*, 771–780.

Sussman, H. M., & McNeilage, P. F. Hemispheric specialization for speech production and perception in stutterers. *Neuropsychologia*, 1975, *13*, 19–27.

Toscher, M., & Rupp, R. A study of the central auditory processes in stutterers using the Synthetic Sentence Identification (SSI) test battery. *Journal of Speech and Hearing Research*, 1978, *21*, 779–792.

Travis, L. E. *Speech pathology.* New York: Appleton–Century, 1931.

Wada, J., & Rasmussen, T. Intracarotid injection of sodium amytal for the lateralization of cerebral speech dominance: Experimental and clinical observation. *Journal of Neurosurgery*, 1960, *17*, 266–282.

Zurif, E. B., & Bryden, M. P. Familial handedness and left–right differences in auditory and visual perception. *Neuropsychologia*, 1969, *7*, 179–187.

Chapter 6

Laryngeal Dynamics of Stutterers

Martin R. Adams
Frances Jackson Freeman
Edward G. Conture

LARYNGEAL ONSET AND REACTION TIME OF STUTTERERS

Martin R. Adams

Historically, there have been periods when the larynx was singled out for attention as an organ that played a central, if not exclusive, role in stuttering (Yates, 1800/1939; Hunt, 1861, Kenyon, 1943). Since this line of inquiry turned up little of significance in the past, one may ask why it should be pursued again. The main reason is because new and more sophisticated measuring devices have been developed. Specifically, workers have borrowed more probing experimental paradigms and more acute sensing instruments from speech science and medicine for the purpose of reopening investigation into the laryngeal behavior of stutterers and the role of the larynx in stuttering.

This area of research has, for the most part, taken three distinct directions. There have been (1) studies of stutterers' voice onset (VOT), voice initiation (VIT), and speech initiation (SIT) times; (2) electromyographic investigations of stutterers' laryngeal muscle activity; and (3) fiberoptic studies in which it has been possible to view the larynx during moments of stuttering. In this chapter, each of these three avenues of inquiry will be reviewed regarding their respective methodologies, instrumentation, and findings.[1]

VOICE ONSET TIMES (VOT)
Methodologies and instrumentation

Traditionally, VOT has been defined as the time that elapses from the release of the consonant burst to the onset of periodic glottal vibration for the production of the vowel that follows the consonant (Lisker & Abramson, 1964) in such simple consonant–vowel syllables as /pʌ, bʌ, tʌ, dʌ, kʌ, gʌ/. VOT begins when the transition is made from consonant implosion to plosion and ends with the commencement of voicing for the following vowel. Thus, we are able to measure VOT with any instrument that (1) reliably senses and records the end of consonantal implosion; (2) reliably senses and records the initiation of glottal vibration for phonation; and (3) provides some means of determining the time lapse between these two events. Over the years, three methods have emerged as ideally suited to perform these functions. The first involves sound spectrography. Two samples of spectrograms are presented, along with explanatory comments in Figure 6-1. The second involves detecting the sizeable rise in intra-oral air pressure that occurs during the implosion phase of stop consonant production. By placing a pressure-sensing device in a speaker's mouth, we can determine when implosion has reached its peak. The subsequent drop in pressure would reflect the release of the articulatory constriction (plosion) that is integral to the consonant's production. If, at the same time, we are recording the subject's voice, then we have a way of establishing the time lapse between the start of the pressure drop or consonantal release (plosion) and the subsequent initiation of phonation. By definition, that is VOT. Figure 6-2 displays the rise (implosion) and fall (plosion) of intra-oral air pressure and the initiation of voicing. The time elapsed between the start of the pressure drop and the start of phonation is VOT. In a similar way, the third method determines VOT through the combined use of X-ray motion pictures and a voice recorder. With the former, you can see the start of the consonantal release on the X-ray film, and the voice recorder tells us when phonation starts. The difference between these two events, expressed in temporal units, is VOT.

Findings

Measurements and comparisons of the VOTs of stutterers and normal speaking control subjects began in the early 1970s. Armed with a sound spectrograph or an equivalent device, investigators were able to assess stutterers' and nonstutterers' VOTs during the fluent productions of simple, isolated CV syllables, during the generation of longer syllable sequences (e.g., /əputətætəkit/), and during the production of stop

FIGURE 6-1. Segments extracted from larger spectrographic displays for clarity of presentation. The segment on the left is for the phrase /tu it/; the one on the right for /tʌf/. Both segments were isolated for analysis out of a subject's oral reading. In each segment, "a" marks the location of the long, sharp vertical line that represents the point of transition from implosion to plosion for /t/. The symbol "b" locates the point of appearance of clearly identifiable, short, regular vertical striations that mark the onset of voicing for the vowels /u/ and /ʌ/, respectively. The distance between "a" and "b", when converted to milliseconds, is VOT. *

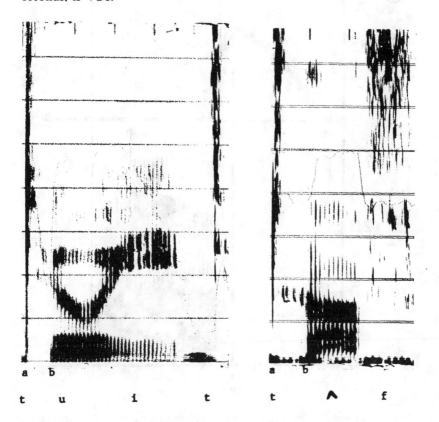

*The faint, ragged vertical lines between "a" and "b" represent the turbulence generated by the explosion of /t/.

FIGURE 6-2. Display of voice onset time derived from the combined use of a pressure sensor and a spectrograph. The curve at the top left of the display is the gradient for intraoral air pressure. Point "a, " where the curve starts downward, represents the drop in pressure that occurs with the transition from implosion to plosion in the production of stop consonants. Point "b" marks the onset of voicing. The distance between "a" and "b, " converted from millimeters to milliseconds, is VOT. *

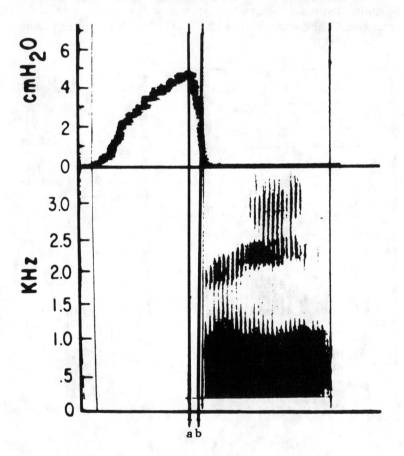

*Reproduced from Agnello, J. "Laryngeal and Articulatory Dynamics of Dysfluency Interpreted within a Vocal Tract Model" in L. M. Webster and L. Furst (Eds.), *Vocal Tract Dynamics and Dysfluency*. New York: Speech and Hearing Institute, 1975, with the kind permission of J. Agnello and L. M. Webster.

consonant plus vowel combinations in continuous oral reading. In the latter case, all phonetic contexts that involved *intra*syllabic stop consonant plus vowel combinations were analyzed. The results of studies of stutterers' and normals' VOT s are set forth in summary form in Table 6-1.

TABLE 6-1. Summary of studies comparing the voice onset times (VOT) of stutterers and normals. The experimenter(s) are cited in column 1. Column 2 describes the methodology for measuring VOT. Column 3 provides information on the subjects tested, and column 4 sets out the results of between group comparisons.

(1)	(2)	(3)	(4)
Agnello and Wingate (1972)[2]	Pressure-sensor and voice-recorder; CV utterances.	Matched groups of 12 adult stutterers and 12 normals.	Stutterers' VOTs were longer.
Wendell (1973)[3]	Spectrographic analysis of CVs.	Matched groups of 12 child stutterers and 12 normals.	Stutterers' VOTs were longer.
Hillman and Gilbert (1977)	Spectrographic analysis of CVs taken from oral reading.	Matched groups of 10 adult stutterers and 10 normals.	Stutterers' VOTs were longer ($p < .05$).
Metz, Conture, and and Caruso (1979)	Spectrographic analysis of 18 different sound clusters in words.	Five young adult stutterers and five normals.	Stutterers' VOTs were longer on only 6 of the 18 clusters ($p < .05$).
Zimmerman (1980)	X-ray motion picture and voice recorder; three CVC words.	Six adult stutterers and seven normals.	Stutterers' VOTs were longer.
Watson and Alfonso (1982)	Spectrographic analysis of three contiguous vowel + consonant + vowel + consonant sequences (e.g., /əputətætəkit/.	Eight adult stutterers, age- and sex-matched with eight normals.	No significant between-group differences in VOT ($p < .05$).

[2,3] A report by Agnello, Wingate, and Wendell (1974) was, in fact, based on a pooling of the separate sets of data from the Agnello and Wingate, and Wendell studies cited above (J. Agnello, personal communication, 1982).

VOICE AND SPEECH INITIATION TIMES (VIT AND SIT)

On superficial examination, one might believe that VOT and VIT are, in actuality, the same phenomenon. That is not the case. VOT is a within syllable period, the boundaries of which are defined by articulatory and phonatory events; it is measured *after* an utterance has started. In contrast, VIT is defined as the time lapse between the appearance of some experimenter-controlled external stimulus (e.g., a pure tone or flash of light), and a subject's initiation of glottal vibration for phonation. Thus, VIT represents the time lapse between some nonspeech event and the start of voicing. In a similar fashion, some investigators have required subjects to utter a response of one word or longer, beginning with a voiced sound. These studies are viewed as measuring speech initiation time (SIT).

Methodologies and instrumentation

Though there have been some minor variations across experiments, most VIT/SIT investigations have employed highly similar methods and designs. In a typical project, a subject is presented with a warning signal, waits for the appearance of a cueing stimulus, and then generates a desired response as rapidly as possible. This sequence may be repeated up to 100 times. The electrical analog of the cueing stimulus is recorded on one track, and the subject's fluent phonatory (or speech) response on another of a recording device, such as an optical oscillograph. The oscillograph creates a permanent visual display that includes a representation of the onset and offset of the external cue, and the initiation of the subject's voice response. A sample oscillographic tracing with explanatory comments is shown in Figure 6-3. Table 6-2 presents a summary of 17 VIT and SIT studies. Because the data in Tables 6-1 and 6-2 are so similar, they will be interpreted together.

INTERPRETATIONS

An obvious trend is apparent in Tables 6-1 and 6-2. In four of the six VOT studies, stutterers had longer (slower) scores than normal speaking control subjects. In the VIT/SIT investigations that were reviewed, significant slowness among the stutterers was noted unequivocally in 11 of 17 projects. Mixed findings were obtained in two studies (Cullinan & Springer, 1980, McFarlane & Shipley, 1981). Nonsignificant differences were observed between stutterers and control subjects in just 4 of the 17 experiments. From these outcomes we may conclude that stutterers as a group are likely to have slower VOTs and VITs/SITs than matched normal subjects.

FIGURE 6-3. A sample oscillographic tracing taken from a study of stutterers' and normals' VIT (Adams & Hayden, 1976). The external cueing stimulus is shown at the top of the display; the subject's phonation of /ɑ/ at the bottom. The line "a" marks the onset of the cueing stimulus; "b" represents the subject's initiation of voicing. The distance between "a" and "b, " when converted to milliseconds, is VIT.

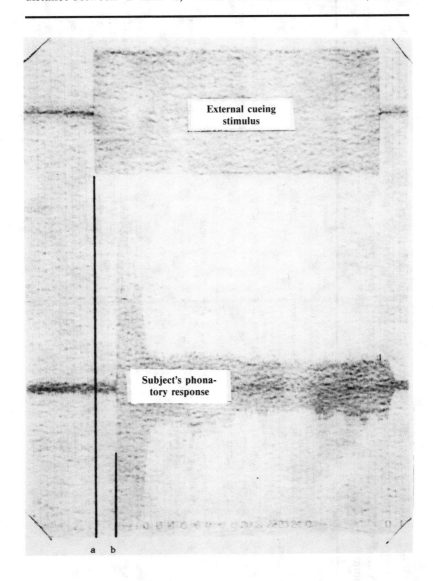

TABLE 6-2. Summary of studies comparing the voice initiation times (VIT) of stutterers and normals. The experimenters are identified in column 1. The second column contains descriptions of the characteristics of the subjects tested. Column 3 cites the external cueing signal(s) used. Subjects' response(s) are provided in column 4. The findings of the experiments are set forth in column 5.

(1) Researcher(s)	(2) Characteristics of subjects tested	(3) External cueing signal(s) used	(4) Subjects' response(s)	(5) Findings
Hayden (1975)*	10 adult stutterers and 10 age- and sex-matched normals	1000 Hz pure tone	Phonated /ɑ/	Stutterers had longer VITs than did the normals, but this difference was judged nonsignificant ($p = .10$).
Adams and Hayden (1976)*	10 adult stutterers and 10 age- and sex-matched normals	1000 Hz pure tone	Phonated /ɑ/	Both groups shortened VIT from the beginning to end of the experiment. Stutterers were slower on two of three comparisons made ($p = .056$ and $.00003$, respectively).
Starkweather, Hirschman, and Tannenbaum (1976)	11 adult stutterers and 11 age- and sex-matched normals	Green light presented on a screen	26 test syllables reflecting a wide range in place and manner of articulation	Both groups shortened their VIT from the beginning to end of the experiment. Stutterers were slower across all test trials ($p = .025$) and across all syllable types investigated ($p = .025$).
Reardon (1977)	5 adult stutterers and 5 sex-matched normals	Auditory stimulus	Phonated /ɑ/ and 6 other test syllables	Stutterers had longer VITs on every utterance ($p < .05$). Stutterers' longest VITs occurred on the six test syllables. Their shortest VITs appeared on the isolated vowel.

(1) Researcher(s)	(2) Characteristics of subjects tested	(3) External cueing signal(s) used	(4) Subjects' response(s)	(5) Findings
Cross, Shadden, and Luper (1979)	10 adult stutterers and 10 age- and sex-matched normals	4000 Hz pure tone presented to each ear in separate conditions	Phonated /ʌ/	No difference in stutterers' VIT when test tone was presented to left as compared to the right ear ($p = .05$). Overall, stutterers were slower than the normals ($p = .004$).
Cross and Luper (1979)	9 stutterers each, at ages 5 and 7 years + 9 adults; age- and sex-matched with like numbers of normals	1000 Hz pure tone	Phonated /ʌ/	In both groups, VIT shortened as age increased. At all three age levels studied, stutterers were slower than normals ($p = .0012$).
Lewis, Ingham, and Gervens (1979)	10 adult stutterers and a like number of normals	1000 Hz pure tone, and a light flash; presented in separate conditions	Phonate an isolated vowel	Stutterers were slower than the normals in both the auditory and visual cueing conditions.
Prosek, Montgomery, Walden, and Schwartz (1979)*[+]	10 adult stutterers and 10 age- and sex-matched normals	Light flash, a 1000 Hz pure tone, and spoken words; presented in separate conditions	16 VC words (e.g., "ape")	Stutterers were slower than the normals in all cueing conditions.

(Continued)

TABLE 6-2. (Continued) Summary of studies comparing the voice initiation times (VIT) of stutterers and normals. The experimenters are identified in column 1. The second column contains descriptions of the characteristics of the subjects tested. Column 3 cites the external cueing signal(s) used. Subjects' response(s) are provided in column 4. The findings of the experiments are set forth in column 5.

(1) Researcher(s)	(2) Characteristics of subjects tested	(3) External cueing signal(s) used	(4) Subjects' response(s)	(5) Findings
Cross, J., and Cooke (1979)*	8 adult stutterers and 8 normal speakers	A visual stimulus, and an auditory stimulus, presented in separate conditions	Phonated /a/	Stutterers were slower than the normals across all experimental conditions. The greatest difference between groups appeared in the auditory-vocal response condition.
Adler and Starkweather (1979)*	A group of stutterers and a group of non-stutterers	A visual stimulus	A laryngeal gesture	The stutterers were slower than the control subjects in all experimental conditions.
Cullinan and Springer (1980)*	11 child stutterers with articulation and language problems; 9 "pure" stutterers; 20 age- and sex-matched normal children	1000 Hz pure tone	Phonated /a/	The two groups of stutterers combined, had slower VITs than did the normals ($p = .05$). However, this difference was a function of the extreme slowness of the stutterers with the associated articulation and language problems. VIT did not differ between the "pure" stutterers and the normals.
McFarlane and Shipley (1981)*	12 adult stutterers matched for age, sex, and educational level, with 12 normals	Light flash presented simultaneously to both eyes; 1000-Hz tone presented to each ear in separate conditions	Phonated /bæ/	Combined data for all three conditions (i.e., visual; left ear; right ear) revealed no difference between groups for VIT ($p > .05$). However, stutterers did evidence significant slowness in both the left ear and right ear conditions ($p = .05$).

(1) Researcher(s)	(2) Characteristics of subjects tested	(3) External cueing signal(s) used	(4) Subjects' response(s)	(5) Findings
Murphy and Baumgartner (1981)	6 child stutterers and 7 normal speaking children	1000 Hz tone	Phonated /ɑ/	No differences were found between the groups.
Venkatagiri (1981)*	10 adult stutterers and 10 age- and sex-matched normals	1000 Hz pure tone	Phonated /ɑ/	No differences were found between the groups.
Reich, Till, and Goldsmith (1981)*+	13 adult stutterers and 13 age-matched normals	1000 Hz pure tone	Phonated /ɑ/ and the word "upper"	Stutterers were slower than the normals on the isolated vowel production and on the word's production.
Watson and Alfonso (1982)*	8 adult stutterers and 8 age- and sex-matched normals	1000 Hz pure tone, and a light flash presented in separate conditions	Phonated /ɑ/, and a nonsense syllable phrase	No differences were found between groups in either condition, for either the vowel or the nonsense syllable phrase response.
Hayden, Adams, and Jordahl (1982)+	10 adult stutterers and 10 sex-matched normal adults	1000 Hz pure tone	Production of 9 sentences, all beginning with a vowel (e.g., "Almonds are nuts.")	Stutterers were slower than the normals ($p = .08$).

*Studies carrying this symbol were actually larger in scope, involving other dependent variables in addition to VIT. However, only those portions of these investigations that dealt directly with voice initiation have been included in this summary table.

+ Investigations carrying this symbol required subjects to make a speech response of one word or longer. In each case, the test utterance began with a voiced sound. These studies are viewed herein as involving the measurement of speech initiation time (SIT).

Beyond this broad interpretation, Tables 6-1 and 6-2 tell us even more. For instance, stutterers' slowness in VOT cuts across productions of isolated CV syllables to prose material being read aloud (Hillman & Gilbert, 1977). Likewise, stutterers' slowness in producing isolated vowels (VIT) appears also to be present in the production of single words (Reich, Till, & Goldsmith, 1981), and sentence length utterances that are initiated with vowels (SIT; Hayden, Adams, & Jordahl, 1982). Furthermore, stutterers' lag in VIT does not seem to be a function of the ear to which an auditory cueing signal is presented (Cross, Shadden, & Luper, 1979), or of the sensory modality that is stimulated. Remember, significant VIT disparities between stutterers and normals were observed under separate conditions of auditory and visual stimulation (Lewis, Ingham, & Gervens, 1979; Cross & Cooke, 1979).

As impressive as these findings are, they need to be interpreted cautiously. After all, voice production is a function of respiratory and laryngeal behaviors *and* their integration. If a subject exhibits slowness in starting voicing, does that lag reflect an abnormal respiratory event, some anomalous glottal response, a combination of the two, or perhaps a breakdown in the coordination of exhalation and laryngeal activity? Here is where we must exercise restraint because the VOT, VIT, and SIT data under review cannot provide an answer to this question. The fact is, these three measures only reflect the time it has taken an individual to organize, coordinate, and commence behavior. The point to be made here is that the data at hand cannot be used to prove the existence of a laryngeal component in stuttering or a laryngeal cause for any presumed disorder.

Shortly after the completion of the first several VOT and VIT experiments, there was considerable conjecture that the slowness was caused by an individual's history of stuttering. In other words, having spent years as a stutterer, a person would be quite likely to approach speech or speech-like acts (such as the production of an isolated vowel or a CV syllable) with an excess of muscular tension in the larynx. Such muscular tension, a result of a history of stuttering, might then act to retard VOT and VIT.

At least two predictions flow from this framework. First, we could forecast that young stutterers, with relatively short histories of stuttering, would be *less* likely to approach speech and speech-like acts with excess muscular tension. With less tension, these children ought to generate VOT and VIT values that would be indistinguishable from those produced by matched normal youngsters. Second, it should also follow that young stutterers would have shorter VOT and VIT values as compared to adult stutterers because the children had briefer histories of stuttering, and hence, had less time to develop higher levels of muscular tension in the larynx.

The results of studies cited in Tables 6-1 and 6-2 fail to bear out these predictions; both VOT and VIT scores for young stutterers were slower than those of control subjects (Wendell, 1973; Cross & Luper, 1979). It was also shown that stutterers' VIT *improved* with age (Cross & Luper, 1979). Neither of these findings would be likely if stuttering were the cause of the slowness. Rather, such slowness probably antedated or coincided with the onset of the disorder. Indeed, it is even possible that difficulty in quickly initiating voicing is one of the immediate causes of stutterers' repetitions and prolongations of articulatory gestures (Adams, 1974), viewed here and elsewhere as core characteristics of stuttering (Wingate, 1964).

The next explanation that was developed pertained only to VIT. In this account, stutterers' slowness is causally related to a specific defect in the *auditory* system that retards the reception or processing of stimuli used to cue vocal responses. Needless to say, this interpretation was abandoned when stutterers were found to have slower than normal VIT s to visual signals as well (Starkweather, Hirschman, & Tannenbaum, 1976).

Noting this slowness in both auditory and visual stimulation, thought was given to attributing it to some *central* disturbance that would reduce the speed with which stutterers organized and started transmitting neural signals to the periphery for voice production. Inherent in this formulation is the idea that stutterers' neural organization and transmission are both *normal* with the exception of the speed with which they take place. Were this true, then it is possible that stutterers might exhibit time lags in responding to other signals, *regardless* of whether the response elicited was related or unrelated to speech.

Recently, some experimenters have measured stutterers' reaction times for nonspeech tasks, such as button pressing, by using lights and/or tones (cf. Luper & Cross, 1978; Prosek, Montgomery, Walden, & Schwartz, 1979; Reich et al., 1981). Stutterers' neural reaction times have also been assessed (McFarlane & Prins, 1978). There are only a few of these investigations and their findings are mixed. Therefore, it would be premature to interpret them at this point.

Finally, in a recent review article, Adams (1981) offered an elaboration on the position that stutterers may be slow to organize and transmit *normal* neural commands to their musculature. Specifically, it was suggested that in addition to integrating and sending commands more slowly, stutterers may also send *inappropriate* commands to the periphery. This would activate muscles in ways that could delay voicing.

For example, neural commands may raise the level of tonus or the amount of contraction in those intrinsic laryngeal muscles that determine glottal width which would also inhibit the rapid onset of voicing. It is interesting to note that stutterers' VIT s and SIT s improve when voicing and speech are initiated in synchrony with a rhythmic stimulus (Hayden, Adams, & Jordahl, 1982; Hayden, Jordahl, & Adams, 1982). This finding is provocative because we have known for years that rhythmic speech improves fluency. Perhaps rhythm enhances fluency by helping a speaker with the timing of events that are integral to speech production (Brayton & Conture, 1978; Hayden, Jordahl, & Adams, 1982). Such an event could be voice initiation.

Prior to 1972 there was little contemporary interest in the laryngeal aspects of stuttering. However, repeated findings of longer VOT s, VIT s, and SIT s in stutterers have rendered more credible the possibility that there is laryngeal involvement in the disorder. As a result of these developments, workers began to design and conduct more sophisticated and penetrating investigations into the role the larynx might play in stuttering. Nowhere is this more evident than in the electromyographic and fiberoptic studies to be covered next.

NOTE

[1] There also have been a few isolated studies of stutterers' laryngeal behavior that do not fall within any of the three groups of research just cited. For this reason and because of space limitations, these experiments will not be reviewed. Omission, however, does not imply criticism of this fine work.

REFERENCES

Adams, M. The speech production abilities of stutterers: Recent, ongoing and future research. *Journal of Fluency Disorders,* 1981, *6,* 311–326.

Adams, M. A physiologic and aerodynamic interpretation of fluent and stuttered speech. *Journal of Fluency Disorders,* 1974, *1,* 35–47.

Adams, M., & Hayden, P. The ability of stutterers and nonstutterers to initiate and terminate phonation of an isolated vowel. *Journal of Speech and Hearing Research,* 1976, *19,* 290–296.

Adler, J., & Starkweather, W. *Oral and laryngeal reaction times in stutterers.* Paper presented at the annual convention of the American Speech-Language-Hearing Association, Atlanta, 1979.

Agnello, J. Laryngeal and articulatory dynamics of dysfluency interpreted within a vocal tract model. In L. M. Webster & L. Furst (Eds.), *Vocal tract dynamics and dysfluency.* New York: Speech and Hearing Institute, 1975.

Agnello, J., & Wingate, M. *Acoustical and physiological aspects of stuttered speech.* Paper presented at the annual convention of the American Speech and Hearing Association; San Francisco, 1972.

Agnello, J., Wingate, M., & Wendell, M. *Voice onset and voice termination times of children and adult stutterers.* Paper presented at the annual convention of the Acoustical Society of America, St. Louis, 1974.

Brayton, E., & Conture, E. Effects of noise and rhythmic stimulation on the speech of stutterers. *Journal of Speech and Hearing Research,* 1978, *21,* 285–294.

Cross, D., & Luper, H. Voice reaction times of stuttering and nonstuttering children and adults. *Journal of Fluency Disorders,* 1979, *4,* 59–78.

Cross, D., Shadden, B., & Luper, H. Effects of stimulus ear presentation on the voice reaction times of adult stutterers and nonstutterers. *Journal of Fluency Disorders,* 1979, *4,* 45–58.

Cross, J., & Cooke, P. *Vocal and manual reaction times of adult stutterers and nonstutterers.* Paper presented at the annual convention of the American Speech–Language–Hearing Association, Atlanta, 1979.

Cullinan, W., & Springer, M. Voice initiation and termination times in stuttering and nonstuttering children. *Journal of Speech and Hearing Research,* 1980, *23,* 344–360.

Hayden, P. *The effects of masking and pacing on stutterers' and nonstutterers' voice and speech initiation times.* Unpublished, PhD dissertation, Purdue University, 1975.

Hayden, P., Adams, M., & Jordahl, N. The effects of pacing and masking on stutterers' and nonstutterers' speech initiation times. *Journal of Fluency Disorders,* 1982, *7,* 9–20.

Hayden, P., Jordahl, N., & Adams, M. Stutterers' voice initiation times during conditions of novel stimulation. *Journal of Fluency Disorders,* 1982, *7,* 1–8.

Hillman, R., & Gilbert, H. Voice onset times for voiceless stop consonants in the fluent reading of stutterers and nonstutterers. *Journal of the Acoustical Society of America,* 1977, *61,* 610–611.

Hunt, J. *Stammering and stuttering: Their nature and treatment.* New York: Hafner, 1861.

Kenyon, E. The etiology of stammering: The psychophysiologic facts which concern the production of speech sounds and of stammering. *Journal of Speech Disorders,* 1943, *8,* 347–348.

Lewis, J., Ingham, R., & Gervens, A. *Voice initiation and termination times in stutterers and normal speakers.* Paper presented at the annual convention of the American Speech–Language–Hearing Association, Atlanta, 1979.

Lisker, L., & Abramsom, A. A cross language study of voicing in initial stops: Acoustical measurements. *Word,* 1964, *20,* 384–422.

Luper, H., & Cross, D. Relation between finger reaction time and voice reaction time in stuttering and nonstuttering children and adults. Paper presented at the annual convention of the American Speech–Language–Hearing Association, San Francisco, 1978.

McFarlane, S., & Prins, D. Neural response time of stutterers and nonstutterers in selected oral motor tasks. *Journal of Speech and Hearing Research,* 1978, *21,* 768–778.

McFarlane, S., & Shipley, K. Latency of vocalization onset for stutterers and nonstutterers under conditions of auditory and visual cueing. *Journal of Speech and Hearing Research,* 1981, *46,* 307–311.

Metz, D., Conture, E., & Caruso, A. Voice onset time, frication, and aspiration during stutterers' fluent speech. *Journal of Speech and Hearing Research,* 1979, *22,* 649–656.

Murphy, M., & Baumgartner, J. Voice initiation and termination time in stuttering and nonstuttering children. *Journal of Fluency Disorders,* 1981, *6,* 257–264.

Prosek, R., Montgomery, A., Walden, B., & Schwartz, E. Reaction time measures of stutterers and nonstutterers. *Journal of Fluency Disorders,* 1979, *4,* 269–278.

Reardon, J. *Temporal characteristics of stutterers' and nonstutterers' voice initiation and termination.* Paper presented at the annual convention of the American Speech and Hearing Association, Chicago, 1977.

Reich, A., Till, J., & Goldsmith, H. Laryngeal and manual reaction times of stuttering and nonstuttering adults. *Journal of Speech and Hearing Research,* 1981, *24,* 192–196.

Starkweather, C., Hirschman, P., & Tannenbaum, R. Latency of vocalization onset: Stutterers vs. nonstutterers. *Journal of Speech and Hearing Research,* 1976, *19,* 481–492.

Venkatagiri, H. Reaction time for voiced and whispered /a/ in stutterers and nonstutterers. *Journal of Fluency Disorders,* 1981, *6,* 265–271.

Watson, B., & Alfonso, P. A comparison of LRT and VOT values between stutterers and nonstutterers. *Journal of Fluency Disorders,* 1982, *7,* 219–241.

Wendell, M. *A study of voice onset time and voice termination in stuttering and non-stuttering children.* Unpublished Master's thesis, University of Cincinnati, 1973.

Wingate, M. Standard definition of stuttering. *Journal of Speech and Hearing Disorders,* 1964, *29,* 484–489.

Yates (first name unknown), cited in Klingbeil, G. The historical background of the modern speech clinic. *Journal of Speech Disorders,* 1939, *4,* 115–131.

Zimmerman, G. Articulatory dynamics of fluent utterances of stutterers and nonstutterers. *Journal of Speech and Hearing Research,* 1980, *23,* 95–107.

LARYNGEAL MUSCLE ACTIVITY OF STUTTERERS
Frances Jackson Freeman

Electromyographic (EMG) studies of stuttering are important because they provide information about a different level of the speech production process. In contrast to studies of structural movements, which describe the effects of contraction and relaxation of groups of muscles, and to perceptual, acoustic, and aerodynamic studies, which describe the results of dynamic movements of a number of structures, EMG studies describe patterns of muscle contraction and relaxation.

Understanding EMG research requires knowledge of the technique.[1] The electromyograph amplifies and records the minute electrical voltages generated each time a motor unit "fires" in response to a neural impulse. As motor units fire more rapidly or as many motor units fire in close succession, electrical activity in a muscle or muscle group increases. EMG recordings reflect the level of contractile activity in muscle tissue and the variations in this activity over time.

When EMG recordings are combined with other information, such as acoustic analyses of the speech produced, and knowledge of the anatomy and physiology of the muscles under study, some inferences may be made regarding movements and/or levels of muscle tension. The inferential nature of such statements must always be stressed, since EMG does not, and indeed cannot directly measure either movements or tension.[2]

While electromyography has been used for over 40 years, its most valuable applications to speech are recent, dating primarily from the late 1960s. The reason for this delay is largely related to the electrodes, the sensory devices that "pick-up" the minute electrical signals. The earliest, and still most commonly used, electrodes are metal discs that are attached to the skin surface over muscles of interest. While these noninvasive, surface-placed disc electrodes are useful for superficial muscles, they have limited value for the study of muscles located some distance from the skin surface, or for very small muscles.

Most of the muscles of speech (with the notable exception of the obicularis oris) fall into the latter category and are not easily studied using surface electrodes. In the case of the larynx, not only are intrinsic laryngeal muscles small and deep, but the larynx moves vertically within the neck as we swallow, speak, and breathe. Thus, the distance between muscles of interest and surface-placed electrodes is constantly changing. Further, the larger, more superficial muscles of the neck generate strong electrical currents that obscure electrical activity of the smaller, deeper, intrinsic laryngeal muscles. For these reasons, surface electrodes have not proven a valid or reliable method for study of intrinsic laryngeal muscles.[3]

Attempts to devise methods for study of deeper muscles led to the development of concentric needle electrodes. While these can be placed in speech muscles, they are rigid and tend to move within the muscle if the muscle moves (as both the tongue and the larynx move in speech). Such movements affect the reliability of recordings and sometimes cause pain.

Development of in-dwelling, hooked-wire electrodes (Basmajian & Steko, 1963) was the innovation that made possible a still-expanding revolution in speech research. Nonirritating and flexible hooked-wires can be inserted (via a carrier needle) into deep, relatively small speech muscles, and will, under most circumstances, remain in place as the needle is removed and as these muscles contract and related structures move. Fortuitously, development of hooked-wire electrodes coincided with development of computer systems that allow acquisition and efficient management of large quantities of data. Thus, it has become increasingly feasible to use multiple electrodes to study simultaneous activity of several muscles, a factor of significance in understanding a complex process such as speech.

ELECTROMYOGRAPHY IN STUTTERING RESEARCH

Most of the early EMG studies conducted with stutterers were designed to investigate basic neurophysiological differences between stutterers and nonstutterers (Morley, 1937; Steer, 1937; Travis, 1934). More recent experiments have focused on "the moment of stuttering" and compared EMG patterns during fluent utterances with those generated during stuttering. A systematic review of literature bearing on stutterers' respiration and articulation exceeds the scope of this section. Similarly, reports of EMG biofeedback treatment of stuttering (even those with a laryngeal placement site) can not be systematically reviewed. However, selected investigations (Fibiger, 1971, 1972, 1977; Platt & Basili, 1973; Sheehan & Voas, 1954) are discussed in relation to the laryngeal studies.

A number of studies of stuttering have attempted to use electromyography as an index of psychological status, for example arousal, anxiety, vigilance, anticipation, or expectancy. In these studies, the distinction between physiological muscle tension and the psychological condition of "being tense" is typically ignored. The relationship between EMG recordings and such psychological states is poorly defined, in part because of difficulties inherent in defining the latter. Interpreting EMG recordings as evidence of a given psychological state, such as anticipation or expectancy is fraught with problems. A critique (Freeman, 1979b) of the work of McLean and Cooper (1978) deals at length with the technical and theoretical pitfalls inherent in such an approach.

One study, which did not directly measure intrinsic laryngeal muscle activity, does offer valuable insight into general throat area muscle activity related to stuttering. Shrum (1967) used silver disc surface electrodes to record from several sites including two bilateral masseter (jaw) muscle sites, two bilateral platysma (neck) muscle sites, and one leg muscle site. He measured the duration of muscle activity from moment A, when muscle activity was elevated over the resting state, to moment B when initiation of phonation was recorded. He found that the interval between moments A and B (duration of prephonatory muscle activity) was significantly longer for stutterers than for nonstutterers. For stutterers, this interval was longest before words on which they stuttered, shorter before words on which they "expected" to stutter (but did not), and shortest before words spoken without anticipation or stuttering. Shrum interpreted these findings as indicating that stutterers began to tense earlier than nonstutterers. An alternate interpretation is that initiation of phonation was delayed in stutterers. This second interpretation of Shrum's findings is consistent with recent research demonstrating longer VOTs and slower initiation of phonation (discussed previously in this chapter).

Intrinsic laryngeal muscle activity in stuttering

For technical reasons already discussed, the only valid and reliable EMG studies of intrinsic laryngeal muscle activity are those that have employed hooked-wire electrodes. Understanding the normal functions of intrinsic and extrinsic laryngeal muscles was a primary goal of some of the earliest hooked-wire EMG studies of speech (Hirose & Gay, 1972; Shipp & McGlone, 1972). The knowledge and skill gained in these normative studies set the stage in the early 1970s for pioneering investigations of laryngeal muscle activity in stuttering.

It is important to recognize, however, that acquisition and analysis of reliable, valid laryngeal EMG data is a complex and time-consuming process, requiring the skills of a number of specialists, including engineers, programmers, laryngologists, and phoneticians. Few laboratories presently have the necessary instrumentation and support staff. Even though a typical EMG study involves less than six subjects, many months are required for collection and analysis of data. For example, Freeman (1977) collected data on the first of her four subjects in 1972, and Shapiro (1980) on his first subject in 1977. At this writing they are still completing some analyses. The small number of published studies of intrinsic laryngeal muscle activity in stuttering (four) and the limited number of stuttering subjects (eight), is understandable, if regrettable.

The methodology employed by Freeman, Shapiro, and their colleagues at Haskins Laboratories has been described in detail in a number of publications (Freeman, 1977; Freeman & Ushijima, 1978; Hirose & Gay, 1972; Shapiro, 1980). Freeman and Shapiro each studied four stutterers. Both used in-dwelling hooked-wire electrodes (except for some orbicularis oris recordings), and both attempted to record simultaneously from five intrinsic laryngeal muscles and from three to four articulator muscles. The number of reliable, verifiable recordings obtained for analyses varied. The subjects studied, and the verifiable recordings by muscle are summarized in Table 6-3.

Most of what we presently know about intrinsic laryngeal muscle activity in stuttering is based on results from eight stutterers, with a total of 40 verifiable recordings (17 from articulator muscles, 22 from intrinsic laryngeal muscles, and 1 from an extrinsic laryngeal muscle). However, recordings from the posterior cricoarytenoid muscle were obtained from only three subjects, and all statements regarding laryngeal abductor-adductor reciprocity in stuttering are based on data from these three subjects. Three significant findings have emerged from these studies and form the basis for the following discussion.

TABLE 6-3. Muscles and Subjects in Studies of Laryngeal Muscle Activity in Stutterers

MUSCLE	F 1	F 2	F 3	F 4	S 1	S 2	S 3	S 4	TOTALS
Orbicularis Oris	X	X	X	X+	X+	X+	X+	X+	8
Superior Longitudinal	X		X	X	X	X	X		6
Inferior Longitudinal	X								1
Genioglossus	X	X							2
Upper Tract Totals	F = 10				S = 7				17
Sternohyoid			X						1
Posterior Cricoarytenoid	X*			X*		X*			3*
Interarytenoid		X	X			X	X	X	5
Lateral Cricoarytenoid	X	X	X	X					4
Vocalis	X	X	X	X	X		X	X	7
Cricothyroid			X				X	X	3
Laryngeal Totals	F = 14				S = 9				23
Totals	7	5	7	5	3	4	5	4	40

NOTE:

F = Subjects of Freeman and Ushijima (1978); S = subjects of Shapiro (1980); * = insertion critical for study of abductor-adductor reciprocity; + = paint-on electrodes (all others are hooked-wire).

1. Levels of muscle activity. Stuttered speech (i.e., speech in which frequent perceived stutterings occurred) was accompanied by higher levels of muscle activity than was speech which contained little or no perceived stuttering. This finding was somewhat more pronounced for laryngeal than for articulator muscles. However, since laryngeal muscles were studied more carefully, this result could be biased.

The highest levels of muscle activity were associated with perceived stutterings and with disrupted coordination between agonist–antagonist laryngeal muscles. Patterns of muscle activity were similar to those reported by Sheehan and Voas (1954) in that the levels of muscle activity dropped dramatically at the moment a stuttered word was finally uttered (when the block terminated). It is impossible to say, however, if activity dropped because the block was terminated or if termination of the block was achieved because the level of muscle activity diminished.

2. Disruption of coordinated muscle activity. In those subjects (three in total) from whom recordings were obtained from the laryngeal abductor (posterior cricoarytenoid) and from at least one adductor muscle (lateral cricoarytenoid, vocalis, or interarytenoid), it was possible to study coordination of functional antagonists. In normal speakers, these muscles act with reciprocity. That is, when the abductor contracts, the adductors relax and vice versa. For the most part, perceived stutterings were accompanied by cocontraction (disruption of reciprocity) of these muscles. However, Shapiro's subject produced some disfluencies in which laryngeal cocontraction was not evident.

Freeman (1977) has argued that disruption of reciprocity in laryngeal abductor and adductor muscles results in a temporary breakdown in the ongoing process of speech production (or, in other words, a physiological block). She hypothesized that the extent to which such disruption (physiological blocking) will fragment or interrupt speech output is dependent on (1) the duration and intensity of the cocontractions; (2) the locus in the speech sequence of its occurrence (between or within words); and (3) a speaker's facility in developing and using strategies to cope with such disruption.

In evaluating laryngeal cocontraction findings, studies of agonist–antagonist articulator muscles (Fibiger, 1977; Platt & Basili, 1973) also warrant consideration. These studies report cocontraction of agonist–antagonist muscles in the lip and jaw, respectively, during moments of stuttering as well as the occurrence of observable, or measurable, tremor associated with such cocontraction. The pattern of activity (including abductor–adductor cocontraction) observed in one of Freeman's subjects (DM, F 1) could be interpreted as evidence of vocal tremor. Available evidence indicates that disruption of agonist–antagonist reciprocity (physiological blocking) of both laryngeal and articulator muscles is often associated with stuttered speech. When such cocontraction is of sufficient duration and intensity, tremor may result.

3. Evidence of abnormal muscle activity during perceptually fluent utterances. Both Freeman and Shapiro also found evidence of abnormal muscle activity during "perceptually fluent" utterances of stutterers. While most perceived stutterings (identified by listeners) were accompanied by disruptions in the normal coordination of muscle activity, similar disruptions also occurred in the speech sequence when listeners did not perceive stuttering. Freeman (1977) found that 7 of 26 perceptually fluent utterances of the word "syllable" showed positive, rather than expected negative, correlations between activity of laryngeal abductor (posterior cricoarytenoid) and adductor (interarytenoid) muscles. A post hoc examination revealed that a brief period of acoustic silence preceded each of these utterances, and that during these periods abductor–adductor cocontraction occurred. Apparently, these pauses were too brief in duration to trigger listener perception of stuttering. Similarly, Shapiro (1980) published illustrations of (1) abnormal orbicularis oris activity during acoustic silences prior to perceptually fluent utterances, (2) abnormal activity of the cricothyroid muscle during a period of acoustic silence preceding an utterance, and (3) abnormal activity of the posterior cricoarytenoid during the utterance of an all-voiced, perceptually fluent word.

These findings strongly suggest that the stutterer, while speaking, experiences many moments of disruption of normal coordination (physiological blocks). Depending on a number of factors, including the nature, intensity, duration, and timing of the disruption, its effects may or may not result in audible or perceptible stuttering. In some cases, a disruption occurring at the onset of a word may simply result in a slight delay in the initiation of the word, a pause too brief to be identified as a disfluency. In other cases, the only result may be a shift in fundamental frequency, a voicing break, fry phonation, or an abnormally long voice onset time.

The preceding description of laryngeal disruptions during the "fluent" speech of stutterers is virtually identical to the perceptible cues of laryngeal origin, described by Adams and Runyan (1981), as distinguishing stutterers' fluency from that of normals. Indeed, the suggestion that stutterers' fluent speech is often characterized by laryngeal motor control disruptions (physiological blocks), too subtle to be perceptually identified as disfluencies, is implicit in most of the studies reviewed in the preceding section of this chapter.

From this perspective, stutterings that listeners identify as disfluencies are only a sampling of the pathophysiological behaviors underlying the disorder and constitute only a fraction of the speech coordination breakdowns (blocks) experienced by stutterers. This "physiological block" hypothesis may also account for the existence of so-called "interiorized" or "closet" stutterers (who consider themselves stutterers, and sometimes seek professional help even though they seldom exhibit stuttering type disfluencies).

While the existence of physiological blocks is consistent with EMG, acoustic, aerodynamic, and fiberoptic studies, strong resistance to the concept is anticipated. Several generations of clinicians have been trained to measure stuttering by counting disfluencies. Many programs for the modification of stuttering depend exclusively on disfluency counts as the measure of improvement. If stuttering is a problem of frequently occurring physiological blocks, only a percentage of which result in listener identified disfluencies, there is much more to evaluating stuttering than counting identified disfluencies, and more to rehabilitation than the elimination of these disfluencies.[4] Acceptance of this concept would dictate that the goal of stuttering therapy be the establishment of fluency, not simply the elimination of overt disfluencies (Adams & Runyan, 1981).

STUDIES OF NONSTUTTERERS
Disruption of agonist–antagonist reciprocity

In terms of muscle activity, "good coordination" occurs when muscles and muscle groups work together to produce the desired effects with a minimum of wasted effort. As described by Sherrington (1909), "reciprocal inhibition" facilitates coordinated movement by agonist muscles through the relaxation of antagonist muscles. Synergist muscles show simultaneous activity, while antagonist muscles are reciprocally active. In general, exceptions to this principle of physiology occur in motor acts that may be described as inefficient or "poorly coordinated. " Specifically, cocontraction of antagonist muscles has been found to occur (1) in physiological stress (created by imposition of high "loads" or resistance; Gellhorn, 1947); (2) in very rapid movements (Goabel & Bouisset, 1966); (3) in the performance of a highly skilled task by untrained subjects (Bratanova, 1966); (4) in infants and young children (Fenges, Gergely, & Toth, 1960; Gater, 1967); (5) in neurological impairment (Kenny & Heaberlin, 1962; Landau & Clare, 1959); and (6) in nonrhythmic performance (Kozmyan, 1965). The parallels between conditions that generate disrupted reciprocity and those in which stuttering is most likely to occur are obvious. Children and those with

TABLE 6-4. Electromyographic Studies of Disfluencies in Normals

STUDY	N	TYPE OF DISFLUENCIES
Freeman (1977)	1[*]	Faked stutterings: 3 levels Mild, Moderate, Severe
Shapiro and DeCicco (1982)	1	Spontaneously occurring: (5 repetitions and 7 prolongations)
Borden, Dorman, Freeman, and Raphael (1977)	2	DAF induced disfluencies

[*] There were two subjects, but a verifiable recording from the PCA was secured from only one, and therefore only data from that subject can be related to abductor-adductor reciprocity.

neurological impairments stutter more frequently than normal adults. Speaking in a "relaxed" easy manner, speaking more slowly, rehearsing or practicing a speech sequence, and speaking in rhythm are all known to reduce stuttering. Indeed, many fluency facilitation techniques may be characterized as antagonist-coordination-facilitation techniques.

Electromyography studies of disfluencies in nonstutterers

EMG studies of disfluencies in normals, summarized in Table 6-4, while limited in number, do offer some valuable information. After finding disruption of laryngeal abductor-adductor reciprocity in stuttering subjects, Freeman (1977) examined "faked" stuttering blocks of a nonstutterer for evidence of similar phenomena. In two instances, while the normal subject was simulating very severe stuttering, cocontraction of laryngeal abductor-adductor muscles occurred. Two differences were noted; the level of activity in the antagonist muscle was lower in the nonstutterer, and the duration of the cocontraction was notably shorter. The brief periods of cocontraction in the nonstutterer coincided with the highest levels of laryngeal muscle activity generated by the subject during the 2-hour recording session. Cocontraction of laryngeal antagonists characterized over 95% of the disfluencies produced by the two stuttering subjects, but less than 1% of the disfluencies simulated by the nonstutterer. However, it is impossible to determine from this study whether abnormal laryngeal behavior distinguishes stutterers from nonstutterers or naturally occurring disfluencies from simulated disfluencies.

Further insight is offered by Shapiro and DeCicco (1982). They analyzed articulator and laryngeal EMG data from a nonstutterer during 12 spontaneously occurring disfluencies. At the articulator level, 8 of the 12 normal disfluencies were characterized by two forms of abnormal muscle activity: (1) excessive muscle activity, and (2) inappropriate bursts of activity. These investigators noted that identical patterns of abnormal articulator muscle activity occurred in stutterers during stuttering (Shapiro, 1980). However, analysis of intrinsic laryngeal muscle activity of this nonstutterer revealed normal, appropriate muscle behavior for all 12 disfluencies. In this case, abnormal laryngeal muscle activity differentiated the disfluencies of stutterers from those of a nonstutterer.

Borden, Dorman, Freeman, and Raphael (1977) placed two nonstuttering subjects under delayed auditory feedback (DAF) in order to study the muscle activity patterns accompanying experimentally induced disfluencies. The main effect of DAF on muscle activity in these normal speakers was to change the timing patterns of muscle activity. Under DAF, intensity levels changed, but there was no predictable pattern. Some muscles showed increases, some showed decreases, and a few remained relatively unchanged. In the articulator muscles (obicularis oris and superior longitudinal), multiple bursts of activity, similar to those noted in stutterers (Shapiro, 1980) and a nonstutterer (Shapiro & DeCicco, 1982) occurred. Instances of disruption of laryngeal abductor–adductor reciprocity (typically bursts of PCA activity during ongoing adductor activity) also occurred with some of the DAF induced disfluencies. However, in stutterers, cocontraction typically occurred prior to or during attempts to initiate voicing. Under DAF, nonstutterers did not show cocontraction coinciding with initiation of voicing. Rather, bursts of PCA activity occurred during prolonged adductor activity that accompanied the increased durations of vocalic segments which characterize speech under DAF. Thus, the loci of abnormal laryngeal muscle activity differed between the disfluencies of stutterers and those of nonstutterers under DAF.

Because of the limitations of data now available on laryngeal muscle activity in stuttering, additional research is necessary. Studies, especially those that combine EMG with fiberoptic, aerodynamic, and acoustic analyses, are needed. It should also be stressed that the search for understanding the disrupted peripheral control of speech production in stuttering does not negate the importance of understanding the neuromotor control processes that underlie peripheral disruptions. Improved understanding of the neurology of phonation and of the role of affective arousal in neural control of phonation are of critical importance.

NOTES

[1] The most widely used "handbook" on EMG is *Muscles Alive* (now in its 4th edition) by John V. Basmajian (1979). The specific applications of EMG to laryngeal research are reviewed by Harris (1982).

[2] The amplitude levels of EMG recordings relate to a number of factors, including load, resistance, distance, and rate of movement. The term tension as used by physiologists refers to measurable properties of load and resistance or "mechanical tension." The complex relationship between EMG and physiological or mechanical tension has been the subject of extensive research (Basmajian, 1979). The term tension has also been used by psychologists and/or speech pathologists to refer to the psychological or emotional state of "being tense." Often there is the assumption that a person who is "tense" will show elevated baseline levels of involuntary muscle activity presumed to be related to the psychological state. However, the precise correlation between EMG and psychological status has not been defined. It should always be remembered that EMG measures electrical voltages produced when muscles contract, it is not a direct measure of tension, either mechanical or psychological.

[3] While surface-placed disc electrodes have limited value for physiological studies of intrinsic laryngeal muscles, they may prove useful for biofeedback treatment of stuttering clients.

[4] It is possible, of course, that disfluency counts may be a valid index of physiological blocks, even though they are not a direct measure of these events. However, as with the use of body temperature as an index for infection, the index may not bear a linear relationship to the underlying problem, and it may not be reliable for all individuals. Further, some treatments may dramatically affect the index (as aspirin with fever) without addressing the underlying problem.

REFERENCES

Adams, M. R., & Runyan, C. M. Stuttering and fluency: Exclusive events or points on a continuum? *Journal of Fluency Disorders,* 1981, *6,* 197–204.

Basmajian, J. V. *Muscles alive,* 4th ed. Baltimore: Williams & Wilkins, 1979.

Basmajian, J. V., & Steko, G. A new bipolar indwelling electrode for electromyography. *Journal of Applied Physiology,* 1963, *17,* 849.

Bratanova, Ts. On bioelectric activity of muscles—Antagonists in the course of elaboration of a motor habit. (Russian text) *Zh. Vvssh. Nerv. Diat. Pavlov.,* 1966, *16,* 411–416 (reported in Basmajian, 1974).

Borden, G., Dorman, M., Freeman, F. J., & Raphael, L. J. Electromyographic changes with delayed auditory feedback of speech. *Journal of Phonetics*, 1977, *5*, 1–8.

Fenges, I., Gergely, C., & Toth, Sz. Clinical and electromyographic studies of "spinal reflexes" in premature and full-term infants. *J. Neurole Neurosurg. and Psychiat.*, 1960, *23*, 63–68.

Fibiger, S. Stuttering explained as a physiological tremor. *Speech Translations Laboratory: Quarterly Progress and Status Report.* Stockholm: Royal Institute of Technology, 1971.

Fibiger, S. Further discussion on stuttering explained as a physiological tremor. *Speech Translations Laboratory: Quarterly Progress and Status Report.* Stockholm: Royal Institute of Technology, 1972.

Fibiger, S. Quantitative electromyographic evaluation of stuttering severity by means of describing the course of muscle activity in the lip-articulatory muscles in connection with labial stop consonants. Interlaken: *Proceedings XVII Congress of Logopedics and Phoniatrics,* pp. 1–14, 1977.

Freeman, F. J. *The stuttering larynx: An electromyographic study of laryngeal muscle activity accompanying stuttering.* Unpublished doctoral dissertation, City University of New York, 1977.

Freeman, F. J. Phonation in stuttering: A review of current research. *Journal of Fluency Disorders,* 1979, *4,* 79–89. (a)

Freeman, F. J. Comments on "Electromyographic indications of laryngeal-area activity during stuttering expectancy," Letter to Editor, *Journal of Fluency Disorders,* 1979, *4,* 299–301. (b)

Gater, V. Studies of the electrical activity of the antagonistic muscles of the arm in normal children aged between 1 and 5 months. *l'Acad. Bul. Sc.,* 1967, *20,* 743–747.

Gellhorn, E. Patterns of muscular activity in man. *Arch. Phys. Med.,* 1947, *28,* 568–574.

Goabel, F., & Bouisset, S. Relation entre l'activite electromyographique integree et la travil mechanique effectue au cours d'un mouvement monoarticulaire simple. *J. de Physiol.,* 1966, *59,* 241.

Harris, K. S. Electromyography as a technique for laryngeal investigation. Bethesda, MD: Conference on the Assessment of Vocal Pathology, National Institutes of Health, April 1979. *American Speech and Hearing Association Report #11,* 1982.

Hirose, H., & Gay, T. The activity of the intrinsic laryngeal muscles in voicing control: An electromyographic study. *Phonetica,* 1972, *25,* 203–213.

Kenny, W., & Heaberlin, P. An electromyographic study of the locomotor pattern of spastic children. *Clin. Orthop.,* 1962, *24,* 139–151.

Kozmyan, E. E. Time relations of excitation and inhibition of antagonist muscles (Russian text). *Zh. Vssh. Nerv. Deiat. Parlor,* 1965, *17,* 125–133 (reported in Basmajian, 1974).

Landau, W., & Clare, M. The plantar reflex in man: With special reference to some conditions where extensors response is unexpectedly absent. *Brain,* 1959, *82,* 321–355.

McLean, A., & Cooper, E. B. Electromyographic indications of laryngeal-area activity during stuttering expectancy. *Journal of Fluency Disorders,* 1978, *3,* 205–219.

Morley, A. An analysis of associative and predisposing factors in the symptomatology of stuttering. *Psychol. Monograph.* 1937, *49,* 50–108.

Platt, L. J., & Basili, A. Jaw tremor during stuttering block. *J. Comm. Disorders, 1973, 6,* 102–109.

Shapiro, A. I. An electromyographic analysis of the fluent and dysfluent utterances of several types of stutterers. *Journal of Fluency Disorders,* 1980, *5,* 203–232.

Shapiro, A. I., & DeCicco, B. A. The relationship between normal dysfluency and stuttering: An old question revisited. *Journal of Fluency Disorders,* 1982, *7,* 109–121.

Sheehan, J. G., & Voas, R. Tension patterns during speech in relation to conflict, anxiety-binding and reinforcement. *Speech Monograph.* 1954, *21,* 272–279.

Sherrington, C. Reciprocal innervation of antagonistic muscles. Fourteenth note. On double reciprocal innervation. *Proc. Royal Soc. B81,* 1909, 249–268.

Shipp, T., & McGlone, R. Laryngeal dynamics associated with voice frequency change. *Journal of Speech and Hearing Research,* 1971, *14,* 761–768.

Shrum, W. *A study of speaking behavior of stutterers and nonstutterers by means of multichannel electromyography.* Unpublished doctoral dissertation, University of Iowa, 1967.

Steer, M. D. Symptomatologies of young stutterers. *Journal of Speech Dis.,* 1937, *2,* 3–13.

Travis, L. Dissociation of the homologous muscle function in stuttering. *Arch. Neuro. Psych.,* 1934, *31,* 127–133.

OBSERVING LARYNGEAL MOVEMENTS OF STUTTERERS
Edward G. Conture

Development of the flexible fiber optic endoscope (fiberscope)—a flexible tube containing bundles of glass or plastic fibers—has had a great impact on otolaryngology, speech science, and speech pathology (cf. Benguerel, Hirose, Sawashima, & Ushijima, 1978; Boraiko, 1979; Brewer & McCall, 1974; Fujimura, 1982; Lawrence, 1982; Sawashima, 1976; Sawashima & Hirose, 1981). The fiberscope contains two bundles of optical glass or plastic strands/fibers with one bundle carrying a "cold," bright light (e.g., xenon) to illuminate the area under investigation and the other bundle returning a color image back for visualization and/or recording (Boyd, 1982). Because a fiberscope can be readily passed through a bodily orifice, routine activities of heretofore inaccessible parts of the body, such as the vocal folds, can be visualized. Its use in the study of laryngeal activity associated with stuttering is the basis of this discussion (Conture, 1977, 1982a, 1983; Conture, McCall, & Brewer, 1977, 1979; Freeman, 1975; Freeman & Ushijima, 1978; Healey & Turton, 1979; Ushijima, Kamiyama, Hirose, & Niimi, 1966; Wolk, 1980).

Methodology and instrumentation

A fiberscope whose diameter is appropriate for insertion into the nasal passages is required. A fiberscope having a diameter of no more than 4 mm is satisfactory for most subjects. Larger diameter fiberscopes are available (approximately 6 mm in diameter), which carry more light for illumination of the larynx; however, they may be too large for subjects with smaller nasal passages. Conversely, smaller diameter fiberscopes

TABLE 6-5. Procedural problems involved with using the fiberscope to study laryngeal behavior during conversational speech of stutterers or other speaker groups. Most such problems make the fiberscope image nonviewable, or so ambiguous as to be unmeasurable, either in a qualitative or quantitative sense.

1. Posterior movement of epiglottis.

2. Mucous/saliva covering the distal end of fiberscope.

3. Lowering of larynx out of the fiberscope's field of illumination.

4. Raising of velum which pulls the fiberscope's distal end up, thus changing the fiberscope's field of illumination and excluding the larynx from it.

5. Pharyngeal constrictor or false vocal fold activity which blocks view of larynx.

6. Large larynx (in both horizontal and vertical dimensions) which "absorbs" too much of fiberscope's light—the "penlight-in-the-Holland-tunnel" effect.

7. Rotation or twisting of fiberscope by examiner (like rolling pencil between index finger and thumb) or side-to-side jostling of fiberscope by movement of lateral pharyngeal walls which makes fiberscope image less than clear.

8. One or both arytenoids or tubercules of corniculates moving partially or completely out of fiberscope's field of illumination or picture itself.

9. Tight adduction or medial compression of arytenoids in such a fashion that it is difficult/impossible to judge their configuration or location.

10. Parallax view of superior surface of vocal folds which makes one side of larynx appear to move faster or with greater degree of excursion than other side, and contributes to false impression of asymmetry of movement. Parallax created by fiberscope being on oblique angle relative to superior surface of vocal folds rather than perpendicular to plane of vocal folds. This is much like viewing the hands of a clock from an angle to the right or left of clock face rather than straight in front of clock face.

11. Intersubject differences in laryngeal structures making measurement landmarks, for example, tubercules of corniculates, less than easy to ascertain. Subtle differences in shapes, tissue coloration, and sizes of laryngeal structures, such as arytenoids, makes them difficult to distinguish from surrounding structures, hence, reliably measure.

(about 2 mm) are available that fit smaller nasal passages such as those of young children. Unfortunately, smaller fiberscopes do not carry sufficient illumination for visualization of the larynx. A "*cold*," (so as not to "heat" and thus damage the fiber optic bundle), bright light source, typically fluorescent or xenon, is used to provide appropriate illumination of the dark laryngeal area. Table 6-5 lists problems that can make fiberscope observations of laryngeal activity nonmeasurable or nonviewable. Either a video or cinematic camera, appropriately interfaced with the fiberscope and a video recorder/reproducer, is also needed to record as well as play back fiberscope images.

Research with the fiberscope creates a number of demands and problems for the speech–language pathologist. Without the collaboration of an otolaryngologist, it is unlikely that fiberscope assessment of stutterers' laryngeal behavior should be undertaken. In addition, insertion of the fiberscope, although requiring neither major nor minor surgery, does involve insertion of a foreign object through the nasal passage. Not all stutterers (or their clinicians) are willing or able to tolerate such a procedure. Another problem which must be solved is the noise of the powerful fan needed to cool the excess heat of the fiberscope's light source. Some means of attenuating this noise must be developed so that acoustic recordings of speech associated with fiberscope views are sufficiently free of such unwanted noise. A means of stopping, starting, and still-framing the videotape or film must also be available for measurements to be made. It is helpful if the film itself has recorded onto it some sort of time code, such as that developed by Mahshie and Conture (1983), which permits correlation of the video image of laryngeal activity with its associated acoustic signal. Various forms of hand or computer-assisted procedures have been developed to analyze this sort of data (cf. Miyazaki, Sekimoto, Ishida, & Sawashima, 1973; Conture, Cudahy, Caruso, Schwartz, Casper, & Brewer, 1982). Thus, much as in high-speed cinematography studies of the larynx that preceded current fiberscope investigations, experimenters who employ the fiberscope have to use fairly specialized, and at times expensive, equipment.

Fiberscope investigations of stuttering

In the mid to late 1960s, the *Zeitgeist* of experimental investigations of stuttering began to turn from environmental studies to those involving genetic/organic/physiological variables. One such early investigation using the fiberscope was completed in Japan by Ushijima et al. (1966) who filmed both inappropriate glottal openings as well as tightly adducted true/false vocal folds during different instances of stuttering. Fujita (1966), using posterior–anterior X-rays of the laryngeal area, also reported nonpredictable openings and closings of the pharyngolaryngeal cavity associated with stuttering. The number of subjects studied and

FIGURE 6-4. Mean percent of videoframes containing each of three categorical judgments of laryngeal behavior: abduction, ABD; intermediate, INT; and adduction, AD associated with adult stutterers' (*N* = 11) instances of stuttering (*n* = 81). The bracket (⊤) on top of the bar indicates one standard deviation (*SD*) above the mean. See Conture, McCall, and Brewer (1977) for further descriptions of categorical judgments. Mean percent and *SD* of nonviewable (NV) videoframes associated with all stuttering are also provided. Similar data are presented for two types of within word speech disfluencies that together made up these 81 stutterings: sound prolongations (*n* = 53) and sound/syllable repetitions (*n* = 28; after Conture, 1982a).

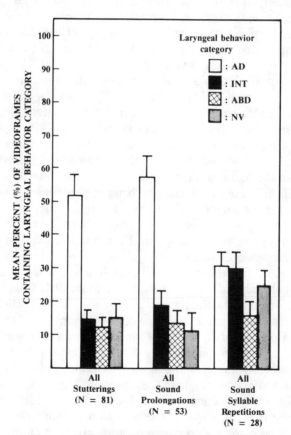

the sample of stutterings assessed limited generalizations of these early findings. Nonetheless, this was ground-breaking research that implicated the larynx in stuttering.

Shortly thereafter, Conture and associates in Syracuse and Freeman and associates at Haskins Laboratories publicly presented their fiberscopic and electromyographic observations of the larynx during stuttering. These presentations culminated in two publications (Conture et al., 1977; Freeman & Ushijima, 1978) and one film (Conture, 1977; for a review of this film see Freeman, 1978). Conture and associates' work focused on fiberscope observations, while that of Freeman and colleagues involved electromyographic studies of stuttering. Conture et al.'s 1977 work indicated that the larynx is often (1) inappropriately, nonpredictably open or (2) inappropriately closed during instances of stuttering. These findings were consistent with those of Ushijima et al. (1966) and, coupled with Freeman and Ushijima's (1978) EMG findings, clearly implicated laryngeal involvement in the disrupted speech physiology that characterizes stuttering.

Conture et al.'s findings further indicated that the nature of such disruption reflects, in large part, the "type" of stuttering observed; that is, sound/syllable repetition versus sound prolongations. Figure 6-4, taken from Conture (1982a), shows that laryngeal behavior was more variable during sound/syllable repetitions than sound prolongations. Moreover, sound/syllable repetitions also contained the greatest number of nonviewable/nonmeasurable videoframes. Too, the variability of laryngeal behavior during fluent speech makes it difficult to characterize the larynx during stuttering. Still, these findings, which are consistent with previous reports, indicate that laryngeal behavior not only differs between stuttering and fluent productions but also between different types of stuttering as well.

If we assume that stuttering for most children who stutter "starts with" sound/syllable repetitions (for example, Johnson, 1959; Conture, 1982), we might wonder how the larynx "acts" during such repetitions produced by adult stutterers. A time-course description of laryngeal behavior from beginning to end of an adult stutterer's sound/syllable repetition is depicted in Figure 6-5. It is apparent that during a sound/syllable repetition, laryngeal behavior is highly variable; the vocal folds open and close throughout the repetition. The larynx is not static; it oscillates between abductory and adductory postures. Preliminary data also suggest that the height of the larynx during stuttering varies. In fact, videofluoroscopic observations of laryngeal height during stuttering (Conture, Gould, & Caruso, 1980) indicate that many repetitions are characterized by a descending or lowering of the larynx compared to

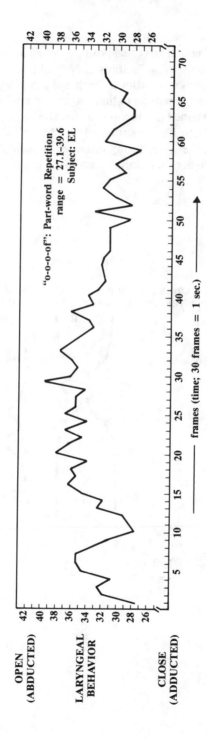

FIGURE 6-5. Time-course description based on computer-assisted measurement (see Conture et al., 1982a for details on measurement procedure) of laryngeal behavior during an adult stutterer's typical sound/syllable repetition ("o-o-o-of"). Units on ordinate are arbitrary, with larger numbers representing increasing laryngeal movement toward complete abduction (as in forced, deep inspiration/inhalation) and smaller numbers indicating movement toward complete adduction (as in vowel production; after Conture, 1982a).

FIGURE 6-6. Vertical laryngeal position (VLP) during adult stutterers' stutterings (Study 1, $N = 7$; Study 2, $N = 6$) using anterior–posterior videofluoroscopic observations. Each subject's VLP values during stuttering were made relative to that subject's mean height of the larynx during three sustained productions of /i/. During stuttering, *Low* VLP = VLP lower than during sustained /i/; *Mid* VLP = VLP equal to or up to 50% higher than during sustained /i/; and *High* VLP = VLP 50% or more higher than during sustained /i/ (after Conture, Gould, & Caruso, 1980).

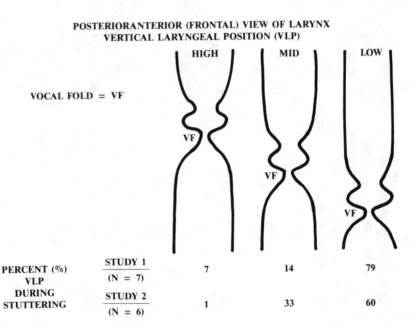

POSTERIORANTERIOR (FRONTAL) VIEW OF LARYNX
VERTICAL LARYNGEAL POSITION (VLP)

		HIGH	MID	LOW
VOCAL FOLD = VF				

PERCENT (%) VLP DURING STUTTERING	STUDY 1 (N = 7)	7	14	79
	STUDY 2 (N = 6)	1	33	60

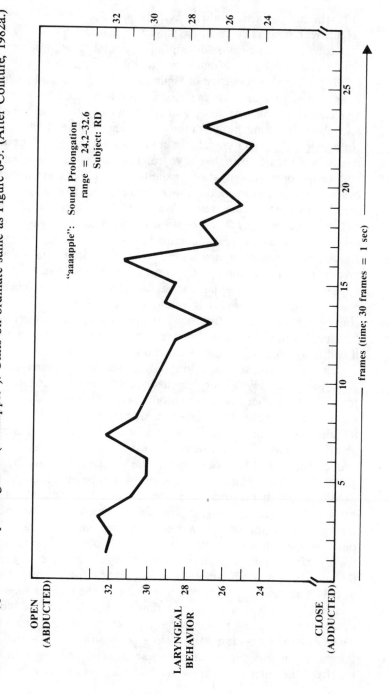

FIGURE 6-7. Time-course description (based on computer-assisted measurement) of laryngeal behavior during an adult stutterer's typical sound prolongation ("aaaapple"). Units on ordinate same as Figure 6-5. (After Conture, 1982a.)

its height during fluent productions of a vowel. Such changes in vertical height, with associated data, are shown in Figure 6-6.

In contrast, a time-course description of a sound prolongation shows that laryngeal behavior is much less variable and the vocal folds more tightly adducted, as depicted in Figure 6-7. For some sound prolongations, the venticular folds are also compressed medially, above the adducted vocal folds, as the epiglottis is "pulled" posteriorly. We have also observed sound prolongations with some stutterers which show constriction of the pharyngeal area at the level of the larynx. The overall relatively static or invariable laryngeal/pharyngeal gesture associated with many sound prolongations is similar to that seen when one closes off the larynx so as to fix the upper torso in order to provide a "platform" for lifting a heavy weight. We believe that stutterers, who point to their throat and say that "the word got stuck here" may not only be sensing excessive laryngeal adduction but aerodynamic back pressures. Readers can gain some appreciation for such sensations by taking a deep breath and then just *thinking* about speaking for 5 to 6 sec. During this imposed delay, before actually speaking, you may note a tendency to close off, constrict, or closely adduct the vocal folds. Such laryngeal constriction may result from an attempt to keep the volume of air "trapped" within the lungs from rushing out prior to the time when it will be needed for speech production.

Conversely, some sound prolongations, particularly those on /s/ and /f/, are associated with widely opened vocal folds. Of course, the vocal folds *should* be abducted during production of these sounds since they are voiceless; however, the degree of abduction is excessive and lasts far too long. Furthermore, a stutterer who senses these extended laryngeal abductions may still describe them in much the same way as overly adducted laryngeal behavior; that is, the stutterer may say "the word got stuck. " To draw an analogy, the larynx may be likened to the flood gates of a dam that regulates the flow of water. The width of the flood gates, or laryngeal opening, determines the amount and rate of flow from a reservoir (the lungs) to a river (the supraglottal vocal tract). When the dam opening is too narrow or completely occluded, water cannot readily exit the reservoir, filling it to near capacity and pressing against the interior of the dam. Similarly, with the vocal folds adducted, there would be an increase in subglottal pressure on the inferior side of the vocal folds as well as minimal or no flow through the vocal folds during the stutterer's inaudible prolongation. In contrast, when the dam opening becomes too wide—and "fixes" in that position—the water flows through in an unregulated, unmanageable "rush" creating a torrent in the river. The latter situation would be analogous to the larynx during audible prolongations on sounds such as /s/. Finally, suppose the flood gates opened and closed in an erratic, nonpredictable fashion. The water would be emitted in spurts or short bursts of varying lengths. This latter situation may be analogous to laryngeal function during sound/syllable repetitions.

While perhaps oversimplified, this three-part analogy clarifies the important role of the larynx in the regulation of the smooth forward-flowing behavior we call "fluent" speech. If speech is to be produced and perceived as normally fluent, the laryngeal "regulatory valve" can neither be too wide nor too narrow, but must be opened/closed to a precise degree at precise moments. Although there is no credible evidence to support claims that the larynx *causes* stuttering, there is ample evidence to support the notion that the larynx plays an important role in the disturbed speech physiology that characterizes its instances.

Electroglottographic (EGG) observations of young stutterers' fluency

Use of the fiberscope is a problem with children, particularly the very young child who is just beginning to stutter. With such small children, procedures that are noninvasive (ones that *do not* enter a bodily orifice or penetrate the outer skin) as well as nonintrusive (ones that *do not* restrict or interfere with natural speech production movements/gestures) are preferable, if not the only means of approach. In terms of studying youngsters' laryngeal behavior during speech, the electroglottograph (EGG) appears ideally suited (see Childers, Moore, Naik, Larar, & Krishnamurthy, 1983; Fourcin, 1981; Ng & Rothenberg, 1982; Rothenberg, 1981 for details on EGG methodology/theory).

Figure 6-8 shows some of our preliminary EGG findings with a 4-year, 10-month-old male stutterer and a 4-year, 9-month-old male normally fluent speaker. Although the EGG traces of these children differ in a number of ways (for example, durations of sound segments) which we are just starting to understand, we would like to focus on the *shape* of the individual glottal pulses of the EGG waveform in the perceptually fluent production of the word-medial vowel /ɛ/ in "again." Note that the young stutterer's EGG waveform is nearly triangular or sawtooth in shape, whereas the young normally fluent child's EGG waveform is more rounded or arched and more nearly sinusoidal. Using other analysis methodologies, we can determine that the stuttering youngster's glottal vibratory cycle is open for approximately 30% and closed for about 70% of the glottal cycle, while the normally fluent youngster's is approximately 50% open and 50% closed per glottal cycle. For this one young stutterer, this suggests a greater degree of vocal fold tension than for

FIGURE 6-8. Inverse vocal fold contact area (IVFCA; see Rothenberg, 1981) waveforms with associated sound spectrograms of a young stutterer (male; age = 4 years 10 months) and normally fluent speaker's (male; age = 4 years 9 months) *fluent* production of word "again" in phrase "say pick again." The top part (toward the spectrogram) of the EGG waveform represents "open" vocal folds with the bottom part (toward the time axis) of the EGG waveform representing "closed." Phonetic segmentations of sound spectrographic and EGG signals are approximations to actual onsets, offsets, and durations of sound segments in the word "again" and are presented for relative comparison purposes only.

IVFCA WAVEFORMS WITH SPECTROGRAMS FOR STUTTERING AND NORMALLY FLUENT SUBJECTS

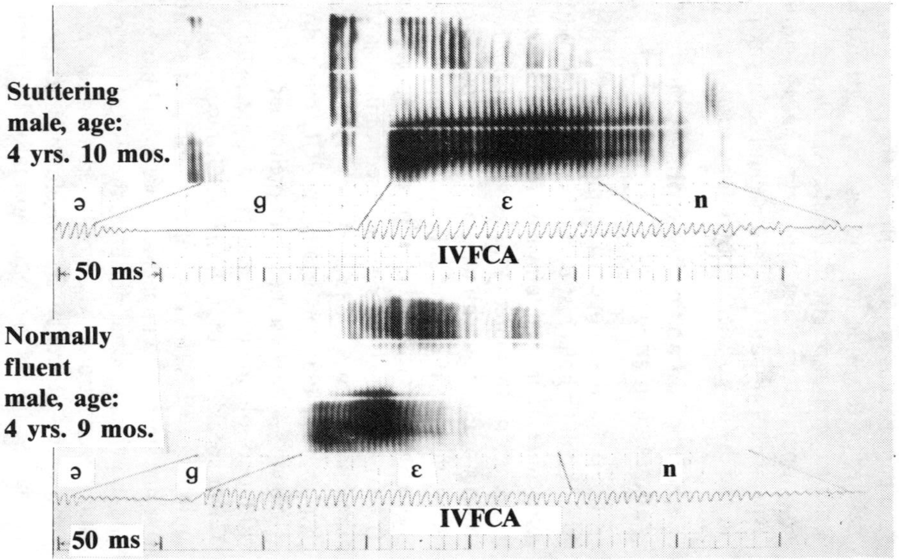

the normally fluent youngster. Some of our other preliminary EGG findings with young stutterers suggest that such excessive or inappropriate vocal fold adduction is most noticeable at the transitions between sounds. Thus, young stutterers may have a tendency to "tighten" or adduct their vocal folds when they move from consonant to vowel or vowel to consonant, regardless of the voicing characteristics of the consonant. Needless to say, much more EGG research with children who stutter needs to be completed before the exact number, nature, and variability of these subtle laryngeal disruptions are known.

Will these preliminary findings be confirmed as we continue to assess more and more children who stutter in more and more speaking situations? At this point, of course, we cannot answer that question, but our findings do suggest that some young stutterers may be using more glottal adduction per glottal cycle than their normally fluent peers, which may also be related to our perceptions of some of these children as having a "tight" or "tense" or "restricted" use of the larynx. Conversely, other EGG findings suggest that some youngsters who stutter may also be opening the larynx inappropriately for very brief periods of time during otherwise normally voiced sounds, for example, during the middle of a vowel. Furthermore, we believe we have observed, with the fiberscope, such brief, generally imperceptible-to-the-ear, laryngeal openings in the fluent speech of some adult stutterers. Because of the very short durations of these laryngeal openings, we have not been able to develop a methodology that accurately and reliably quantifies these fiberscopic observations of sudden, brief laryngeal openings in the otherwise fluent speech of adult stutterers.

While the precise nature and number of these apparent EGG aberrancies await continued research, they strongly suggest that, at the least, some young stutterers' vocal folds are excessively tense throughout speech (during fluent as well as stuttered aspects) and that some young stutterers may have subtle difficulties in controlling and stabilizing laryngeal gestures for fluent speech production. It is not farfetched to envision the day when speech–language pathologists will routinely use advances in technology such as EGG to differentially diagnose stutterers from normally fluent youngsters, as well as differentiate between those young stutterers who may or may not need immediate remediation.

ACKNOWLEDGMENT

The research in Part 3 of this chapter was supported in part by NINCDS Grant (NS 14351) and Contract (N01-N-0-2331) to Syracuse University. Special appreciation is extended to Dr. David W. Brewer for his aid in collection and interpretation of fiber optic laryngeal data and to Anthony Caruso, James Mahshie, and Howard Schwartz for their assistance with data reduction and analysis.

REFERENCES

Boraiko, A. Harnessing light by a thread. *National Geographic,* 1979, *156,* 516–535.

Boyd, W. *Fiber Optics Communications, Experiments & Projects.* Indianapolis, IN: Howard W. Sams, 1982.

Benguerel, A., Hirose, H., Sawashima, M., & Ushijima, T. Laryngeal control in French stop production: A fiberoptic, acoustical and EMG study. *Folia Phoniatrica,* 1978, *30,* 175–198.

Brewer, D., & McCall, G. Visible laryngeal changes during voice therapy: Fiberoptic study. *Annuals of Otology, Rhinology and Laryngology,* 1974, *83,* 423–427.

Childers, D., Moore, G., Naik, J., Larar, J., & Krishnamurthy, A. Assessment of laryngeal function by simultaneous, synchronized measurement of speech, electroglottography and ultra-high speed film. *Eleventh Symposium: Care of the Professional Voice.* New York: Voice Foundation, 1983.

Conture, E. *Laryngeal behavior associated with stuttering* [16mm color sound film]. Syracuse, NY: Syracuse University Film Rental Center, 1977.

Conture, E., McCall, G., & Brewer, D. Laryngeal behavior during stuttering. *Journal of Speech and Hearing Research,* 1977, *20,* 661–668.

Conture, E., McCall, G., & Brewer, D. Author's reply to Healey and Turton's comments, *Journal of Speech and Hearing Research,* 1979, *22,* 413–415.

Conture, E., Gould, L., & Caruso, A. *The descent of the larynx during stuttering.* Paper presented at the convention of the American Speech-Language-Hearing Association, Detroit, 1980.

Conture, E. *Stuttering.* Englewood Cliffs, NJ: Prentice-Hall, 1982.

Conture, E. *Laryngeal behavior during stuttering.* Final Report of Grant NS 14351, U.S. Department of Health, Education and Welfare, National Institutes of Health, National Institute of Neurological Communicative Disorder and Stroke, 1982. (a)

Conture, E. *A further study of laryngeal behavior during stuttering.* Manuscript submitted for publication, 1983.

Conture, E., Cudahy, E., Caruso, A., Schwartz, H., Casper, J., & Brewer, D. Computer-assisted measure of videotape data: A description and case study. *Tenth Symposium: Care of the Professional Voice.* New York; Voice Foundation, 1982.

Fourcin, A. Laryngographic characteristics of phonatory function. In C. Ludlow, & M. Hart (Eds.), *Proceedings of the Conference on the Assessment of Vocal Pathology.* Rockville, MD: ASHA Reports *11,* 1981.

Freeman, F. Fluency and phonation. In M. Webster & L. Furst (Eds.), *Vocal tract dynamics and dysfluency,* 229–266. New York: Speech and Hearing Institute, 1975.

Freeman, F. Film review: Laryngeal behavior associated with stuttering [16-mm color film produced by Edward G. Conture]. *Journal of Fluency Disorders,* 1978, *3,* 229–231.

Freeman, F., & Ushijima, T. Laryngeal muscle activity during stuttering. *Journal of Speech and Hearing Research,* 1978, *21,* 538–562.

Fujimura, O. Fiberoptic observation and measurement of vocal fold movement. In C. Ludlow & M. Hart (Eds.), *Proceedings of the Conference on the Assessment of Vocal Phonology.* ASHA Reports 11, Rockville, MD: American Speech-Language-Hearing Association, 1982.

Fujita, K. Pathophysiology of the larynx from the viewpoint of phonation. *Journal Japanese Society of Otorhinolaryngology,* 1966, *69,* 459.

Healey, C., & Turton, L. Comments on "Laryngeal behavior during stuttering." *Journal of Speech and Hearing Research,* 1979, *22,* 412–413.

Johnson, W. *The onset of stuttering.* Minneapolis: University of Minnesota Press, 1959.

Lawrence, V. (Ed.) *Transcripts of the Tenth Symposium: Care of the Professional Voice* New York: Voice Foundation, 1982.

Mahshie, J., & Conture, E. Deaf speakers' laryngeal behavior. *Journal of Speech and Hearing Research*, 1983, *26*, 550–559.

Miyazaki, S., Sekimoto, S., Ishida, H., & Sawashima, M. A computerized method of frame-by-frame film analysis for fiberscopic measurement of the glottis. *Annual Bulletin 7*, Research Institute of Logopedics and Phoniatrics, University of Tokyo, 1973.

Ng, R., & Rothenberg, M. A matched delay approach to substantive linear phase high-pass filtering. *IEEE Transactions on Circuits and Systems,* 1982, CAS-29, *8*, 584–587.

Rothenberg, M. Some relations between glottal air flow and vocal fold contact area. In C. Ludlow & M. Hart (Eds.), *Proceedings of the Conference on the Assessment of Vocal Pathology*. Rockville, MD: ASHA Reports 11, 1981.

Sawashima, M. Fiberoptic observations of the larynx and other speech. In M. Sawashima & F. Cooper (Eds.), *Dynamic aspects of speech production*. Tokyo, Japan: University of Tokyo Press, 1976.

Sawashima, M., & Hirose, H. Abduction–adduction of the glottis in speech and voice production. In K. Stevens & M. Hirano (Eds.), *Vocal fold physiology*. Tokyo, Japan: University of Tokyo Press, 1981.

Ushijima, R., Kamiyama, G., Hirose, H., & Nimi, S. *Articulatory movements of the larynx during stuttering* [Film]. Produced at the Research Institute of Logopedics and Phoniatrics, Faculty of Medicine, University of Tokyo, Japan, 1966.

Wolk, L. Vocal tract dynamics in a single adult stutterer. Paper presented at the Convention of the American Speech-Language-Hearing Association, Detroit, 1980.

Chapter 7

Articulatory Dynamics of Stutterers

Gerald Zimmermann

BEWARE "UNDERSTANDING STUTTERING"

This book resembles Eisenson's Symposium (1958) in which several "experts" were asked to write about their theories and treatment of stuttering. It was in this symposium that Johnson cited the allegory of the six blind men studying different portions of an elephant, all coming to different conclusions about what it was they had investigated (see Figure 7-1). The resemblance between this book, Eisenson's, and many others derives neither from coincidence nor from a lack of originality by the authors and editors. Rather, it reflects the lack of progress in coming to an understanding of stuttering and its treatment. The lack of progress is attributable to the constraints on our thinking pointed out to us by Johnson. Johnson suggested that even if the men studying the elephant were not blinded, their views would still be constrained by their experiences and interests. They would still have come to different conclusions about the different parts of the elephant—about what to measure and how to interpret their measurements. This may seem obvious, perhaps trivial. It reflects, however, a critical error in our approach to stuttering. It reflects the fact that we have not come to any agreement on why we should be asking questions about different parts of the elephant or even why we are asking questions. It is not clear what the blind men wanted to accomplish by studying the elephant, as it is often not clear what investigators are trying to accomplish by studying certain aspects of stuttering or stutterers. By being explicit about the purpose of our studies we can argue and come to some agreement about the importance of a given purpose and the suitability of our vocabulary and methods for accomplishing it.

FIGURE 7-1. The elephant and the wise men.

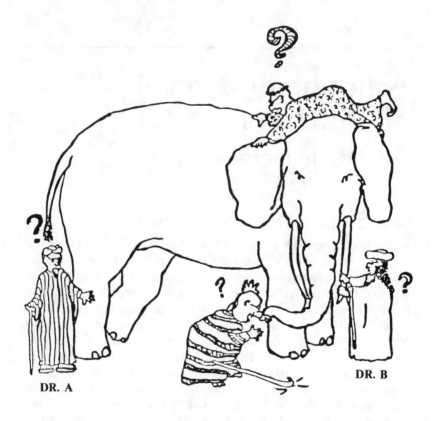

DR. A   DR. B

WHAT STATUS "STUTTERING"?

The parable chosen by Johnson, however, may have been seriously misleading. The allegory between stuttering and the elephant implies that stuttering can be viewed as something of an entity, with several parts that can be investigated as if they were independent of one another. Certainly, Johnson did not believe this, but the construct of stuttering has enjoyed such status.

This view of stuttering as a divisible entity has had dramatic consequences. It has led people to try to identify or define stuttering as if it had some real existence: that it was quantifiable or measurable, and it could be investigated as if it had discrete parts. This view has drawn us away from focusing on the behaviors of stuttering as the results of an interaction of an individual with certain organismic/biological attributes and specific environmental conditions.

It is not playing semantic games to point out how viewing stuttering as a discrete entity has very different implications than viewing stuttering only as a perceptually reliable perceptual category. In fact, the case has been made that stuttering does not warrant definition other than as a diagnostic category (Zimmermann & Kelso, 1982), which is important only because it demarcates a significant difference from normal which can impede communication and which is held in low esteem by the culture. This view leads us away from seeking simplistic, univariate causes of "stuttering" and the identification of biological and environmental conditions that are associated with behavior breakdown and with becoming diagnosed a stutterer.

Many questions already have been asked about this diagnostic category. Differences between those who fall within and outside this diagnostic category have long been used to draw inferences about the causation of the disorder rather than about the cause for being diagnosed as a stutterer. An obvious example is the status given to observed differences in "voicing." Differences between stutterers and nonstutterers in certain aspects of voice control have often been reported. Conclusions have been drawn about stuttering being a disorder of phonatory control. The only proper conclusion to be drawn from such designs is that the differences found are correlated with the diagnostic category of stuttering. Once this conclusion is drawn one can then pose other questions about the biological–behavioral development of phonatory control and the role of phonatory behavior in fluency breakdown. The differences shown between stutterers and nonstutterers in phonatory control may reflect differences in the control or coordination processes that are directly related to the increased likelihood of speech breakdown, or these differences might be the result of some compensatory strategy that the stutterers develop to avoid behavior breakdown. The issue then becomes, for what are they compensating? In no case, however, can such differences be raised to causal status without major leaps of logic like that of the insect trainer who trained insects to jump when they heard a tone, cut off the insects' legs and, finding they could no longer jump, concluded they heard with their legs (Lowentin, 1983). While such logic has led clinicians to train easy voice onsets and make other manipulations of the phonatory mechanism, therapeutic success is not support for the identification of a "causal" agent.

DESCRIPTION VERSUS EXPLANATION

Figure 7-2 depicts a simplified view of the relationship between different descriptors and explanations for stuttering. On the right of the figure are descriptors that have been used to categorize events associated

FIGURE 7-2. Description (clues) and Explanation.

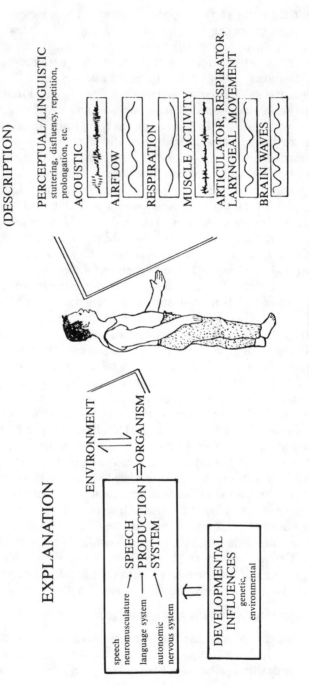

with differences between groups of stutterers and nonstutterers. Differences in these dependent variables have led investigators to raise these variables to causal status. That is, differences in voice onset times have led to the hypothesis that laryngeal behaviors are the core behaviors in stuttering; differences in number of repetitions and prolongations have led to these behaviors acquiring definitional status as the core behaviors in stuttering; analyses of acoustic events have led investigators to attribute stuttering to a defect in coarticulation. Recordings of muscle activity have led to theories of stuttering as a disorder of cocontraction of agonist and antagonist muscles. The study of other observables has led to other explanations. Such "explanations" seek an understanding in terms of seductive unitary causes rather than focusing attention on organism-environment interactions, which are necessary to account for the very simple as well as the complex behaviors of all biological systems. It is only after a great deal of time and energy is spent confusing description for explanation that rational approaches emerge (see Freeman, 1979).

Differences between stutterers and nonstutterers may have differential significance for theoretic (explanatory) and therapeutic (clinical) enterprises. However, the question would still remain why the speech production-perception systems of stutterers seem more susceptible to breakdown even at the youngest ages studied. Even if there were no differences found in the environmental conditions of stutterers and nonstutterers we would still be faced with determining whether stutterers responded differently to identical environmental changes or events than nonstutterers. It may be that the effects of a given event on the production-perception system of a stutterer are different from its effects on a nonstutterer. *The point is that experimental designs which seek to isolate differences between stutterers and nonstutterers have not, and cannot, on the basis of these differences, lead to conclusions about causal events. They can only lead to hypotheses and investigations of the conditions associated with the development of these differences.*

AN EXAMPLE OF UNDERSTANDING CAUSATION

An example of a search for "significant causes" and a search for a theory may be instructive. The example, borrowed from David Bohm (1977), forces a distinction between an association and a causal relationship between events. It furthermore points out the need to agree upon a level of explanation or an account that we will accept before we begin to argue about what approach to take.

The disease malaria was first associated with damp night air. The hypothesis did not explain the known facts very well, however. Another hypothesis was raised suggesting that mosquitoes carried something from the blood of a sick person to the blood of a healthy person, something which caused malaria. This could explain why damp places could exist without malaria, provided that none with the disease lived in the neighborhood. Thus, a hypothesis had been developed that could fit the wide range of facts known about malaria. To verify this hypothesis, experiments were needed to eliminate the possibility that mosquitoes were incidently associated with the disease, while damp air was one of the "real" causes. An experiment was done and only those who were bitten by the malaria-carrying mosquitoes, independent of damp air, contracted malaria. The true causes therefore, had to be something transmitted by the *Anopheles* mosquito from the blood of a sick person to that of a healthy person. Later a specific bacterium was isolated. This shows how to search for an improved explanation of some phenomenon, in this case a constellation of symptoms and facts surrounding their development, helped to uncover what Bohm calls the "significant causes;" it also shows how the isolation of antecedent conditions can lead to the control of a disease. Finally, this case demonstrates how a constellation of symptoms can have different explanations depending upon which descriptors one chooses. These descriptors are often the result of observation rather than precursors to observation of a particular phenomenon.

The analogy to stuttering, I hope, is obvious. The toxic agent, carried by the *Anopheles* mosquito, might be either an environmental or an organismic condition. The constellation of symptoms analogous to the diagnostic class malaria is the constellation of symptoms associated with the diagnostic class of stuttering. The analogy holds insofar as a myriad of conditions surrounding the development and maintenance of stuttering have been posed but appears to break down insofar as no single significant cause, either environmental/developmental or organismic, has been isolated. The same principles may hold for accounting for both malaria and stuttering.

While the identification of the significant causes of stuttering might be more complex in that there may be more significant causes and in that the diagnostic category may not reflect a homogeneous group in terms of these causes, the same logic may hold. That is, for a given individual an account of the presence of diagnostic category "stuttering" might depend on the identification of those conditions, both environmental/developmental and organismic, which are sufficient to make him fall into the stuttering classification. The account must involve, according to Bohm, significant causes: those conditions or events which, in the context of interest, have appreciable influence on the effect in question, that is, those which influence whether an individual is called a stutterer or not. What the significant causes are cannot be determined a priori but must be decided by careful observation and study. Much of the problem with the schools of thought in the area of stuttering is that certain conditions are ruled out a priori as not significant either implicitly or explicitly. For instance, those who proselytize a learning theoretic view often disregard the organismic variables as significant to the development or maintenance of behavior breakdown associated with stuttering.

The question of which variables, events, or conditions are significant to the development of stuttering, or whether there are any variables, events, or conditions that are universally related to its development, is an experimental question and one that has singularly important implications for both theories and therapies.

A PHYSIOLOGICAL APPROACH

For numerous reasons, academic, sociological, and economic, we have focused on an analysis of the function of the speech mechanism of those diagnosed as stutterers. A brief discussion of our work and its alleged significance follows. Our task is similar to the task that von Bertalanffy (1949) has assigned to biology. The task is to establish laws governing order and organization within a living system. We must account for the breakdowns in order and organization.

It needs to be clear from the outset that the approach finally suggested herein is not a physiological theory of stuttering and does not suggest a cause for stuttering. Rather, we are interested in the identification of (1) physiological conditions that are associated with the breakdown in fluent speech; and (2) those conditions among diagnosed stutterers which make them more susceptible to breakdowns in speech fluency than those not so diagnosed. It may be that stutterers have inherently different speech production–perception systems or that they are affected differently by environmental influences. If behaviors associated with stuttering are like most other behaviors a complete account of who will and who will not be diagnosed as a stutterer will incorporate organismic (biological) and environmental conditions. What will be left to argue over, and what this book is about, is which conditions may be most significant in the development and maintenance of behaviors associated with the stuttering label and which factors may be most useful for changing these behaviors. Few would disagree that both organismic and environmental factors play a role in the development and maintenance of the behavior.

A model of behavior breakdown and an explanation for the diagnosis of stuttering should emerge from an account of the regularities and deviations from regularity of the speech production system and from an account of the perceptual consequences of those deviations. Although our focus is on the principles of operation of the speech production system, "understanding of the nature of stuttering" must also involve the identification of the developmental/environmental conditions associated with the development of speech as well as the identification of the biological conditions that may differentiate those who are at risk to stutter from those who are not.

It is important to recognize that a physiological approach or physiological description of the differences between stutterer and nonstutterer is not the only useful level of description. We focus on this description, however, because we believe that to understand stuttering is to identify the conditions (biological and environmental) that lead to the breakdown in behaviors of the speech production system. Thus, while many descriptions of differences between stutterers and nonstutterers may be useful and while many explanations may be offered, all such explanations should be interfaced with knowledge and theories of perceptual–motor control. Recognizing that speech breakdowns, or any behavioral breakdowns for that matter, are often contextually (environmentally) conditioned, it is apparent that the effect of the environment, or how the speaker/actor perceives the environment, plays a critical role in achieving or maintaining stability in the production process. From this point of view the perceptual aspects of interactions are probably critical to a full account of speech breakdown or the behaviors associated with stuttering. The evaluation and modification of these speaker–environment interactions (perception, attitudes, etc.) warrant a great deal of discussion and research.

Potentially significant differences have been found in variables that are associated with environmental conditions as well as those that are associated with the physiological makeup of stutterers and nonstutterers. We chose to study the physiological aspects because (1) evidence from hundreds of studies (reviewed by Bloodstein, 1975; St. Louis, 1979; Van Riper, 1982) shows differences in speech and nonspeech behaviors in these groups, even in fluent productions and even at the youngest ages studied; (2) the familial nature of stuttering is not attributable to environmental–cultural factors alone (Kidd, Heimbuch, & Records, 1981); (3) the prospects for early identification and for the development of an index of risk for stuttering seem best in the physiological domain.

Initial attempts at describing the movements of articulators of stutterers was based on the belief that any explanation of speech breakdown, whatever one's point of view, must ultimately be consistent with physiological principles underlying speech production. Rather than focusing at the level of a perceptual–linguistic description, we sought a vocabulary that was conducive to understanding speech and its pathologies in terms of motor control processes. Following the arguments of Moll, Zimmermann, and Smith (1977) the movements of stutterers' articulators were approached in the same way that movement physiologists have approached analysis of other movement system such as gait (Grillner, 1975), locust flight (Wilson, 1961), scallop swimming (Mellon, 1969), and mastication and swallowing in cat, monkey, and man (Lund, McLachlan, & Dellow, 1971). When we began, an important issue was whether certain kinematic (movement-related) characteristics of the perceptually fluent speech of stutterers were different in degree or kind from those of nonstutterers. We were also interested in the patterns of articulator events that may be related to the initiation and completion of a perceptually judged "block."

The focus on parameters such as velocity, displacement, and duration of movement and the coordination or timing between articulator events was motivated by the possibility of relating these events to underlying neurophysiological processes. The study of perceptually fluent events arose from the presupposition that differences found in even the motorically most simple speech-related task might lead us to develop hypothoses and theories about the inherent character or nature of the production mechanism that was associated with stuttering.

These studies revealed unexpected differences in the movement patterns in perceptually fluent utterances of stutterers and nonstutterers (Zimmermann, 1980a). Furthermore, results revealed that disfluent events were associated with particular patterns that preceded and followed them (Zimmermann, 1980b). These findings led to speculation about the association between disfluent events and aberrant activation of brainstem pathways that physiologically link the articulators (Zimmermann, 1980c; Zimmermann, Smith, & Hanley, 1982). Specifically, it was suggested that lower velocities and displacements and longer durations in the movements of stutterers are associated with processes that keep activation of brainstem pathways below "threshold" level during perceptually fluent speech (Zimmermann, 1980c).

Based on such kinematic analyses we have speculated about physiological processes that may be involved in speech breakdown. Bernstein (1967) proposed that the onset of any movement is preceded by preliminary tuning of the excitability of all participating sensory and motor elements. Tuning, or biasing, facilitates or inhibits the excitability of certain pools of motorneurons and thereby alters the relationships among groups of muscles and determines the kind of behavior they will promote. Tuning sets the stage for groups of muscles to act as functional units called "coordinative structures" which are activated by the appropriate triggering signals (Easton, 1972; Fowler, Rubin, Remez, & Turvey, 1978). Such muscle groupings are formed to accomplish an intended goal, but certain properties of the coordinative structures may be manipulated to give them versatility and adaptiveness.

If movement is the result of an interaction among tuning or reflex excitability, peripheral biomechanics of coordinative structures, and triggering signals to these muscle groups, an analytic framework for speech breakdown emerges. Incoordination may occur when either tuning or triggering inputs are aberrant. The excessive tension noted in some stutterers prior to speech (Van Riper, 1982), the aberrant position of articulators preceding oscillatory or tonic activity of the articulators (Zimmermann, 1980b), and the fact that most stuttering occurs on initial gestures (Hahn, 1942; Johnson & Brown, 1935) indicate that the period before speech movements may be a time in which aberrant inputs are likely to occur in stutterers.

There is evidence that tuning occurs before speech movements. Based on a study by Netsell and Abbs (1975), McClean (1977) measured muscle activity associated with mechanically induced stretch to the corner of the mouth prior to muscle contractions in speech. McClean reported systematic increases in peripheral reflex amplitudes as a function of the interval between mechanical stimulation and the onset of voluntary muscle contraction. Such systematic modulation of activity suggests that neural events are altered just prior to articulatory movement. Smith and Luschei (1983) found that the stutterers they investigated fell on the ends of the continuum of reflex amplitude on a task involving articulation or an oral reflex. The most severe stutterers had the largest reflex. A very mild, well-controlled stutterer had only a minimal reflex.

The role of reflex activity associated with stuttering-like behavior has been demonstrated for other movement systems. Afferent input has been shown to disrupt ongoing behavior and lead to oscillatory movements under the proper conditions (Brown, Rack, & Ross, 1982a, b; Stein & Oguztoreli, 1976). Interestingly, Brown and colleagues described conditions under which subjects reported they were "losing control" as their thumb tremor built to large amplitude oscillations. The interaction of reflex activity and the force imposed by a subject seemed important to the development of these large oscillations. Both the behavioral (oscillatory) and perceptual (losing control) descriptions make the analogy to behaviors associated with stuttering compelling.

A MODEL OF BREAKDOWN: THE INTERACTION OF INFORMATION AND ACTION

Information from afferent channels other than kinesthetic, tactile, or proprioceptive may influence speech production and be related to speech breakdown. The effects of delayed auditory feedback (DAF) on speech have been of interest to researchers concerned with stuttering and offer a convenient point of departure for more general models of behavior breakdown. Most explanations have employed explanatory constructs involving servosystem analogs of speech production. The finding that maximal speech disturbance occurs with a delay interval of about 200 ms has been interpreted to suggest that this interval either is related to the duration of input units (syllables) or that it reflects a critical delay between afferent and efferent signals in the servosystem underlying speech (Fairbanks, 1955).

The servosystem metaphor used to account for DAF effects has been of tremendous utility in motivating research into sensory motor processes. However, it carries a great deal of theoretical baggage that may not be essential for the analysis of the functional relationship between inputs and outputs of the system (Kelso, Holt, Kugler, & Turvey, 1981). To track down this functional relationship, we asked whether there was a systematic association between the occurrence of speech breakdowns under DAF and the relationship between information coming in the ear and activity of the articulators (Zimmermann, Forrest, & Kelso, 1980). Cinefluorographic investigations showed that breakdowns in movements were associated with the arrival of auditory information that specified gestures incompatible with those about to be produced by the speaker (Figure 7-3). For example, a breakdown (a stoppage and/or change of direction of movement) was likely to occur if an acoustic signal associated with upward movement of the tongue tip or jaw occurred at the very beginning or just prior to a downward movement of the jaw or tongue in a CV gesture (see Figure 7-3). To the extent that the delay signal ended before the onset of an incompatible CV gesture, the destabilizing associations between acoustic and production were thought to decrease. The tentative conclusions are that the slowing and durational changes of speech gestures usually observed under DAF reflect an adaptive strategy of the system to minimize the probabilities of these perturbating relations; the breakdowns in coordination or fluency that do occur reflect responses to unexpected perturbing relationships between incoming auditory information and speech production events.

This interpretation can be related to results from animal studies on the function relationships between sensory and motor events. Lund and

FIGURE 7-3. The relationship between breakdown, delayed auditory information, and movement for the utterance /p'æt/ in the context " ... like pat and mat" in the 200-ms delay condition. Point 1 represents the point of perturbation of lower lip and jaw movement at the beginning of the downward (CV) gesture in /pæt/. The delayed feedback occurring at point 1 is associated with the onset of upward movement of the lip and jaw for the VC gesture in /lɑik/. The incompatibility between the information associated with upward movement in the delayed auditory signal and the CV gesture /p æ/ is thought to be a condition associated with articulatory breakdown (from Zimmermann, Kelso, & Forrest, 1980).

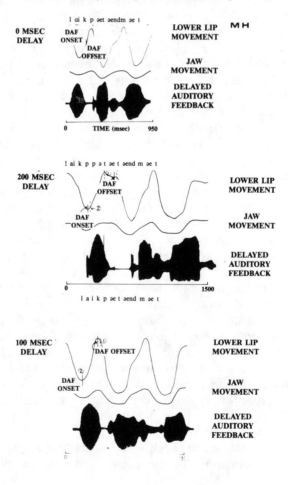

co-workers (1971) demonstrated that the effects of electrical stimulation of the upper lip on chewing were different when stimulation occurred at different phases of the chewing cycle in rabbits. Similarly, Forssberg, Grillner, and Rossignol (1977) showed that the effect of a stimulus to the paw of a cat during walking depends on the phase of locomotion in which it is presented. These and other studies illustrate that changes in relationships between sensory information and motor output allow responses to adapt to changing behavioral contexts. In terms of the DAF effect, acoustic information has perturbing (breakdown) effects only when it occurs at particular phases of a speech gesture. Hence, the same information, acoustic signal, will have different effects at different times in the speech production process.

There is nothing special about acoustic information leading to breakdown. The acoustic channel is only one of several channels of afferent information that may lead to perturbation of speech. We suspect, however, that the type of relationship demonstrated between sensory/perceptual information, phase of production, and behavioral breakdown may be critical to a physiological account of the behaviors associated with stuttering. In addition, autonomic activity, which may operate over a different time scale, may also be associated with fluency breakdown. Autonomic stimulation has been shown to affect the blood supply to striated muscle (Marshall, 1976) and also to affect reflex activity (Chase, Torii & Nakamura, 1970).

The speech breakdowns of stutterers, as well as those of nonstutterers, may be a result of irregularities in the relationship between sensory and perceptual events and movement. It may be that (1) stutterers manifest more aberrant relationships because of more variable motorics, or (2) they have "low thresholds" for breakdown but the same pattern of motor output. Speech breakdowns may be associated with irregular productions or irregular afferent inputs or some combination. Also, general states or levels of an organism's arousal may also play a significant role insofar as such arousal is reflected in the operation of the neuromotor system for speech. Whether stutterers have intrinsically different speech production–perception systems is still open to question. Whether they do or not, we still must know, for a full account, the environmental/developmental conditions and their physiological effects that lead to fluency breakdowns and the diagnosis of stuttering. At present, our view is that if there are differences in the operations of the speech production systems in stutterers and nonstutterers, and our best bet is that there are, an analysis of how the system operates is critical to the identification of significant causes of fluency breakdown and will serve as a partial account of why some people become diagnosed as stutterers and others not.

THERAPEUTIC CONSIDERATIONS

The effects of specific therapeutic procedures can also be analyzed within the proposed framework. Regardless of the numerous theoretical and practical approaches taken to therapy (operant, systematic desensitization, counterconditioning, fluency training, personality/attitudinal, psychodynamic, etc.) there may be only a limited number of ways to affect inputs to motorneuron pools and hence change behavior. For example, one may (a) alter the background activity and/or reflex excitability of pathways involved in speech gestures; (b) alter the absolute inputs to the muscles involved in a coordinative structure or to specific agonist muscles (Greene, 1972; Kots, 1977); or (c) some combination of these. From this perspective, each approach to therapy implicitly emphasizes some aspect of these potential changes in inputs to motorneuron pools. For example, systematic desensitization stresses the deconditioning or extinction of emotional reactions. Presumably its therapeutic effect is to decrease autonomic inputs to the motorneuron pool, thereby altering the reflex excitability of pathways involved in speech production. Procedures that use relaxation in a counterconditioning framework stress the learning of new relaxation responses to supplant responses involved in increases in muscle tension. Such procedures may have their effect by reducing background activity of motorneuron pools. Operant or fluency therapies that stress the modification of specific speech gestures may alter the relative or absolute levels of triggering inputs to muscle groups involved in speech gestures. Though these and other effects may be inferred from the various treatment procedures, the efficiency of each technique should be empirically determined. We believe that different therapies can have many common effects when evaluated at the motor unit or movement level but will differ in their efficiencies.

There are logical and empirical grounds for suggesting certain goals for therapy. If stutterers possess the necessary organization or coordinative structures for relatively fluent production, as evidenced by their perceptually fluent speech, one must wonder how the necessary conditions may be maintained for the coordinative structure to operate within relatively fluent limits. A number of lines of evidence suggest that it may not be efficient to try to change the pattern of coordination or timing among muscles involved in a movement. From studies of animal locomotion, Boylls (1975) stated that parameters associated with the relative timing of a gesture are the least modulable movement parameters. Changing the amount of input to a specific muscle in a group of muscles involved in a gesture also changes the relative timing among muscle actions. The view is consistent with the evidence on the stability of timing relationships shown in locomotion. The stability of timing relationships, among articulators, has been well established in the speech literature (Kozhevnikov & Chistovich, 1965; Zimmermann, Kelso, & Lander, 1980; Zimmermann & Rettaliata, 1981).

According to Boylls (1975), the more easily modulable movement parameters are those related to alterations in absolute inputs, rather than relative inputs, to muscles involved in a gesture. Absolute changes in muscle inputs are associated with changes in "metrical" parameters, such as velocity, displacement, and acceleration, while timing among muscles and structures are held constant. This view suggests that therapy methods designed to modify the absolute levels of input to all of the muscles involved in a speech gesture may be more efficient than those focusing on the modification of isolated muscles or structures.

REFERENCES

Bernstein, N. *The coordination and regulation of movements*. London: Pergamon, 1967.

Bloodstein, O. *A handbook on stuttering*. Easter Seal Society for Crippled Children and Adults, 1975.

Bohm, D. Science as perception–communication. In F. R. Suppe (Ed.), *The structure of scientific theories*. Urbana: University of Illinois Press, 1977.

Brown, T. I. N., Rack, P. M. H., & Ross, H. F. Forces generated at the thumb interphalangeal joint during imposed sinusoidal movement. *Journal of Physiology*, 1982, *332*, 69–85. (a)

Brown, T. I. N., Rack, P. M. H., & Ross, H. F. Different types of tremor in the human thumb, *Journal of Physiology*, 1982, *332*, 113–123. (b)

Boylls, C. C. *A theory of cerebellum function with applications to locomotion. II. The relation of anterior lobe climbing fiber function to locomotor behavior in the cat*. COINS (Technical Report 76-1), University of Massachusetts, 1975.

Chase, M. H., Nakamura, Y., & Torii, S. Afferent vagal modulation on brainstem somatic reflex activity. *Experimental Neurology*, 1970a, *27*, 534–544.

Chase, M. H., Torii, S., & Nakamura, Y. The influence of vagal afferent fiber activity on masticatory reflexes. *Experimental Neurology*, 1970b, *27*, 545–553.

Eisenson, J. *Stuttering: A symposium*. New York: Harper, 1958.

Easton, T. A. On the normal use of reflexes. *American Scientist*, 1972, *60*, 591–599.

Fairbanks, G. Selective vocal effects of delayed auditory feedback. *Journal of Speech and Hearing Disorders*, 1955, *20*, 333–346.

Forssberg, H., Grillner, S., & Rossignol, S. Phasic gain control of reflexes from the dorsum of the paw during spinal locomotion. *Brain Research*, 1977, *132*, 121–139.

Fowler, C., Rubin, C., Remez, R., & Turvey, M. Implications for speech production of a general theory of action. In B. Butterworth (Ed.), *Language production*. New York: Academic Press, 1978.

Freeman, F. Phonation in stuttering: A review of current research. *Journal of Fluency Disorders*, 1979, *4*, 74–89.

Greene, P. H. Problems of organization of motor systems. In R. Rosen & F. Snell (Eds.), *Progress in theoretical biology,* Vol. 2 (pp. 304–332). New York: Academic Press, 1972.

Grillner, S. Locomotion in vertebrates: Central mechanisms and reflex interaction. *Physiology Reviews,* 1975, *55,* 247–304.

Hahn, E. A study of the relationship between stuttering occurence and grammatical factors in oral reading. *Journal of Speech and Hearing Disorders,* 1942, *7,* 329–335.

Hegde, M. N. Antecedents of fluent and dysfluent oral readings: A descriptive analysis. *Journal of Fluency Disorders,* 1982, *7,* 323–341.

Johnson, W., & Brown, S. F. Stuttering in relation to various speech sounds. *Quarterly Journal of Speech,* 1935, *21,* 481–496.

Johnston, T. D. Contrasting approaches to a theory of learning. *The Behavioral and Brain Sciences,* 1981, *4,* 1.

Johnston, T., & Turvey, M. T. A sketch of an ecological metatheory for theories of learning. In G. H. Bower (Ed.), *The psychology of learning and motivation.* New York: Academic Press, 1980.

Kelso, J. A. S., Holt, K. G., Kugler, P. N., & Turvey, M. T. On the concept of coordinative structure as dissipative structure. II. Empirical line of convergence. In G. E. Stelmach (Ed.), *Tutorials in motor behavior.* Amsterdam: North-Holland, 1980.

Kidd, K., Heimbuch, R., & Records, M. A. Vertical transmission of susceptibility to stuttering with sex modified expression. *Proceedings of the National Academy of Science,* 1981, *78,* 606–610.

Kots, Ya. M. *The organization of voluntary movement: Neurophysiological mechanisms.* New York: Plenum, 1977.

Kozhenikov, V. A., & Chistovich, L. A. Rech' ,*Artikulyatsiya i Vospriyatiye* [Speech: Articulation and perception]. Washington, D.C.: Joint Publications Research Service, Vol. 30, p. 543, 1966.

Lowentin, K. C. The corpse in the elevator. *The New York Review,* January 20, 1982.

Lund, J., McLachlan, R., & Dellow, P. A lateral jaw movement reflex. *Experimental Neurology,* 1971, *31,* 189–199.

McClean, N. Effects of auditory masking on lip movements during speech. *Journal of Speech and Hearing Research,* 1977, *20,* 731–741.

Marshall, J. M. The influence of the sympathetic nervous system on the microcirculation of skeletal muscle. *Journal of Physiology.* 1976, *258,* 118–119P.

Mellon, D. The reflex control of rhythmic motor output during swimming in the scallop. *Verlerchende Physiologie,* 1969, *62,* 318–336.

Moll, K., Zimmermann, G. N., & Smith, A. The study of speech production as a human neuromotor system. In M. Sawashima & F. Cooper (Eds.), *Dynamic aspects of speech production.* Tokyo: University of Tokyo Press, 1977.

Netsell, R., & Abbs, J. Modulations of perioral reflex sensitivity during speech movements. *Journal of Acoustical Society of America* (Suppl.), 1975, *S41.*

Smith, A., & Luschei, E. Assessment of oral–motor reflexes in stutterers and normal speakers: Preliminary observations. *Journal of Speech and Hearing Research,* 1983, *26,* 322–328.

Stein, R., & Oguztoreli, M. Tremor and other oscillations in neuromuscular systems. *Biology of Cybernetics,* 1976, *22,* 147–157.

St. Louis, K. O. Linguistic and motor aspects of stuttering. In N. Tass (Ed.), *Speech and language: Advances in basic research and practice.* New York: Academic Press, 1979.

Van Riper, C. *The nature of stuttering.* Englewood Cliffs, NJ: Prentice-Hall, 1971.

von Bertalanffy, Ludwig. *Problems of life.* London: Wats, 1949.

Wilson, D. M. The central control of flight in a locust. *Journal of Experimental Biology,* 1961, *38,* 471–490.

Zimmermann, G. N. Articulatory dynamics of simple, "fluent" utterances of stutterers and nonstutterers. *Journal of Speech and Hearing Research,* 1980, *23,* 95–107. (a)

Zimmermann, G. N. Articulatory behaviors associated with stuttering: A cineradiographic analysis. *Journal of Speech and Hearing Research,* 1980, *23,* 108–121. (b)

Zimmermann, G. N. Stuttering: A disorder of movement. *Journal of Speech and Hearing Research,* 1980, *23,* 122–136. (c)

Zimmermann, G. N., Forrest, K., & Kelso, J. A. S. Delayed auditory feedback: A reinterpretation (Abstract). Acoustical Society Meeting, Los Angeles (1980) (manuscript submitted).

Zimmermann, G. N., & Kelso, J. A. S. Remarks on the "causal" basis of stuttering. *The Proceedings of Van Riper Lecture Series,* April 1-2, 1982, Kalamazoo, MI (in press).

Zimmermann, G. N., Kelso, J. A. S., & Lander, L. Articulatory behavior pre and post full mouth tooth extraction and alveoloplasty: A cinefluorographic study. *Journal of Speech and Hearing Research,* 1980, *23,* 630–645.

Zimmermann, G. N., & Rettaliata, P. Articulatory patterns of adventitiously deaf speakers: Implications for the role of auditory information in speech production. *Journal of Speech and Hearing Research,* 1981, *24,* 169–178.

Zimmermann, G. N., Smith, A. C., & Hanley, J. M. Stuttering: In need of a unifying conceptual framework. *Journal of Speech and Hearing Research,* 1981, *46,* 25–31.

Theoretical perspectives of stuttering

Chapter 8

Stuttering as a Genetic Disorder

Kenneth K. Kidd

INTRODUCTION

Stuttering runs in families. While that fact has been known for centuries, its explanation is still not fully understood, even though the possibility of some hereditary involvement is immediately suggested for any trait or disorder that is observed to run in families. Genetic involvement is self-evident for such traits as hair color and stature and for disorders that involve a biochemical abnormality. But there is also increasing evidence of genetic involvement among such behavioral disorders as stuttering, dyslexia, Tourette syndrome (Pauls & Kidd, 1981; Scarr & Kidd, 1983), as well as such major psychiatric disorders as schizophrenia (Gottesman & Shields, 1982) and manic-depressive illness (Gershon et al., 1976).

The statement that heredity can affect behavior does not negate the importance of environmental factors; behavioral traits are obviously affected by learning and by an individual's psychosocial environment. This chapter argues that complex behavioral disorders, such as stuttering, are not determined by nature or by nurture, but by both. The important research objectives are to determine the magnitude and relevance of both genetic and environmental factors and to identify the interactions that determine which individuals develop stuttering and which do not. The argument to be presented is that an inherited neurologic susceptibility underlies most cases of stuttering.

It is possible to formulate specific hypotheses about how genes and environment might interact to produce family patterns seen for stuttering. Several analyses, most based on a large set of family data collected in the Yale Family Study of Stuttering, are discussed and their implications for identifying the causes of stuttering are considered. First, however, we briefly consider genetic variation among individuals and patterns of genetic transmission and interaction with the environment in human development.

GENETIC VARIATION AMONG INDIVIDUALS

Genes influence development along common lines; we all develop as recognizably human. At the same time, because of numerous differences in the genes among individuals, each individual develops along a slightly different pathway. Such differences among individuals probably extend to different levels of susceptibility for behavioral disorders. But genes are not wholly deterministic; the pathway from a fertilized egg to an intact adult organism is complex, dependent on many environmental factors, and influenced in its course by variation in the environment.

One needs only to look around to realize that there is considerable genetic variation among humans. Differences in natural hair color, stature, and skin color are all consequences of *normal* genetic variation. During the last 20 years, we have learned that normal genetic variation is far more extensive than had been thought. The variation we see in everyday encounters is but the tip of the iceberg. Whenever a metabolic system or a developmental process is studied closely, genetically determined variation is found among normal individuals. Each human is unique mostly because each has a unique genetic blueprint, except for identical twins.

Each individual's genetic constitution (genotype) is determined when a sperm fertilizes an egg. Exactly how information in DNA determines the way in which that original single cell divides and its descendants differentiate into the numerous complex systems of a human being is largely unknown. Numerous examples of genetic effects on development and normal function are relatively well understood, but these are merely glimpses of a continuous process. Ignorance of detail, though, should not be confused with gross ignorance; the outline of the overall process is reasonably clear. Among other things, it is clear that developmental processes vary slightly from individual to individual and that such variation is partly a result of normal genetic differences (variation) among individuals. The concept that genetic differences underlie normal variation is an important one and is well documented (Cavalli-Sforza & Bodmer, 1971; Harris, 1975).

The human brain is the most complex of all human organs, and its structure is largely determined by genetic information. We do not yet know enough to correlate human brain anatomy with genetic variation among individuals. While all normal human brains are largely alike, they also differ in numerous small details. Genetic information is important in controlling brain function, too. There is evidence that over twice as many genes are involved in brain function as are involved, for example, in liver function—between 100,000 and 200,000 compared to about 50,000 (Hahn et al., 1982; Kaplan & Finch, 1982). Although we do not yet know what those 100,000-plus genes are, neuroscientists have identified some enzymes that control metabolism of neurotransmitters, the chemical messengers that carry nerve impulses between neurons, and geneticists have identified inherited differences for some of these enzymes (see, e.g., Weinshilboum, 1981). Because concentrations of neurotransmitters can affect the strength of impulses transmitted from one nerve to another, different individuals are likely to be genetically programmed to function differently in different parts of their brains. Consequently, such genetic variation probably affects speech to some degree. Indeed, we know that many recognized genetic disorders with neurologic and/or muscular effects do disturb fluent speech. Whether some genetic variation may affect only speech or whether stuttering might be a specific manifestation of such genetic variation is not yet known.

CLASSICAL PATTERNS OF INHERITANCE

Controlled breeding experiments, such as were used by Mendel with garden peas to discover his laws of inheritance, are not available for studies of human traits. Since even full siblings differ for many gene loci, it has been difficult to identify and isolate the effects of differences at a single gene locus. Furthermore, simple autosomal dominant or autosomal recessive modes of inheritance, such as were described by Mendel, are not commonly seen in human traits. Since such simple modes of inheritance are largely irrelevant to behavioral genetics in humans or to the genetics of stuttering, they will not be considered further. Interested readers should consult a good introductory textbook of genetics.

GENE–ENVIRONMENT INTERACTION IN DEVELOPMENT

The genetic information that governs the complex interactions of development is encoded in DNA (deoxyribonucleic acid, the genetic material). It is clear, however, that realization of a function specified by any segment of DNA (i.e., any gene) is directly dependent on the metabolic system of the cell, which, in turn, is dependent on the functioning of the whole organism. Indeed, not only the biological environment but also the physical and social environments required for an organism's development are necessary for the expression of many phenotypes. There can be no controversy over whether genetic constitution or environment is more important; both are essential. The development of an organism occurs only through the joint action of a genetic blueprint and the necessary environmental conditions which allow that genetic information to be expressed.

The relationship of genotype (the genetic constitution) to phenotype (the appearance; all observable characteristics) in human development is extremely complex and only three points will be made here: (1) Different genotypes can, and usually do, produce different phenotypes; (2) different genotypes can, and often do, produce phenotypes that are indistinguishable; and (3) the same genotype is often capable of producing more than one phenotype, depending on environmental conditions. A concept that accounts for such gene–environment interactions is the reaction range, which provides a basis for formulating a general model for the inheritance of stuttering.

Reaction range refers to the quantitatively and qualitatively different phenotypes that can develop from the same genotype under varying environmental conditions (Gottesman, 1963; Lewontin, 1974). A given genotype is believed to have a specific range. In one individual some phenotype within that range will result, but which phenotype develops will be determined by environmental interactions that occur throughout development. It is not correct, however, to say that heredity sets the limits on development while environment determines the extent of development. Both are half-truths because they ignore the interdependence that results from the constant transactions between genotype and environment during development.

There are no general laws of reaction range that can predict the development of individuals. As Hirsch (1971, p. 94) has said,

> The more varied the conditions, the more diverse might be the phenotypes developed from any one genotype. Of course, different genotypes should not be expected to have the same norm of reaction; unfortunately psychology's attention was diverted from appreciating this basic fact of biology by half a century of misguided environmentalism. Just as we see that, except for monozygotes [monozygous, or identical twins], no two human faces are alike, so we must expect norms of reaction to show genotypic uniqueness....Extreme environmentalists were wrong to hope that one law or set of laws described universal features of modifiability. Extreme hereditarians were wrong to ignore the norm of reaction.

Not all "non-genetic" variation is attributable to "environmental" factors. Chance is ever present and can be partly responsible for phenotypic variation. Consider that there are many times as many neurons in the brain as there are genes controlling their growth and development. Certainly, which neuron forms a synapse with which other neuron must be a function of chance. The genes specify certain rules that are followed in forming neural connections but do not specify all individual connections. Variation among people in thought patterns, coordination of movement, and so forth, may reflect, in part, this element of chance in the development of each individual's brain.

DATA RELEVANT TO GENETICS AND STUTTERING

Three types of data can give information on the importance of genetic variation in determining who is and who is not susceptible to stuttering: adoption studies, twin studies, and family studies. Each has strengths and weaknesses.

Adoption studies

Genetic studies of behavioral traits are always confounded by environment—the more closely related two people are, the more similar, on average, are their environments. An ideal adoption study completely severs the cultural link between biological relatives. If the frequency of stuttering among, for instance, adopted-away children of a biological parent who stutters is higher than among adopted offspring of a non-stutterer, then the shared genes must be responsible. Since stuttering has often been considered to be culturally determined, data from an adoption study would be one way to demonstrate that the increased frequencies of stuttering in relatives of stutterers are due to shared genes. Unfortunately, no such data are available, partly because an adoption study is very difficult to design properly.

Twin studies

Twin studies have been used for decades to study genetic factors in behavior. The logic is deceptively simple. Identical twins are essentially one individual cloned; both have exactly the same genetic makeup. Fraternal twins are no more alike genetically than any two siblings; they just happened to be conceived at the same time. Thus, these two types of twins can be used for a type of experiment that controls for complex genetic determination and for gene–environment interaction. If behavior is more similar in identical twins than in fraternal twins, the greater genetic similarity of the identical twins seems a likely cause.

Most early investigations of stuttering in twins focused on the possibility of an increased prevalence among twins as compared to single-tons. The rates of stuttering reported among different twin groups varied widely from 1.9% (Graf, 1955) to 20% (Nelson et al., 1945). The data were often not collected in a systematic manner, the twins' zygosity (monozygous (MZ) = identical; dizygous (DZ) = fraternal) was usually not precisely determined, and the sexes of the pairs were rarely given. Such deficiencies render most twin concordance studies of little value in quantifying familial frequencies. For example, Nelson et al. (1945) reported that 9 of 10 monozygotic (MZ) pairs and 2 of 30 dizygotic (DZ) pairs were concordant for stuttering. While consistent with the frequencies reported by Andrews and Harris (1964) for siblings, these concordances are not sex specific and, hence, provide little useful information.

Howie (1981) conducted a twin study of 30 same-sex twin pairs: 21 male pairs (12 MZ, 9 DZ) and 9 female pairs (5 MZ, 4 DZ). Pairwise concordance for stuttering was significantly higher in MZ twins (58-63%, depending on diagnostic criteria for stuttering) than in DZ twins (13-19%). The more meaningful proband concordances were about 75% for both male and female MZ twins, but were only 45% for male DZ twins and 0% (all 4 pairs discordant) for female DZ twins. The interclass correlation of total disfluency scores was also significantly higher in MZ twins (.67) than DZ twins (−.09) (Howie, 1981).

In an Italian population, pairwise concordances for stuttering were 83% for MZ twins (12 pairs) and 10.5% for DZ twins (19 pairs) (Godai et al., 1976). Eight of the nine male MZ pairs were concordant as were two of the three female MZ pairs. All nine male DZ pairs were discordant, one of the two female DZ pairs was concordant, and among the eight unlike-sex pairs, both stuttered in one, the male stuttered in four, and the female stuttered in three.

Though these two studies report concordances that differ numerically, the numbers involved are quite small, and their findings seem to be in broad general agreement. Moreover, it is exceedingly difficult to be certain that a twin study gives unbiased concordances unless a systematic study is done of twin pairs already identified. Neither of these studies used a twin registry, and it is possible that MZ pairs that were concordant were more likely to "volunteer" or otherwise come to the attention of investigators. Thus, high concordances may be an artifact of biased ascertainment. While both studies yielded results compatible with genetic hypotheses, the data provide only limited support for genetic hypotheses.

The twin data do, however, clearly demonstrate that nongenetic factors can be important in the development of stuttering. Since monozygotic twins are genetically identical but are not always concordant for stuttering, identical genotypes may develop into a person who stutters OR into a person who does not stutter. The twin studies do not indicate what nongenetic factor(s) might be involved.

Family studies

One disadvantage of adoption and twin data is that even when they suggest the involvement of genetic factors, they can provide little information on the number of genes involved or on the forms of interaction with the environment. Data on complete families provide such information. The major weakness in family data is that nongenetic cultural transmission is largely impossible to exclude as an alternative hypothesis. A "classic" example of this problem is the report on the X family (Gray, 1940). Because stuttering occurred through several generations in one branch of the family but did not occur at all in another large branch, this family was used to support Johnson's (1955) hypothesis that stuttering was culturally determined. Casual examination of the pedigree shows that it is also completely compatible with a genetic hypothesis. This case also illustrates a basic scientific principle: compatibility of data with a hypothesis does not prove that hypothesis; a different hypothesis may be equally compatible with the data. Because the bulk of data on the genetics of stuttering comes from the Yale Family Study of Stuttering, that study is used as a framework for discussing all the family data on stuttering and its interpretations.

THE YALE FAMILY STUDY OF STUTTERING

The Yale Family Study of Stuttering has been in progress since 1973. Initial results from this study are now available, but these new data do not completely elucidate the role of genetic factors in the etiology of stuttering. Even the existence of relevant genetic factors has yet to be established beyond all doubt. However, we now have a much clearer understanding of the multifaceted problems involved, and some important new findings have been made. In the remainder of this chapter, the results from the Yale Family Study are reviewed in conjunction with other relevant studies.

Family studies have been used for many years in discussions about genetic factors in the etiology of stuttering. Most studies were anecdotal or were limited to reports of positive family history. While familial concentration of stutterers was reasonably well documented, no genetic conclusions were possible. Before more rigorous genetic analyses could be done, a large number of complete pedigrees of stutterers was needed. The pedigrees published by Gray (1940) and Kant and Ahuja (1970) were not collected in a carefully defined manner that allowed statistical evaluation. The Yale study was designed to collect data suitable for testing genetic hypotheses.

Methods

Information has been collected on over 600 stutterers and several thousand of their first-degree relatives. The majority of those individuals contacted to participate in the study were diagnosed as stutterers by trained clinicians and were initially referred to us by speech–language pathologists. These stutterers, who first bring a family to our attention, are called probands. We are concerned that every proband has a confirmed diagnosis of stuttering; however, we have not required that the proband has to have been enrolled in therapy or to stutter currently. Any stutterer with known mental retardation, epilepsy, cerebral palsy, or neurologic disorders that might be associated with a higher incidence of stuttering or suggestive of generalized neurologic dysfunction has not been accepted. All probands not excluded by the above criteria have been included in the study, without regard to family size or knowledge of stuttering in the family. We also discussed with all referring clinicians our concern that they *not* refer only "familial" stutterers to us. Since we wanted to learn with what frequency relatives were stutterers, it would have seriously biased our data if we preferentially studied families already known to have stuttering relatives.

We asked about each proband's ethnic origins and about the country of origin of each of the four grandparents. We have included in the analyses only families of European descent. We employed this restriction to eliminate a possible source of genetic heterogeneity. Since gene frequency is a parameter in genetic models and different ethnic groups often have different gene frequencies, it is obviously incorrect to analyze data on an ethnically mixed population. This control should also decrease cultural differences.

Approximately half of our data sample was collected by standardized interview of the proband (or in the case of a child, the proband's parent) and half by a self-report questionnaire. Two definitions of stuttering were used; one for the proband and one for family members. First, stuttering in the proband required a diagnosis by a speech–language pathologist. (A direct diagnosis by the interviewer was not possible if the proband no longer stuttered or stuttered in only a few specific situations, or if the self-report form was used.) Individuals with questionable diagnoses, such as cluttering or spastic dysphonia, were not included in the analyses. Although individual speech–language pathologists may have slightly different definitions of stuttering, their diagnoses were considered to be conservative and reliable. In the majority of active stutterers (especially adults), diagnosis is relatively straightforward and does not present the difficulties encountered in diagnosing a disorder such as schizophrenia.

Stuttering in other family members, if not previously diagnosed by a speech–language pathologist, was defined as excessive repetitions or prolongations or "having trouble getting the word out." Such symptoms reported by a proband usually coincided with the proband's identification of a relative as a "stutterer" or "stammerer." When it was not possible to obtain specific information on stuttering symptoms (e.g., for a parent who had stuttered only as a child), we accepted the classi- fication conveyed from relatives through the proband. Additional information on subject selection criteria and ascertainment has been described by Kidd and Records (1979) and Seider et al. (1982).

In 1979, approximately 5 years after the beginning of the study, a follow-up study was conducted. Questionnaires were obtained from 145 families who had indicated that there were children in the family under age 14 at the time of the initial interview. These questionnaires provided more current information about new onsets of, or recoveries from, stuttering or about the development or improvement of other speech and language problems. Information about the fluency status of any other first-degree relative of a proband was also obtained. A stutterer was always defined as one who had ever stuttered or ever stammered, and included those individuals who were reported to have stuttered only as children for a period greater than 6 consecutive months.

Detailed pedigrees were collected for the families of all of the more than 600 probands, including information on speech patterns for every family member. This information included reports on concomitant speech and language problems, therapy histories, age of stuttering onset, and age of recovery. Though some pedigrees were more extensive than others, each pedigree included all first-degree relatives of the proband— parents, brothers and sisters, and children—and our initial analyses have been limited to that subset of data. Two examples from among the larger pedigrees collected are shown in Figure 8-1.

Prevalence and sex effect

Stuttering is a disorder believed to affect roughly 1% of the popu- lation at any given time. Unfortunately, there are few studies that allow good estimates of the lifetime prevalence. However, the preponderance of affected males over affected females is well documented. Van Riper (1971) reviewed 18 studies which show a sex ratio among stutterers ranging from 2:1 (males:females) to 5:1. This difference between the sexes appears to hold in all cultures and races. Interestingly, most studies do not present lifetime prevalence data by sex. In fact, most studies of stuttering report point prevalence rather than lifetime incidence of "ever- stuttered." For a transitory trait with variable age of onset and duration, true lifetime incidence is difficult to assess reliably.

Preliminary data from the Yale Family Study of Stuttering were used by Kidd, Kidd, and Records (1978) to examine several possible explana- tions of the sex difference among stutterers. A more recent tabulation of data, based only on families of adult probands but showing the same

FIGURE 8-1. Selected pedigrees of stutterers. In these standard pedigree drawings a square represents a male and a circle, a female. Filled-in symbols indicate "ever-stuttered." Horizontal lines connecting individuals below their symbols indicates a marriage; a break in that line indicates that marriage terminated by death or divorce. The marriage line is connected to the sibship line which connects all children of that marriage (full siblings) above their symbols. The arrow indicates the proband, the person who first came to our attention.

FAMILY 49

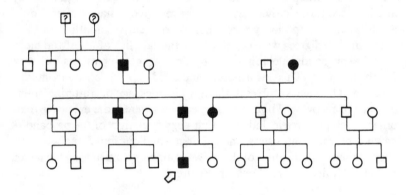

FAMILY 22

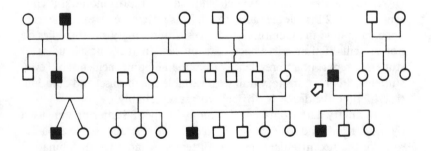

TABLE 8-1. Frequencies of stutterers among relatives of adult stutterers categorized by sex (from Kidd, 1983)

Relatives:	Male Probands:	Female Probands:
Fathers	.184 ± .023	.204 ± .040
Mothers	.044 ± .012	.117 ± .032
Brothers	.194 ± .021	.231 ± .041
Sisters	.041 ± .012	.128 ± .029

The frequencies are given with their binomial standard errors. Because there were fewer families identified through female probands, the numbers of relatives of female probands are smaller and the standard errors correspondingly larger. Statistical analyses show that the frequencies in the second column are significantly higher than those in the first. The frequencies among male relatives are also significantly higher than among female relatives.

sex effects, is shown in Table 8-1. Two points are demonstrated in these data: (1) males are more susceptible (biologically?) to stuttering and (2) relatives, of both sexes, are at higher risk of stuttering if the family is originally found (ascertained) through a female proband.

Familial concentration

Several studies have shown that the risk for stuttering among relatives of a stutterer is markedly elevated above that of the general population or of nonstuttering control groups (Andrews & Harris, 1964; Kant & Ahuja, 1970; Wepman, 1939). In the more than 20 pertinent studies compiled by Van Riper (1971), the proportion of stutterers with a family history of stuttering ranged from 24 to 80%, with a median of 42%. With few exceptions, those studies did not report the number or frequency of affected relatives or their relationship to the proband. A number of these studies used matched control groups; for example, Andrews and Harris (1964) found a family history of stuttering for 38% of the stutterers but only 1.4% of the controls. Furthermore, among 30 of the stutterers with a positive family history, 13 were reported to have had no direct contact with the stuttering relative, suggesting that imitation or social learning probably did not play a major role in the etiology of the disorder, at least in these cases.

A positive family history, even with a control group, conveys little useful genetic information, since it is also a function of total family size, a variable largely independent of the genetics of a disorder. For example, a stutterer in a large family may have several dozen first cousins. If only one of them were also a stutterer, the degree of familiality would be quite low. Yet, such a stutterer would be classified as having a positive family history. So too, would a stutterer with only four first cousins, two of whom were also stutterers, but in this case, the degree of familial concentration would be much higher. These quantitative aspects of a family history of stuttering are important in trying to determine whether there is a significant difference between families of stutterers and nonstutterers and, if there is, what might cause it.

Progress toward sex-specific quantification of familial concentration started in the early 1960s. Wingate (1964) reported that 21% of males ($n = 32$) who had stuttered had relatives in their immediate families who also stuttered, all of whom were males. Of 18 female stutterers, 33% reported other stutterers in their immediate families, 67% of whom were males. Andrews and Harris (1964) also found that female probands have a higher frequency of affected relatives of both sexes than do male probands. Kay (1964), however, was the first to calculate risks for first-degree relatives by sex of proband and relative. His calculations indicated significant differences for male and female relatives, with frequencies similar to those in Table 8-1.

The Yale data on 2,035 relatives of 397 unrelated adult stutterers confirmed the reports of earlier studies and quantified a strong familial concentration (Kidd, Heimbuch, & Records, 1981). An initial question asked of these data was whether or not vertical transmission exists; does having a stuttering parent increase the risk of offspring stuttering? Evidence of vertical transmission is a prerequisite to most genetic hypotheses. Our analysis divided the families into subsets. Families of adult probands were first classified by whether the proband was a male or a female. Both groups of families were then classified according to stuttering in the proband's parents: (1) N, neither parent ever-stuttered; (2) F, father ever-stuttered; (3) M, mother ever-stuttered; and (4) B, both parents ever-stuttered. Tables 8-2 and 8-3 show the frequencies of stutterers among siblings and children of the probands in the two most frequent types of families. The frequency of stuttering increases markedly if the father of the proband also stuttered.

The data also suggest that the sex difference involves a transmittable component. A lower overall incidence among females in conjunction with a higher incidence of affected relatives of female stuttering probands suggests that more factors promoting stuttering are required for a female to stutter and that families of female probands have more of those factors since they have more affected members. A full analysis

TABLE 8-2. Risk to siblings and children of adult MALE stutterers according to family type

	Family Type	
	N **(78%)**	**F** **(17%)**
Brothers	.174 ± .022	.236 ± .057
Sisters	.022 ± .009	.100 ± .039
Sons	.214 ± .041	.350 ± .107
Daughters	.093 ± .029	.095 ± .064

Frequencies of relatives who ever-stuttered are presented for families in which neither parent of the proband had ever stuttered (type N for Neither) and families in which the father but not the mother had ever stuttered (type F for Father). The percentages of these two family types are given at the top of each column. Families in which the mother only, or in which both parents had ever-stuttered occurred in small percentages and are not tabulated here because there were few total relatives.

of the data showed that this pattern of distribution within families is statistically significant and supports stuttering's vertical transmission and sex-modified expression within families (Kidd et al., 1981).

Genetic hypothesis

One of the difficulties with genetic studies of stuttering is that a gene product such as an enzyme or a structural protein cannot be directly measured. In the absence of an ability to measure a gene product and in the absence of a clear, simple pattern of genetic transmission, one can only proceed by posing specific hypotheses pertinent to genetic transmission and testing them against the data. This is done with the hope that one can reject all but one hypothesis or can learn enough to formulate new hypotheses and collect new data for testing. Unfortunately, one can never prove such hypotheses; the scientific method only permits hypotheses to be disproved.

In studying the genetics of stuttering, several different genetic hypotheses have been considered. The data in Tables 8-1, 8-2, and 8-3 do not fit any simple Mendelian hypothesis. The near equality of the

TABLE 8-3. Risk to siblings and children of adult FEMALE stuttering probands according to family type.

	Family Type	
	N (70%)	F (19%)
Brothers	.176 ± .044	.333 ± .096
Sisters	.088 ± .030	.167 ± .076
Sons	.333 ± .058	0.0 ± .152
Daughters	.093 ± .029	.095 ± .064

Frequencies of ever-stuttering among relatives of female probands are presented for families in which neither parent of the proband had ever stuttered (type N for Neither) and families in which the father but not the mother of the proband had ever-stuttered (type F for Father). The percentages of these two family types are given at the top of each column. Families in which the mother only, or in which both parents had ever-stuttered occurred in small percentages and are not tabulated here because there were few total relatives. The numbers of relatives in the second column are already quite small; note that the risks for sons of these female stuttering probands are not significantly different.

frequencies of stuttering among both siblings and offspring of stutterers is not compatible with simple autosomal recessive inheritance. The frequencies of stuttering among relatives are too low to be compatible with autosomal dominant inheritance. X-linked inheritance is not compatible with the high frequency of father-to-son "transmission" of stuttering. As noted earlier in the chapter, more sophisticated genetic models which can account for gene–environment interaction are required. Two such models have been applied (Kidd et al., 1978; Kidd, 1980), and both account for the data even though they are extremely different. Having two equally plausible but different models does not mean that genetic hypotheses should be dismissed. It means that we have not yet developed the necessary statistical power or have not considered our data in a way that allows us to discriminate among alternative hypotheses. Both of these models suggest that the genetic component is much more important than the nongenetic component in determining whether an individual will stutter or not.

We will consider in detail one of those models, the model which postulates that a single major genetic locus determines the inheritance of an innate susceptibility to stuttering. The single-major-locus model (Figure 8-2) consists of three genotypes, each with sex-specific probabilities of being affected (Kidd & Spence, 1976). The probabilities reflect nongenetic variation that determines the liability distribution around each genotype mean. A sex-specific threshold, then, divides the total distribution into those who do and those who do not stutter. In this model gene–environment interaction is evident from two directions. Genetically normal individuals (genotype S_1S_1 in Figure 8-2) could be affected if they have a sufficiently exacerbating environment. Alternatively, even homozygotes for the predisposing allele (genotype S_2S_2 in Figure 8-2) could be unaffected in a sufficiently ameliorating environment. As graphed for one sex in Figure 8-2, the heterozygotes (genotype S_1S_2) would have a sufficiently stressful environment to be above the threshold and would stutter about 5% of the time. In contrast, homozygotes would have a sufficiently benign or ameliorating environment to be below the threshold about 5% of the time and would not stutter. The positions of the modes, thresholds, and the allele frequencies can be varied to find the best explanation of the data. Note that if the overlap of the distributions were negligible and the threshold fell between the heterozygote and one of the homozygotes, this model would depict a classic dominant or recessive mode of inheritance.

Results for this single-major-locus hypothesis applied to the Yale data are given in Table 8-4. This solution accounts for family data quite well. The gene frequency is estimated at 4%—not a rare gene, but not a common one either. Most individuals in the general population lack the gene. According to the model about 8% of the population is heterozygous and less than 2 in 1,000 are homozygous. The penetrances, the probabilities that individuals with particular genotypes will ever stutter, differ for males and females and account for the sex effect observed in the data. Both male and female penetrances are virtually zero for homozygotes for the normal genotype; both are one (or 100%) for homozygotes for the stuttering genotype. A striking sex difference is predicted for heterozygotes: penetrance is about 40% for a heterozygous male but only 11% for a heterozygous female. These parameter values predict a lifetime prevalence of ever stuttering in childhood at around 4% for males and 1% for females, approximately the values

FIGURE 8-2. A simplified graphical representation of the single-major-locus model. The "high-susceptibility" form of the gene (allele) is represented by S_2; the normal (allele) by S_1. Individuals will have one of three genetic types—S_1S_1, S_1S_2, or S_2S_2. These genotypes exist in the population in the frequencies p^2, $2pq$, and q^2, respectively, where $q=1-p$ is the frequency of the S_2 form of the gene. Each genotype has an average liability (M), but individuals with that genotype are distributed around that value because of nongenetic (environmental) factors. The standard deviation of that distribution is measured by ε. Individuals whose susceptibility is above the threshold (T) are affected. In this example some individuals with high genetic susceptibility will be unaffected while some with only moderate genetic susceptibility will be above the threshold and affected. (Modified from Kidd, 1980.)

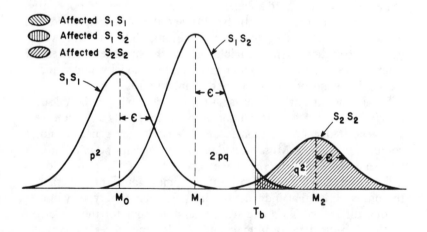

TABLE 8-4. Single-Major-Locus Analysis of Stuttering Estimates of Genetic Parameters

	Genotypes		
	NN	NS	SS
Male Penetrances	.005	.378 ± .025	1.0
Female Penetrances	<.001	.107 ± .019	1.0
q = frequency of S = .040 ± .007			

reported. These findings, however, do not constitute proof that a single genetic locus is responsible for stuttering. While these findings may be encouraging for genetic hypotheses in general, the question of how susceptibility to stutter is actually determined and transmitted is left unanswered.

Though severity of symptoms, by one measure, appears to be unrelated to transmission of stuttering (Kidd et al., 1980), *severity* defined in some other way might be correlated with susceptibility and help resolve current uncertainty over alternative genetic models. An obvious candidate is persistence of stuttering vs. recovery. The breakdown of ever-stuttered relatives in our study according to recovery is presented in Table 8-5. Analyses of these and additional data found no consistent pattern of recovery or persistence among relatives related to severity for either general model of transmission we have proposed (Kidd, 1980; Kidd et al., 1978) or other genetic models (Cox & Kidd, 1983). The data indicate that persistently stuttering probands have an excess of same-sex siblings whose stuttering also persists. This finding may be the result of nongenetic factors affecting recovery or may be attributable to an ascertainment bias of some sort. Additional work on this question is clearly needed.

Nongenetic hypotheses

While the family data provide the strongest evidence for genetic inheritance of susceptibility, the case can be made stronger if nongenetic forms of transmission are examined and can be shown to be incompatible with the data. We have tested several cultural hypotheses for stuttering and

TABLE 8-5. Recovered and Persistent Stutterers among Relatives of Adult Persistent Probands: The frequencies show significant heterogeneity

Relatives of Male Probands

Relationship to Proband	Total Ever Stuttered	Number Recovered	Percentage Recovered
Fathers	46	25	54
Mothers	13	9	69
Brothers	60	16	27
Sisters	10	6	60

Relatives of Female Probands

Relationship to Proband	Total Ever Stuttered	Number Recovered	Percentage Recovered
Fathers	19	10	53
Mothers	12	10	83
Brothers	23	11	48
Sisters	14	5	36

found none that was compatible with the transmission pattern in the data. Direct mimicry of behavior is excluded because most stutterers had no stuttering model (Kidd et al., 1978; Kidd & Records, 1979). Both mimicry and transmission of attitudes about speech are argued against by analyses that show that stutterers occur randomly within sibships; stutterers show no differences from their nonstuttering siblings with respect to birth rank, age separation, and so forth (Gladstien et al., 1981). As mentioned earlier, we also found that one measure of severity is not related to the degree of familial concentration (Kidd et al., 1980). This finding argues against cultural transmission hypotheses which predict severity of stuttering would be positively correlated with frequency of stutterers among relatives.

As part of our effort to obtain more extensive data on nongenetic factors, we have interviewed all individuals in a few extended families that contain several stutterers and/or recovered stutterers. These data show that stutterers and their nonstuttering siblings have similar impressions of their parents, similar levels of anxiety, and so forth (Cox, 1982). The only differences found seem to result from stuttering (e.g., more problems in school for stutterers) rather than cause stuttering (e.g., onset was during preschool years). Thus, a wide range of nongenetic hypotheses are excluded by the Yale data.

SUMMARY AND FUTURE DIRECTIONS

Our analyses of these family data show that stuttering among relatives occurs in a pattern indicating vertical transmission of a susceptibility to stutter with sex-modified expression.

Several genetic hypotheses can be tested with the data available from families of stutterers. Simple genetic models can be rejected easily, but several that allow environmental interaction and sex differences are consistent with these data. Many hypotheses of nongenetic causation of stuttering cannot be formulated in a way that permits them to be tested; however, all such hypotheses that have been tested have been rejected.

Our analyses have shown several factors to be significantly associated with stuttering. (1) Significantly more males stutter than females. (2) If at least one parent ever stuttered, the familial risk is significantly increased. (3) If the proband is a female, the familial risk is also significantly increased. We have concluded that (1) an inherited genetic susceptibility, possibly necessary but certainly not sufficient, is a major factor in stuttering; and (2) females are more resistant to an inherited susceptibility to stutter (more resilient) than males.

We do not yet understand what causes stuttering, but we can more clearly state some of the questions that need to be answered: (1) What are the transmitted factors? (2) If they are genes, how many different loci are involved? (3) Can different statistical analyses yield more specific answers as to possible genetic mechanisms? (4) In what ways are females more resistant to transmitted factors of stuttering susceptibility? (5) Why do some stutterers recover and others persist? (6) Can a person's susceptibility be detected or revealed by testing? (7) Can the transmitted component of stuttering susceptibility be demonstrated as a genetic factor in a more compelling manner? We are now in the process of examining some of these questions.

One important consequence of these findings affects research aimed at identifying environmental (sociocultural) factors that *cause* stuttering. Such research should be designed to control for differences in inherited susceptibility. Similar environmental factors present for two children, one with high inherited susceptibility and one without, can result in one developing stuttering while the other continues to have fluent speech. Since this possibility is clearly plausible, special research designs are needed to identify relevant nongenetic factors.

REFERENCES

Andrews, G., & Harris, M. M. *The syndrome of stuttering.* Clinics in Developmental Med., No. 17, London: Spastics Society Medical Education and Information Unit/Heinemann, 1964.

Cavalli-Sforza, L. L., & Bodmer, W. F. *The genetics of human populations.* San Francisco: Freeman, 1971.

Cox, N. J. *A genetic study of stuttering.* Doctoral thesis in Human Genetics, Yale University, 1982.

Cox, N. J., & Kidd, K. K. Can recovery from stuttering be considered a genetically milder subtype of stuttering? *Behavior Genetics,* 1983, *13,* 129-139.

Gershon, E. S., Bunney, W. E., Leckman, J. F., Van Eedewegh, M., & DeBauche, B. A. The inheritance of affective disorders: A review of data and of hypotheses. *Behavior Genetics,* 1976, *6,* 3.

Gladstien, K., Seider, R. A., & Kidd, K. K. Analysis of sibship patterns of stutterers. *Journal of Speech and Hearing Research,* 1981, *24,* 460-462.

Gottesman, I. I. Genetic aspects of intelligent behavior. In N. Ellis (Ed.), *Handbook of mental deficiency* (pp. 253-296). New York: McGraw-Hill, 1966.

Gottesman, I. I., & Shields, J. *Schizophrenia, the epigenetic puzzle.* Cambridge: Cambridge University Press, 1982.

Gray, M. The X family: A clinical and laboratory study of "stuttering" family. *Journal of Speech Disorders,* 1940, *5,* 343-348.

Hahn, W. E., Van Ness, J., & Chaudhari, N. Overview of the molecular genetics of mouse brain. In F. O. Schmitt, S. J. Bird, & F. E. Bloom (Eds.), *Molecular genetic neuroscience* (pp. 323-334). New York: Raven Press, 1982.

Harris, H. *The principles of human biochemical genetics.* Oxford: North-Holland, 1976.

Hirsch, J. Behavior-genetic analysis and its biosocial consequences. In R. Cancro (Ed.), *Intelligence: Genetics and environmental influences* (pp. 23-29). New York: Grune & Stratton, 1971.

Johnson, W. A study of the onset and development of stuttering. In W. Johnson & R. Leutenegger (Eds.), *Stuttering in children and adults.* Minneapolis: University of Minnesota Press, 1955.

Johnson, W. *The onset of stuttering. Research findings and implications.* Minneapolis: University of Minnesota Press, 1959.

Kant, K., & Ahuja, Y. R. Inheritance of stuttering. *Acta medica auxologica,* 1970, *2,* 179-191.

Kaplan, B. B., & Finch, C. E. The sequence complexity of brain ribonucleic acids. In I. R. Brown (Ed.), *Molecular approaches to neurobiology* (pp. 71-98). New York: Academic Press, 1982.

Kay, D. W. K. The genetics of stuttering. In G. Andrews & M. M. Harris (Eds.), *The syndrome of stuttering.* London: Heinemann, 1964.

Kidd, K. K. Genetic models of stuttering. *Journal of Fluency Disorders,* 1980, *5,* 187-201.

Kidd, K. K. Recent developments in the genetics of stuttering. In C. L. Ludlow and J. A. Cooper (Ed.), *The genetic aspects of speech and language disorders.* New York: Academic Press, 1983, in press.

Kidd, K. K., Heimbuch, R. C., & Records, M. A. Vertical transmission of susceptibility to stuttering with sex-modified expression. *Proceedings of the National Academy of Sciences, USA,* 1981, *78,* 606-610.

Kidd, K. K., Kidd, J. R., & Records, M. A. The possible causes of the sex ratio in stuttering and its implication. *Journal of Fluency Disorders,* 1978, *3,* 13-23.

Kidd, K. K., Oehlert, G., Heimbuch, R. C., Records, M. A., & Webster, R. L. Familial stuttering patterns are not related to one measure of severity. *Journal of Speech and Hearing Research,* 1980, *23,* 539-545.

Kidd, K. K., & Records, M. A. Genetic methodologies for the study of speech. In X. O. Breakefield (Ed.), *Neurogenetics: Genetic approaches to the nervous system* (pp. 311-344). New York: Elsevier/North-Holland, 1979.

Kidd, K. K., & Spence, M. A. Genetic analyses of pyloric stenosis suggesting a specific maternal effect. *Journal of Medical Genetics,* 1976, *13,* 290-294.

Lenneberg, E. H. A biological perspective of language. In R. C. Oldfield & J. C. Marshall (Eds.), *Language* (pp. 32-47). Baltimore: Penguin, 1976.

Lewontin, R. C. The analysis of variance and the analysis of causes. *American Journal of Human Genetics,* 1974, *26,* 400-411.

Pauls, D. L., & Kidd, K. K. Genetics of childhood behavior disorders. In B. B. Lahey & A. E. Kazdin (Eds.), *Advances in clinical child psychology* (pp. 331-362). New York: Plenum, 1981.

Scarr, S., & Kidd, K. K. Developmental Behavior Genetics. In J. J. Campos & M. M. Haith (Eds.), *Manual of child psychology.* New York: Wiley, 1983.

Seider, R. A., Gladstien, K. L., & Kidd, K. K. Recovery and persistence of stuttering among relatives of stutterers. *Journal of Speech and Hearing Disorders,* 1983, *48,* 402-409.

Smeraldi, E., Negri, F., Heimbuch, R. C., & Kidd, K. K. Familial patterns and possible modes of inheritance of primary affective disorders. *Journal of Affective Disorders,* 1981, *3,* 785-793.

Van Riper, C. *The nature of stuttering.* Englewood Cliffs, NJ: Prentice-Hall, 1971.

Wepman, J. M. Familial incidence in stammering. *Journal of Speech Disorders,* 1939, *4,* 199-204.

Wingate, M. E. Recovery from stuttering. *Journal of Speech and Hearing Disorders,* 1964, *29,* 312-321.

Chapter 9

Stuttering as an Anticipatory Struggle Disorder

Oliver Bloodstein

A NOTE ON METHODOLOGY

In this chapter we will be reviewing a good number of research investigations that bear on the validity of the anticipatory struggle hypothesis. Some of the best evidence for the hypothesis consists of clinical observations, however, and we will not neglect these either. The use of such clinical evidence calls for a stringent appraisal of its scientific merit.

Let us first state the case against clinical observations as forcefully as we can. The use of such evidence is notorious for its limitations. It lends itself to subjectivity, distortion, and self-delusion. Clinical observations can be invoked to support almost any theory or therapy of stuttering. Objective laboratory experimentation is the way of science, and its superiority as a method of obtaining reliable knowledge is so well established that we employ any other approach at considerable peril.

In the face of such an indictment, with which almost everyone would agree, can anything be said in defense of clinical observation? Let us make an attempt. The collection, analysis, and interpretation of experimental data on stuttering are not immune to bias and error, as is shown by the frequency with which findings from different studies have appeared hopelessly conflicting. Nor is it grossly unfair to say that a good deal of the most expertly conducted laboratory research on stuttering has amounted to the unassailable verification of the self-evident or trivial. This is because the more important questions about stuttering are not always conveniently answered by laboratory studies.

This being the case, clinical observations based on the experience of many workers can be ignored only at the risk of gaps in knowledge and distortions of perspective. Who could, with absolute confidence, disagree with this judgment?

Perhaps the point to be made is that we who treat speech disorders are more like physicians than physicists with respect to the importance of clinical observation for what we do. A physicist struck by an apple while napping under a tree might be excused for overlooking the implications for celestial mechanics. But a physician cannot afford to overlook what other physicians have observed clinically about symptoms of disease. Nor can we in our profession ignore all the observable features of stuttering that have not yet been the subjects of laboratory investigation or do not lend themselves to it.

Rather than dismiss all clinical observations categorically, it would seem wiser to differentiate those that have genuine merit from those that do not. Valid clinical observations are descriptions, not inferences. "All stutterers are fluent when they sing" is not an observation. Neither is "He stuttered on 'Mississippi' because he thought he was going to." On the other hand, "Some stutterers speak fluently when they pretend to be angry" is a good example of genuine clinical observation which we cannot afford to overlook. Good clinical observations are capable of verification. The best ones are those that have been repeatedly corroborated by other workers.

In summary, we may draw two conclusions. First, we need a balance of experimental research and systematic clinical observation for the sake of the deepest possible insight into stuttering. Second, neither methodology of seeking knowledge will lead to the truth automatically. Both make severe demands on the wisdom of the seeker.

STATEMENT OF THE THEORY

The anticipatory struggle hypothesis is first and foremost a cognitive theory of stuttering. It holds that stuttering stems largely from early speech experiences which infect a child's system of beliefs with the conviction that speech is difficult. A theory in all probability as old as stuttering itself, it has been advanced in crude form by every stutterer who ever observed that he could say any word in the language except when it was important for him to say it fluently, or he thought of it as a difficult word, or was expecting to stutter. What is missing from such casual statements of the theory is any attempt to explain why a stutterer's belief that a word is difficult should make it so. If this lack is not glaringly obvious at first glance, it is perhaps only because most of us have experienced similar effects on a small scale in such activities as typing, writing, or the playing of musical instruments, to say nothing of speech itself. Nevertheless, such an explanation is required.

Wendell Johnson's writings gave wide currency to the explanation that stuttering is essentially nothing but the effort to avoid stuttering, and originates as the effort to avoid normal childhood disfluency (see Johnson, 1967). This certainly explains how a belief in the difficulty of producing speech fluently might lead to stuttering, but it is suitable only for Johnson's own distinctive form of anticipatory struggle theory, which asserts that stuttering results from parents' misdiagnoses of their children's normal speech hesitancies as stuttering.

An alternative model, which permits a much wider array of etiological possibilities, is the view that stuttering is the reflection of tension and fragmentation in speech. Whenever we are overwhelmed by the difficulty of a complex, automatic, serially ordered motor activity, we are likely, first, to initiate the activity with excessive tension, and second, to fragment the activity— that is, to break it up into manageable segments, and especially to repeat the first part of the activity until we gain the conviction to execute it as a whole. All of the surface features of stuttering, whether repetition, prolongation, hard attack on sound, or stoppage, may be viewed as manifestations of underlying tension and fragmentation in the initiation of speech units. On this assumption, it is clear that virtually any imaginable kind of speech pressure or chronic speech failure in childhood might lead to stuttering.

LEARNING VERSUS HEREDITY IN STUTTERING

At the present time we are witnessing the revival of interest in constitutional and genetic influences on stuttering, an area of research which had been neglected for many years. Now the anticipatory struggle hypothesis clearly rests on the premise that stuttering is learned behavior, so it would be well for us to address the general question of environmental influences on stuttering before going on to specific evidence in support of the hypothesis.

Several independent sources of evidence can be adduced to show that environmental influences are capable of playing a decisive role in stuttering. To begin with, there are the findings from anthropological studies by Lemert (1953), Stewart (1960), and Morgenstern (reported by Johnson, 1967) which suggest that stuttering tends to flourish in cultures that impose heavy competitive pressures for achievement and conformity. Perhaps more telling is the very marked decline in the prevalence of stuttering that has taken place in the United States during recent decades (Van Riper, 1982, p. 49). This observation, revealing how stuttering may vary from era to era, is not well documented, but the agreement on it among clinicians of long experience is difficult to ignore. Even more conclusive evidence of the influence of environment comes from studies of stuttering in identical twins. Although the concordance of stuttering in monozygotic twins is quite high, cases in which only one member of the pair stutters are relatively common (Howie, 1981; Luchsinger, 1959). The discordant cases, of course, can only be due to differences in environment. Equally conclusive are the findings of Kidd and his colleagues. These workers applied a genetic model that made it possible for them to predict with considerable accuracy the proportions of stutterers' mothers, fathers, sisters, and brothers who would prove to be stutterers (Kidd, Heimbuch, & Records, 1981). This model assumed that stuttering is the product of an interaction between genes and environmental factors. The same findings that speak for the influence of heredity, then, also underscore the power of the environment.

Since the days when speech pathology was very young, there has been a tacit assumption that we will one day discover whether stuttering is an organic or functional disorder. Perhaps what we have been learning above all from recent genetic studies of stuttering is that we have been asking a nonsensical question. The effects of heredity, environment, physical makeup, and learning are probably inextricably interwoven in most cases of stuttering, as they are in so many other human traits.

THE INFLUENCE OF BELIEFS ON STUTTERING

Both as children and adults, persistent stutterers are victimized by a proliferation of morbid beliefs. The incipient belief in the difficulty of speech that stutterers first verbalize in early childhood by saying "I can't talk" or "I can't say it" soon develops into a specific self-concept as a stutterer. This in turn gives rise eventually to the assumptions that certain words, sounds, or "letters" are difficult to say, that listeners and situations are threatening, that stutterers are helpless to talk in any other way, and that stuttering is something to be hidden or avoided at all costs. Such beliefs are familiar to virtually all who have worked clinically with stutterers. What we are considering here is the theory that these beliefs not only result from, but also cause and serve to perpetuate and maintain, stuttering.

It is self-evident that if a stutterer could forget that he was a stutterer, this whole system of beliefs would instantly vanish. For all practical purposes, then, we can reduce the anticipatory struggle hypothesis to the prediction that if a stutterer were to forget that he was a stutterer, he would have no further difficulty with his speech. On this prediction the theory stands or falls. Evidence that it is true would seem to constitute the most direct possible support for the theory.

Under ordinary conditions, to forget that one is a stutterer is a very difficult thing to do. Yet such forgetting does appear to take place in varying degrees, and the stuttering does seem to disappear as a result. The most striking examples are those relatively rare "born-again" experiences in which stutterers either emerge from a religious reawakening convinced that they will never stutter again, or so narrowly escape from a life-threatening situation that their self-concepts as stutterers recede into comparative insignificance. An example of the first is known to the author through direct personal observation and a case of the second has been described by Tawadros (1957). Other examples have been reported informally, but such cases are unfortunately not well documented.

More adequately documented is the observation that stuttering can be made to disappear temporarily by suggestion. The effects of hypnotic suggestion have been reliably reported by Moore (1946), who conducted a clinical study of hypnosis with 40 stutterers, and by many others in observations of a more general sort going back to the last century. The effect of powerful nonhypnotic suggestion is best illustrated by a multitude of reports of at least temporary recovery from stuttering due to therapies whose effects could only have derived from the stutterer's faith in the outcome. A good example is the use of tongue surgery in the 19th century (Burdin, 1940).

Also well attested are the brief intervals of fluency stutterers experience when they forget for the moment that they are stutterers because they are carried away by excitement, enthusiasm, or anger, or because they are distracted by surprise or by fear of bodily harm (Bloodstein, 1950). In the same category are such situations as acting a part in a play, assuming an unaccustomed role, impersonating someone else, or speaking in a dialect, all of which are likely to result in fluency (Bloodstein, 1950). The well-known fact that virtually any change that stutterers make in their usual speech patterns results in immediate fluency appears to be due in large measure to the same "masquerade" effect that is exemplified by the act of impersonating someone else, "putting on" a role, or the like. It is possible to suggest other factors that may contribute to certain changes in speech pattern, but the masquerade effect encompasses all of them.

Finally, it may be appropriate to mention those revealing instances in which the vagaries of English spelling induce stutterers to "forget" that words beginning with certain sounds are difficult for them to say. To cite a well-known example, stutterers who are unable to say words beginning with *f* may have little difficulty with *photo*.

We have been discussing conditions under which stutterers appear to speak fluently because they forget their self-concepts as stutterers and their belief in the difficulty of speech. Conversely, stuttering seems to increase when stutterers are made more conscious of their speech difficulty or their roles as speakers. For example, they often have great difficulty when speaking on the telephone, which reduces them to a voice. They almost always stutter when asked to repeat what they have said when the listener has failed to hear it. Outside the speech clinic their stuttering has often been observed to increase noticeably when they unexpectedly discover that the person they are speaking to is a speech pathologist.

THE RELATION OF STUTTERING TO ANTICIPATORY EVENTS

The hypothesis that stuttering results from a belief in the difficulty of speech would seem to call for the occurrence of some kind of anticipatory reaction prior to stuttering, but the question of how to identify this reaction has been a source of confusion. For Johnson, the anticipation of stuttering was defined by the ability of stutterers to indicate accurately by a signal the word on which they were about to stutter. Most of the stutterers who served as subjects in early studies of anticipation by Johnson and his colleagues were able to predict the occurrence of their stutterings with considerable accuracy (Knott, Johnson, & Webster, 1937; Milisen, 1938; Van Riper, 1936). The accuracy was not perfect, but Johnson theorized that the anticipation of stuttering could sometimes occur on a low level of consciousness. The subjects of these studies were adults. Much later, Silverman and Williams (1972) found that stuttering children were far more variable in their ability to predict the occurrence of their stutterings; about half were able to predict less than 50%.

In other research, measures of autonomic arousal just prior to the block have suggested the presence of anticipation. It has been found that blocks are often preceded by a rise in pulse rate, vasoconstriction, disturbed breathing, increased electrical skin conductance, and motor disturbances (Brutten, 1963; Ickes & Pierce, 1973; Kurshev, 1968, 1969; Tanberg, 1955; Van Riper, 1936). Again, these are evidently not universal findings. Futhermore, they appear to be indications of anxiety rather than merely anticipation of difficulty. In subjects with high levels of anxiety about stuttering, we would naturally expect anticipation of stuttering to be accompanied by physiological arousal. But the anticipatory struggle hypothesis does not require the presence of anxiety. It is sufficient that the stutterer possess a certain eccentric system of assumptions about the imagined difficulty of speech and the unusual things that must be done to overcome that difficulty.

Of more consequence for the anticipatory struggle theory is the presence of some type of preparatory activity of the speech musculature prior to stuttering. Such activity has been reported in electromyographic studies by Shrum (1967) and Guitar (1975). In addition, Peters, Love, Otto, Wood, and Benignus (1976) found changes in brain waves preceding subjects' attempts on their difficult words, whether or not they were stuttered. In a spectrographic study, Knox (1975) observed decreased rate, rise in pitch, and eccentric formant transitions on syllables spoken just prior to stuttering.

It is evident that many kinds of anticipatory events are observable in advance of stuttering. Whether any of them can be found in association with all stutterings, and whether they are to be observed in young children as well as adults, are questions to which we do not yet have the answers.

An entirely different approach to the study of anticipation was taken by Goss (1952), who systematically varied the time interval between the exposure of a word and a signal to the stutterer to say it. He found that for intervals between 2 and 10 sec, the longer the time interval the greater was the probability of stuttering. (As the interval decreased below 2 sec there was also a rise in stuttering, as a different kind of pressure apparently asserted itself.) Forte and Schlesinger (1972) observed the same effect in children. The importance of these findings is that they show stuttering to be not merely associated with but functionally dependent on anticipation.

THE ROLE OF STIMULI REPRESENTATIVE OF PAST STUTTERING

Although the anticipatory struggle hypothesis lends itself most readily to formulation in terms of attitudes and beliefs, it can also be framed in terms of observable behavior. In these terms, the theory states that stuttering in its developed form is a response to stimuli representative of past stuttering. To take a concrete example, suppose a stutterer, introducing a friend at a social gathering, blocks severely on the name "Gabriella. " If stuttering is an anticipatory struggle reaction, will he be less likely, equally likely, or more likely to stutter on the name if he has to introduce the friend again a few moments later? The answer is more likely, of course, other things being equal. Coming back to attitudes and beliefs for a moment, he will remember his recent difficulty and will be even more certain than he was before that "Gabriella" is a difficult name for him to say.

So the theory says he will be more likely to block again. What are the facts? Among stutterers and their clinicians, the prevailing impression appears to be that the prediction is correct. It was, in fact, from such experiences as the one with Gabriella that the theory probably arose in the first place. Many stutterers, as is well known, tend to have personal lists of words that cause unusual difficulty. Clinical impression points to memorable past experiences of unusual stuttering or severe social penalties for blocking on these words, as the source of the difficulty. Van Riper (1972, pp. 269, 270) has presented a series of examples from his clinical experience, such as the case of the young woman who could no longer say the word *well* after she had been harshly ridiculed for repeating it as a starting device. Incidents of this kind epitomize stuttering as an anticipatory struggle reaction.

An experimental paradigm of the tendency of stuttering to occur in response to stimuli associated with past speech failures was discovered by Johnson and Millsapps (1937). On subjects' copies of a reading passage they blotted out the words on which the subjects stuttered in successive readings. In subsequent readings the subjects were found to have stuttered to a significant degree on words adjacent to the blots. Johnson and Millsapps inferred that the blots had served as cues representative of past stutterings. This "adjacency" effect, and the interpretation Johnson and Millsapps placed on it, were confirmed in later studies (Brutten & Gray, 1961; Rappaport & Bloodstein, 1971). The effect was also found in children (Avari & Bloodstein, 1974). These demonstrations of the adjacency effect perhaps offer as much evidence of a strictly experimental kind as has yet been possible to obtain in support of the anticipatory struggle hypothesis.

EXPLANATORY POTENTIAL OF THE HYPOTHESIS

Since no theory of stuttering has yet been conclusively proved by a crucial laboratory experiment, and very possibly never will be, the validity of a theory may ultimately have to rest on how well it explains the known phenomena of the disorder and perhaps on how well it enables us to predict phenomena yet unknown. In the preceding sections of this chapter we have already touched on certain aspects of stuttering that are explained particularly well by the anticipatory struggle hypothesis. Here we would like to show that the hypothesis is consistent with all of the many conditions and factors that are known to influence the occurrence of stuttering.

If we begin with the manner in which stuttering is distributed in the speech sequence, the most fundamental fact about it is the consistency effect—the tendency of the stutterer to block on many of the same words from reading to reading of a passage. This shows that the stuttering is in part a response to stimuli in the reading passage, and is probably the best evidence we have of the role that learning plays in the distribution of stutterings.

Next in importance is the fact that the blocks tend to be distributed on different words from stutterer to stutterer (Hendel & Bloodstein, 1973). That is, factors that differ from case to case are far more powerful in determining what words are stuttered than are factors which operate for stutterers as a group. The studies do not indicate what these factors are, but clinical experience strongly suggests that stutterers' personal assumptions about the difficulty of certain words are of major importance in determining the loci of blocks.

Lastly, there are the factors that affect the distribution of blocks for stutterers as a group. These have been investigated extensively (Brown, 1937, 1938, 1945; Brown & Moren, 1942; Danzger & Halpern, 1973; Griggs & Still, 1979; Hahn, 1942a, 1942b; Johnson & Brown, 1935; Lanyon, 1968; Lanyon & Duprez, 1970; Quarrington, 1965; Quarrington, Conway, & Siegel, 1962; Schlesinger, Forte, Fried, & Melkman, 1965; Schlesinger, Melkman, & Levy, 1966; Soderberg, 1962, 1966, 1967, 1971; Taylor, 1966a, 1966b; Wingate, 1967, 1979). As a result of these studies, we know that most stutterers tend to have more difficulty on words beginning with consonants than vowels; on longer words; on content words; on words at the beginning of the sentence; on words of low frequency of occurrence in the language; on words that have high "information value" in the sense that they are difficult to guess from the preceding context; and on words in the sentence that receive the most stress. All of this is consistent with the anticipatory struggle hypothesis. Such attributes of words tend to make them seem difficult or conspicuous. These are consequently the words on which stuttering is most likely to be anticipated.

The myriad conditions under which stuttering increases and decreases in frequency are also readily explained in terms of variations in anticipatory struggle. Most of them involve changes in the amount of communicative pressure of various kinds—the pressure of communicative responsibility, of time, of motor planning of speech, of listener reactions, of concern about social approval, and of audience size. Other conditions involve suggestion, the factor of stutterers' attention to their speech and their role as speakers to which we have already alluded, states of generalized tension, and the role of cues that evoke anticipation of stuttering. The writer has discussed these conditions at length in relation to the anticipatory struggle hypothesis elsewhere (Bloodstein, 1981, pp. 238–287). In general, the conditions under which stuttering is most frequent appear to be those that are most likely to evoke anticipation of stuttering, or in which the social penalties for stuttering are severe.

We have saved for last one additional observation which must be included in any discussion of the variables to which stuttering is related, and that is the locus of stuttering within the word. Blocks occur on the first sound or syllable in over 90% of cases. Occasionally they are to be observed on accented syllables within words, but virtually never on final sounds or syllables. The absence of stuttering from the ends of words enjoys an unusual position among the phenomena of stuttering; it is one of the very few that have the status of a rule. A generalization to which there are only rare exceptions would appear to harbor some information of basic importance about stuttering. In the writer's view, it is the information that the stutterer's belief in the difficulty of speech revolves mainly around the execution of words rather than other units of speech. The stutterer who repeats or prolongs the first sound of a word is hardly having difficulty with the sound, as a moment's thought will show. What the stutterer appears to be doing is fragmenting the word—that is, uttering only the first part of it without the conviction that is necessary to say it as a whole. Note that this explanation is consistent with the factors that influence the distribution of stuttering, which are mainly attributes of words.

It is important to keep in mind that the observations we have discussed in this section are about stuttering in its developed form. When we deal with stuttering in very young children, the picture changes considerably, as we will see.

THE ETIOLOGY OF STUTTERING

We have attempted to show that a great number of facts that we know about stuttering in its fully developed form are in accord with the anticipatory struggle hypothesis. To this may be added evidence that the conditions surrounding the development of the problem in early childhood are such as to instill a belief in the difficulty of speech. The evidence takes a number of different forms.

A large proportion of young stutterers appear to have experiences of speech or language failure before they are observed to stutter. Many have a history of delayed language development (Andrews & Harris, 1964; Berry, 1938; Blood & Seider, 1981; Milisen & Johnson, 1936; Morley, 1957). As a group, they tend to score lower than nonstuttering children on tests of language skill (Kline & Starkweather, 1979; Murray & Reed, 1977; Wall, 1980; Westby, 1979). From 15 to 50% of stuttering children have been reported to have articulatory or other speech defects (Andrews & Harris, 1964; Blood & Seider, 1981; Darley, 1955; Johnson

& Associates, 1959; Kent & Williams, 1963; Morley, 1957; Schindler, 1955; Williams & Silverman, 1968).

Elsewhere the writer has presented clinical accounts of a considerable number of cases of early stuttering in which language difficulties, articulatory defects, cluttering, and other chronic failures in communication appeared to act as provocations to stuttering, particularly in an environment of speech or language pressures (Bloodstein, 1975). A clinical observation of special significance, because of the frequency with which it is corroborated by independent reports from widely scattered speech clinics, is that some children experience episodes of stuttering during periods of therapy for language disorders. Two such cases were the subject of an article by Hall (1977).

In this connection the results of a study by Merits-Patterson and Reed (1981) are well worth pondering. They studied the disfluencies of nine young children who were receiving therapy for delayed language development, nine children with delayed language who were not undergoing therapy, and nine children with normal language development. The children receiving therapy were found to have more word and part-word repetitions than the others. There was no difference between the no therapy language-delayed children and those with normal language.

In sum, there is a considerable body of evidence suggesting that the self-concept as a stutterer has its early source in a more general self-concept as a poor speaker; and that the anticipation of stuttering on specific words originally develops from a more vague and general belief in the difficulty of speech. Without question, much of this evidence is capable of interpretation in other ways. The inferences we have drawn from it, however, are corroborated by other evidence of a quite different kind.

When we examine the stuttering of preschool children, we find that it usually differs in certain respects from that of older children and adults. One of the outstanding differences is the presence of a large amount of word repetition. To be sure, word repetition is a very prominent feature of normal childhood disfluency, too, and so there has long been some confusion over the question of whether it should be defined as stuttering. The best normative data we have, however, shows it to be four times as prevalent in stutterers' as in nonstutterers' speech (Johnson & Associates, 1959, p. 210). These normative data indicate further that word and part-word repetitions form the bulk of the stuttering in 2- to 8-year-old children. In clinical experience with 2- to 4-year-old stutterers, extended repetitions of words are often the essence of the problem. To exclude it as stuttering would, therefore, only seem to create the need to invent another word for abnormal disfluency. To this writer it seems a far simpler solution to say that stuttering and certain types of normal disfluency in early childhood belong on a single continuum, an assumption for which there is considerable evidence (Bloodstein, 1975, pp. 48–56).

The large number of word repetitions in the speech of young stutterers may be telling us something of great significance. In the preceding section we alluded to the fact that repetitions of sounds or syllables obey a rule: They do not occur at the ends of words. There is a parallel rule that applies to word repetitions: With rare exceptions, they do not occur at the ends of syntactic units. Almost invariably, the repeated word is the first word of a sentence, clause, or phrase (Bloodstein, 1974; Bloodstein & Grossman, 1981). For example, we may hear "Squirrels squirrels squirrels eat dirty nuts, " but not "Squirrels eat dirty nuts nuts nuts. " What is the meaning of this rule? By the same reasoning that we applied to sound repetitions, we would have to infer that word repetitions represent a hesitancy in the initiation of syntactic units. Whereas developed stuttering is primarily a difficulty with words, the distribution of early stuttering seems to reflect a more general difficulty that centers on whole utterances or their constituent phrases.

This inference gains additional support from the verification of a prediction that flows from it. If early stuttering does not represent difficulty with words, its distribution in the speech sequence should not be influenced by the various attributes of words that influence developed stuttering, such as their length, grammatical function, and initial sound (consonant versus vowel). Findings obtained so far have tended to confirm this prediction (Bloodstein & Gantwerk, 1967; Bloodstein & Grossman, 1981; Wall, Starkweather, & Harris, 1981).

In conclusion, we infer that stuttering gives several different indications of being an anticipatory struggle reaction even in its earliest manifestations. By the end of the preschool years, however, a significant change takes place in the form of that reaction. By that time persistent stutterers have begun to acquire self-concepts as stutterers. By about age 5, children also begin to have some awareness of language (Prutting, 1979). The stage is thus set for a process of development through which stuttering eventually comes to be dominated by the anticipation of stuttering and a belief in the difficulty of words.

CLINICAL IMPLICATIONS

From a therapeutic point of view, the main lesson of the anticipatory struggle hypothesis is that the way to overcome stuttering completely and permanently is to forget that one is a stutterer. If there were a drug that could make us forget selectively some of what we know, how quickly we might eradicate stuttering, to say nothing of superstition, prejudice, delusions, irrational fears, guilt, and grief. Since we have no such remedy, the lesson of our hypothesis may not appear to have any immediate practical consequences. Yet it does serve to illuminate some fundamental facts about the outcome of all our therapies for stuttering. It explains why essentially any method of treatment seems to have the potential for producing some successes, even some long-lasting ones. It also goes far to explain the large amount of failure that seems to bedevil all therapies. It explains why even anxiety reduction, which some have regarded as a specific remedy for anticipatory struggle, has had its share of frustration. A familiar figure in such therapeutic situations has been the client who has little fear of stuttering, but still stutters because, it is our surmise, he knows he is a stutterer and remembers all of the things he has to do in order to talk.

Experience seems to teach that almost every clinical approach— whether psychotherapy, fear reduction, relaxation, a new way of talking, a new way of stuttering, or anything else—is capable of erasing a self-image as a stutterer in some cases. The key appears to be a deep and unremitting commitment to therapy. With fully developed stuttering, no casual efforts are likely to succeed.

REFERENCES

Andrews, G., & Harris, M. *The syndrome of stuttering*. London: Spastics Society Medical Education and Information Unit in association with Heinemann, 1964.

Avari, D. N., & Bloodstein, O. Adjacency and prediction in school-age stutterers. *Journal of Speech and Hearing Research*, 1974, *17*, 33–40.

Berry, M. F. Developmental history of stuttering children. *Journal of Pediatrics*, 1938, *12*, 209–217.

Blood, G. W., & Seider, R. The concomitant problems of young stutterers. *Journal of Speech and Hearing Disorders*, 1981, *46*, 31–33.

Bloodstein, O. A rating scale study of conditions under which stuttering is reduced or absent. *Journal of Speech and Hearing Disorders*, 1950, *15*, 29–36.

Bloodstein, O. The rules of early stuttering. *Journal of Speech and Hearing Disorders*, 1974, *39*, 379–394.

Bloodstein, O. Stuttering as tension and fragmentation. In J. Eisenson (Ed.), *Stuttering: A second symposium*. New York: Harper & Row, 1975.

Bloodstein, O. *A handbook on stuttering* (3rd ed.). Chicago: National Easter Seal Society, 1981.

Bloodstein, O., & Gantwerk, B. F. Grammatical function in relation to stuttering in young children. *Journal of Speech and Hearing Research*, 1967, *10*, 786–789.

Bloodstein, O., & Grossman, M. Early stutterings: Some aspects of their form and distribution. *Journal of Speech and Hearing Research*, 1981, *24*, 298–302.

Brown, S. F. The influence of grammatical function on the incidence of stuttering. *Journal of Speech Disorders*, 1937, *2*, 207–215.

Brown, S. F. Stuttering with relation to word accent and word position. *Journal of Abnormal and Social Psychology,* 1938, *33,* 112–120.

Brown, S. F. The loci of stutterings in the speech sequence. *Journal of Speech Disorders,* 1945, *10,* 181–192.

Brown, S. F., & Moren, A. The frequency of stuttering in relation to word length during oral reading. *Journal of Speech Disorders,* 1942, *7,* 153–159.

Brutten, E. J. Palmar sweat investigation of disfluency and expectancy adaptation. *Journal of Speech and Hearing Research,* 1963, *6,* 40–48.

Brutten, E. J., & Gray, B. B. Effect of word cue removal on adaptation and adjacency: A clinical paradigm. *Journal of Speech and Hearing Disorders,* 1961, *26,* 385–389.

Burdin, G. The surgical treatment of stammering 1840–1842. *Journal of Speech Disorders,* 1940, *5,* 43–64.

Danzger, M., & Halpern, H. Relation of stuttering to word abstraction, part of speech, word length, and word frequency. *Perceptual and Motor Skills,* 1973, *37,* 959–962.

Darley, F. L. The relationship of parental attitudes and adjustments to the development of stuttering. In W. Johnson (Ed.), *Stuttering in children and adults.* Minneapolis: University of Minnesota Press, 1955.

Forte, M., & Schlesinger, I. M. Stuttering as a function of time of expectation. *Journal of Communication Disorders,* 1972, *5,* 347–358.

Goss, A. E. Stuttering behavior and anxiety theory: I. Stuttering behavior and anxiety as a function of the duration of stimulus words. *Journal of Abnormal and Social Psychology,* 1952, *47,* 38–50.

Griggs, S., & Still, A. W. An analysis of individual differences in words stuttered. *Journal of Speech and Hearing Research,* 1979, *22,* 572–580.

Guitar, B. Reduction of stuttering frequency using analog electromyographic feedback. *Journal of Speech and Hearing Research,* 1975, *18,* 672–685.

Hahn, E. F. A study of the relationship between stuttering occurrence and grammatical factors in oral reading. *Journal of Speech Disorders,* 1942, *7,* 329–335. (a)

Hahn, E. F. A study of the relationship between stuttering occurrence and phonetic factors in oral reading. *Journal of Speech Disorders,* 1942, *7,* 143–151. (b)

Hall, P. K. The occurrence of disfluencies in language-disordered school-age children. *Journal of Speech and Hearing Disorders,* 1977, *42,* 364–369.

Hendel, D., & Bloodstein, O. Consistency in relation to inter-subject congruity in the loci of stutterings. *Journal of Communication Disorders,* 1973, *6,* 37–43.

Howie, P. M. Concordance for stuttering in monozygotic and dizygotic twin pairs. *Journal of Speech and Hearing Research,* 1981, *24,* 317–321.

Ickes, W. K., & Pierce, S. The stuttering moment: A plethysmographic study. *Journal of Communication Disorders,* 1973, *6,* 155–164.

Johnson, W. Stuttering. In W. Johnson, S. F. Brown, J. F. Curtis, C. W. Edney, & J. Keaster (Eds.), *Speech handicapped school children* (3rd ed.). New York: Harper & Row, 1967.

Johnson, W., & Associates. *The onset of stuttering.* Minneapolis: University of Minnesota Press, 1959.

Johnson, W., & Brown, S. F. Stuttering in relation to various speech sounds. *Quarterly Journal of Speech,* 1935, *21,* 481–496.

Johnson, W., & Millsapps, L. S. Studies in the psychology of stuttering: VI. The role of cues representative of stuttering moments during oral reading. *Journal of Speech Disorders,* 1937, *2,* 101–104.

Kent, L. R., & Williams, D. E. Alleged former stutterers in grade two. *Asha,* 1963, *5,* 772.

Kidd, K. K., Heimbuch, R. C., & Records, M. A. Vertical transmission of susceptibility to stuttering with sex-modified expression. *Proceedings of the National Academy of Sciences*, 1981, *78*, 606–610.

Kline, M. L., & Starkweather, C. W. Receptive and expressive language performance in young stutterers. *Asha*, 1979, *21*, 797.

Knott, J. R., Johnson, W., & Webster, M. J. Studies in the psychology of stuttering: II. A quantitative evaluation of expectation of stuttering in relation to the occurrence of stuttering. *Journal of Speech Disorders*, 1937, *2*, 20–22.

Knox, J. A. *Acoustic analysis of stuttering behavior within the context of fluent speech.* Unpublished PhD dissertation, University of Iowa, 1975.

Kurshev, V. A. Study of nonspeech respiration in stutterers. *Zhurnal Nevropatologii i Psikhiatrii*, 1968, *68*, 1840–1841.

Kurshev, V. A. Unconscious reactions in stutterers. *Zhurnal Nevropatologii i Psikhiatrii*, 1969, *69*, 1075–1077.

Lanyon, R. I. Some characteristics of nonfluency in normal speakers and stutterers. *Journal of Abnormal Psychology*, 1968, *73*, 550–555.

Lanyon, R. I., & Duprez, D. A. Nonfluency, information, and word length. *Journal of Abnormal Psychology*, 1970, *76*, 93–97.

Lemert, E. M. Some Indians who stutter. *Journal of Speech and Hearing Disorders*, 1953, *18*, 168–174.

Luchsinger, R. Die Vererbung von Sprach und Stimmstoerungen. *Folia Phoniatrica*, 1959, *11*, 7–64.

Merits-Patterson, R., & Reed, C. G. Disfluencies in the speech of language-delayed children. *Journal of Speech and Hearing Research*, 1981, *24*, 55–58.

Milisen, R. Frequency of stuttering with anticipation of stuttering controlled. *Journal of Speech Disorders*, 1938, *3*, 207–214.

Milisen, R., & Johnson, W. A comparative study of stutterers, former stutterers and normal speakers whose handedness has been changed. *Archives of Speech*, 1936, *1*, 61–86.

Moore, W. E. Hypnosis in a system of therapy for stutterers. *Journal of Speech Disorders*, 1946, *11*, 117–122.

Morley, M. E. *The development and disorders of speech in childhood.* Edinburgh: Livingstone, 1957.

Murray, H. L., & Reed, C. G. Language abilities of preschool stuttering children. *Journal of Fluency Disorders*, 1977, *2*, 171–176.

Peters, R. W., Love, L., Otto, D., Wood, T., & Benignus, V. Cerebral processing of speech and non-speech signals by stutterers. In *Proceedings of the XVI International Congress of Logopedics and Phoniatrics*. Basel: Karger, 1976.

Prutting, C. A. Process\prä̌\, ses\n: The action of moving forward progressively from one point to another on the way to completion. *Journal of Speech and Hearing Disorders*, 1979, *44*, 3–30.

Quarrington, B. Stuttering as a function of the information value and sentence position of words. *Journal of Abnormal Psychology*, 1965, *70*, 221–224.

Quarrington, B., Conway, J., & Siegel, N. An experimental study of some properties of stuttered words. *Journal of Speech and Hearing Research*, 1962, *5*, 387–394.

Rappaport, B., & Bloodstein, O. The role of random blackout cues in the distribution of moments of stuttering. *Journal of Speech and Hearing Research*, 1971, *14*, 874–879.

Schindler, M. D. A study of educational adjustments of stuttering and nonstuttering children. In W. Johnson (Ed.), *Stuttering in children and adults.* Minneapolis: University of Minnesota Press, 1955.

Schlesinger, I. M., Forte, M., Fried, B., & Melkman, R. Stuttering, information load, and response strength. *Journal of Speech and Hearing Disorders,* 1965, *30,* 32-36.

Schlesinger, I. M., Melkman, R., & Levy, R. Word length and frequency as determinants of stuttering. *Psychonomic Science,* 1966, *6,* 255-256.

Shrum, W. *A study of speaking behavior of stutterers and nonstutterers by means of multichannel electromyography.* Unpublished PhD dissertation, University of Iowa, 1967.

Silverman, F. H., & Williams, D. E. Prediction of stuttering by school-age stutterers. *Journal of Speech and Hearing Research,* 1972, *15,* 189-193.

Soderberg, G. A. Phonetic influences upon stuttering. *Journal of Speech and Hearing Research,* 1962, *5,* 315-320.

Soderberg, G. A. The relations of stuttering to word length and word frequency. *Journal of Speech and Hearing Research,* 1966, *9,* 584-589.

Soderberg, G. A. Linguistic factors in stuttering. *Journal of Speech and Hearing Research,* 1967, *10,* 801-810.

Soderberg, G. A. Relations of word information and word length to stuttering disfluencies. *Journal of Communication Disorders,* 1971, *4,* 9-14.

Stewart, J. L. The problem of stuttering in certain North American Indian societies. *Journal of Speech and Hearing Disorders,* 1960, Monograph Supplement 6.

Tanberg, M. C. A study of the role of inhibition in the moment of stuttering. In W. Johnson (Ed.), *Stuttering in children and adults,* Minneapolis; University of Minnesota Press, 1955.

Tawadros, S. M. An experiment in the group psychotherapy of stutterers. *International Journal of Sociometry and Sociatry,* 1957, *1,* 181-189.

Taylor, I. K. The properties of stuttered words. *Journal of Verbal Learning and Verbal Behavior,* 1966, *5,* 112-118. (a)

Taylor, I. K. What words are stuttered? *Psychological Bulletin,* 1966, *65,* 233-242. (b)

Van Riper, C. Study of the thoracic breathing of stutterers during expectancy and occurrence of stuttering spasm. *Journal of Speech Disorders,* 1936, *1,* 61-72.

Van Riper, C. *Speech correction: Principles and methods* (5th ed.). Englewood Cliff, NJ: Prentice-Hall, 1972.

Van Riper, C. *The nature of stuttering* (2nd ed.). Englewood Cliffs, NJ: Prentice-Hall, 1982.

Wall, M. J. A comparison of syntax in young stutterers and nonstutterers. *Journal of Fluency Disorders,* 1980, *5,* 345-352.

Wall, M. J., Starkweather, C. W., & Harris, K. S. The influence of voicing adjustments on the location of stuttering in the spontaneous speech of young child stutterers. *Journal of Fluency Disorders,* 1981, *6,* 299-310.

Westby, C. E. Language performance of stuttering and nonstuttering children. *Journal of Communication Disorders,* 1979, *12,* 133-145.

Williams, D. E., & Silverman, F. H. Note concerning articulation of school-age stutterers. *Perceptual and Motor Skills,* 1968, *27,* 713-714.

Wingate, M. E. Stuttering and word length. *Journal of Speech and Hearing Research,* 1967, *10,* 146-152.

Wingate, M. E. The first three words. *Journal of Speech and Hearing Research,* 1979, *22,* 604-612.

Chapter 10

Stuttering as an Operant Disorder

Janis M. Costello* and
Roger J. Ingham

The nature of stuttering has been described from varying viewpoints (e.g., Bloodstein, 1981), some of which have relied on principles of learning (e.g., Bloodstein, 1972; Brutten, 1975; Johnson, 1959; Sheehan, 1975; Wischner, 1950). Among these, the most well developed and empirically based expositions have addressed the proposition that stuttering may be an operant disorder, hence the concentration of this chapter solely on that corner of learning-based frames of reference. It is the purpose of this chapter to review the research relevant to this proposition and to update and expand upon previous writings on this topic (e.g., Bloodstein, 1981; Costello, 1980; Hegde, 1984; Ingham, 1975, 1984 chap. 9; Ingham & Andrews, 1973b; Martin & Ingham, 1973; Ryan, 1974, 1979; Shames, 1975). In so doing, we shall relate this research to the principles of operant conditioning in order to determine whether stuttering can be regarded as operant behavior.

OPERANT METHODOLOGY AND STUTTERING

The empirically established principles of operant conditioning stem from the discovery that different types of functional relationships exist between observable behaviors and environmental events. Operant behaviors are those responses, or classes of responses, that are controlled

*This chapter was prepared while Janis Costello was a Foundation Fellow at the Cumberland College of Health Sciences, Sydney, Australia.

One look at our reference list indicates why Richard Martin was originally asked to prepare this chapter. Unfortunately, he was unable to do so. We hope that our contribution does justice to the topic that he is so eminently qualified to address, and we dedicate this chapter to him with our thanks for his influence on our professional lives.

TABLE 10-1. The effects on operant behavior of response contingent withdrawal and presentation of positive and negative stimuli.

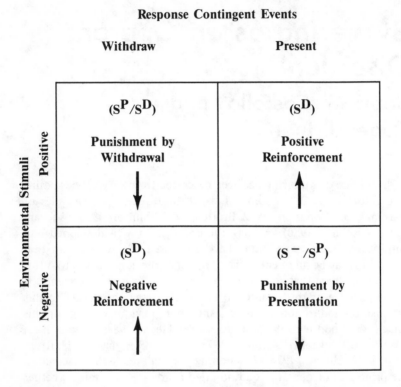

Response Contingent Events

	Withdraw	Present
Positive	(S^P/S^D) Punishment by Withdrawal ↓	(S^D) Positive Reinforcement ↑
Negative	(S^D) Negative Reinforcement ↑	(S^-/S^P) Punishment by Presentation ↓

Environmental Stimuli

NOTE:

Arrows indicate increases or decreases in response frequency occasioned by each procedure. The letter *S* with superscript indicates the labels of classes of antecedent stimuli that are associated with each procedure and act as cues to the subject, also exerting control over response rates.

(changed in frequency or form) by their consequences, that is, by environmental events that follow their occurrence. Table 10-1 illustrates the principles of operant conditioning by showing the various possible response contingent arrangements of stimuli that identify operant behaviors. (Operant principles and within-subject experimental designs are described in more detail in Brookshire [1967b], Costello [1982], Hersen and Barlow [1976], Holland [1967], Holland and Skinner [1961],

Honig [1966], Kazdin [1978], McReynolds [1970], McReynolds & Kearns [1983], and Miller [1982]). Table 10-1 indicates that operant behaviors can be increased and decreased by response contingent manipulation (withdrawal or presentation) of stimuli that are functionally positive or negative *for the particular subject*. In experimental terms, *response contingent* (RC) means that presentation or withdrawal of a stimulus is dependent upon the occurrence of the behavior of interest. Operant behaviors are also reduced in frequency of occurrence by extinction, that is, by not delivering the consequent stimuli that maintain a response. It is also possible for antecedent events, stimuli present during the reinforcement, punishment, or extinction of a behavior, to acquire properties that positively or negatively influence the occurrence of that behavior in the future. Through association with positive reinforcement for a given behavior, a particular stimulus, referred to as a discriminative stimulus (S^D or S^+), may become able to evoke that behavior. Stimuli present during extinction (S^Δ's) or punishment (S^-'s or S^P's) of a given response may signify a low probability of reinforcement or the likelihood of punishment and may thereby reduce rates of responding by their presence. Throughout the remainder of this chapter, published research using stuttering as the dependent variable is examined in the context of each of these definitions of operant behavior.

Punishment by contingent withdrawal

Although positive reinforcement is probably most commonly identified with operant conditioning, the punishment principle has been studied much more extensively in regard to stuttering. And the most thoroughly investigated punishment procedure has been *time-out from positive reinforcement*. The first reported examination of the effects of this procedure was conducted by Haroldson, Martin, and Starr (1968). Based on the assumption that talking is self-reinforcing, four male adult stutterers were individually studied in fifteen 1-hour sessions. In the first two sessions each subject spoke spontaneously during 60-min baserate (A condition) sessions. During the first 40 min of Sessions 3 through 7, the experimenter illuminated a red light for 10 sec after each "moment of stuttering" (B condition). Subjects were instructed beforehand to stop talking when the red light was on. During the last 20 min of these five sessions, the time-out (TO) contingency was withheld while subjects continued to talk (A condition). These alternating periods of baseline and "treatment" tested whether stuttering frequency was consistently modified by the TO condition (an ABAB design). During Sessions 8 through 13 the TO contingency was in effect for the entire session, followed by the repetition of baseline conditions during the last two sessions (14 and 15). The resulting data confirmed the reinforcing properties of talking for these subjects, because the RC 10-sec removal of the opportunity to talk produced a reliable and substantial (at least 88%) reduction in each subject's percentage of words stuttered.

Some variations on the Haroldson et al. (1968) procedure were investigated in subsequent studies. Martin and Berndt (1970) replicated the procedure on a 12-year-old male subject whose stuttering decreased essentially to zero and increased only slightly when TO contingencies were withdrawn. Later, Martin, Kuhl, and Haroldson (1972) used the procedure with even younger stutterers. In this ground-breaking study, two preschool children separately talked with a puppet who "turned off" whenever they stuttered. Not only did their stuttering essentially disappear within the clinic setting and remain at zero when the contingencies were removed, but this improvement generalized to the children's natural environment (measured covertly) and was maintained a year later. Martin and Haroldson (1971) also experimented with peer-presented TO while pairs of adult stuttering subjects talked together in dyads. TO was not effective in this situation, probably because peers presented the TO signal to one another for less than 2% of their stutterings. When the experimenter took over TO presentation, the now-familiar effects of TO occurred immediately for all four subjects. Egolf, Shames, and Seltzer (1971) also experimented with the use of TO during conversational interactions. In their experiment, 10 adults engaged in normal group conversation except that, during the treatment condition, each subject was allowed to talk only until a moment of stuttering occurred, at which time the speaking turn passed to another member of the group. These contingencies produced a 73% mean increase in the number of words spoken per turn and reduced stuttering substantially for 8 of the 10 subjects. Costello (1975) also reported the clinical utility of TO contingencies employed in within-session ABA conditions to establish and maintain clinically significantly reduced stuttering rates for three young adult male clients.

In a treatment comparison study, Martin and Haroldson (1969) compared a brief exposure to TO treatment (eight sessions) to a like amount of "information-attitude therapy" (1969, p. 115) for two groups of 10 adult stutterers. Stuttering, once again, was reliably reduced for the TO subjects, but was unchanged for the other subjects. In a more exacting comparison study, Martin and Haroldson (1979) assessed the differential effects of five procedures commonly reported to reduce stuttering (TO, noise, DAF, wrong, metronome). Not only did TO produce the greatest reduction in stuttering (a 76% reduction from a pretreatment mean of 11.55% words stuttered [%WS] to 2.73% WS), but it was also effective, to some degree, for all 20 subjects. In yet another variation, Martin and Haroldson (1982) compared the effects of experimenter-administered and self-administered TO contingencies and found them equally effective in reducing stuttering; however, self-administered TO appeared to have more generalized effects, since low stuttering rates continued, even during a telephone talking task that was not used in treatment.

One study has assessed the effect of response cost, the contingent withdrawal of a previously awarded positive reinforcer. Halvorson (1971) awarded three adult male stutterers a given number of points on a counter at the beginning of treatment sessions, and then removed one point each time a subject stuttered. For one subject each point was also worth 1¢. Halvorson's data indicate that response cost was a reliably effective punisher.

It would seem, then, that punishment by contingent withdrawal is a remarkably consistent and effective method of reducing stuttering frequency (and, evidently, at no cost to word output). Indeed, the pervasive effectiveness of this contingency has prompted investigations into the nature of the interaction between TO and stuttering. The research of James (1976, 1981c; James & Ingham, 1974) has been largely concerned with this issue. In one experiment James (1976) studied the effects of differing lengths (or assumed intensities) of TO periods. Five groups of nine adult stutterers participated in one session wherein each subject spoke in monologue for a 10-min baseline followed by a 20-min TO treatment condition (with time spent in TO excluded). During treatment each of the experimental groups received TO of differing lengths (1, 5, 10, or 30 sec), while a control group received no TO. As expected, the control group's percent syllables stuttered (%SS) and syllables spoken per minute (SPM) scores did not change appreciably from baseline to treatment, but all TO groups significantly reduced stuttering, with no differences according to TO duration (and no systematic changes in speaking rate). Only 2 of the 36 TO subjects failed to decrease their frequency of stuttering.

In order to appreciate the implications of James' (1976) findings, it should first be recognized that TO is a complex stimulus, composed of at least two dimensions: (1) interruption of speaking and (2) an imposed period of silence. The first can be viewed as *removal of positive reinforcement,* while the second may involve the *presentation of an aversive stimulus.* It is not always clear which is the principal component during the operation of punishment by TO (Leitenberg, 1965). Some research has demonstrated that the duration of TO may be the significant component that influences performance (Ferster & Appel, 1961). Since this was not the case in James' study, these data could be interpreted to mean that *removal* of the opportunity to continue talking (common to all TO conditions in this study), rather than *presentation* of a period of silence, may be the critical variable involved in the TO effect on stuttering.[1]

Another factor which may contribute to the TO effect is an inter-action between TO and subjects' expectancies of a beneficial effect. James and Ingham (1974) studied this factor with 14 male adult stutterers using an ABAB′ or AB′AB experimental design. In the A condition subjects spoke in monologue for 15 min. The B condition, during which a 10-sec TO was presented following each moment of stuttering, was preceded with a placebo tranquilizer and a rather elaborate set of expla-nations designed to lead subjects to expect that TO would reduce stuttering. The B′ condition also involved a 10-sec TO stimulus, but this time minus the "tranquilizer" and accompanied by an explanation calculated to make subjects believe that TO would not modify their stuttering. Subjects' responses to a postexperiment questionnaire indi-cated that 13 of the 14 subjects clearly acquired the desired expectations. In spite of it all, however, both the B and B′ conditions significantly reduced stuttering frequency and to an approximately equivalent extent. Therefore, it was clear that TO's response decelerating capacities were not due to subjects' expectations.

In relation to the previously raised questions regarding the way in which TO works to produce stuttering reductions, James and Ingham (1976) were able to contribute further information from their question-naire data. They asked the same question Adams and Popelka (1971) had asked of their subjects following subjects' exposure to effective TO contingencies: "What were your personal reactions, if any, to the periods of silence you had to observe if you stuttered?" (James & Ingham, 1974, p. 90). In the Adams and Popelka study, six of eight subjects reported that TO allowed them to relax, and only one subject clearly indicated that TO had aversive properties in that it signaled "failure and dis-approval" (Adams & Popelka, 1971, p. 338). For James and Ingham's

---

[1] However, careful inspection of James' data (see p. 210) indicates a tendency for the 30-sec TO period to produce a greater reduction in stuttering than that produced by the shorter TO durations. One wonders whether more subjects, different selected increments in TO durations, longer TO durations, or longer experimental sessions might have shown a relationship between length of TO and amounts of stuttering reduction and thus offered support for the functional role of an aversive component of the TO contingency.

subjects, however, 6 of 14 reacted to TO as an aversive stimulus, while 5 found it more neutral, noting that it gave them "time to think" (p. 92). The aggregate information from both studies suggests that different aspects of TO might be salient for different subjects. This intrepretation may partially explain TO's ameliorative effects across so many subjects (159 subjects across the 14 studies described herein).

One further study conducted by James (1981c) was directed toward, among other things, evaluating the effects of contingent and noncontingent presentation of TO. In this part of the study, two groups of nine adult stutterers spoke in AB conditions within one session. For one group, the baseline condition was followed by the typical RC presentation of a 10-sec period of TO. For the other group, noncontingent TO periods were presented randomly. All contingent TO subjects reduced stuttering (average 46%), while only four non-RC subjects produced very small, possibly random, reductions in stuttering. Only the change for the RC group was significant ($p < .01$), which indicates that the contingency arrangement is critical to the TO effect and militates against the argument that TO (or other response contingent stimuli) gains its effects through distraction (Biggs & Sheehan, 1969).[2] Further evidence in this regard is offered by Ingham and Andrews (1973a). They provided token reinforcement for 12 subjects on the basis of reductions in the response class, percent syllables stuttered. In an ABAB design, tokens were presented noncontingently during A conditions; that is, subjects were given tokens simply for speaking a required number of syllables. This was altered with B conditions of RC token reinforcement wherein 10% or greater decreases in %SS were reinforced by tokens and 10% or greater increases in %SS were punished by the loss of tokens. The group data clearly illustrated the functional role played by RC, in contrast to non-RC, tokens; and later analyses of the data for individual subjects (Ingham, 1975) indicated the tokens to be effective consequences for 9 of the 12 subjects.

In summary, there now exists substantial evidence that stuttering is reduced by the contingent withdrawal of (positive) stimulation, although the precise way in which TO operates has yet to be fully explored. The fact is, however, that stuttering alters under both time-out and response

---

[2] Martin and Ingham (1973) report a similar unpublished study by Martin and Haroldson on two adult stuttering subjects wherein noncontingent and contingent TO were presented, in that order, to each subject during monologue talking. Results were consistent with those of James.

cost procedures in much the same fashion as other operant behaviors (Azrin & Holz, 1966).

Punishment by contingent presentation

The most controversial punishment of stuttering studies involve RC presentation of presumably aversive stimuli. This research was largely prompted by early viewpoints about the etiological effects of aversive stimuli on stuttering (see Siegel, 1970). Following the lead of relevant animal and human experiments, early studies investigated the effects of stuttering-contingent presentation of such unconditioned aversive stimuli as loud noise and shock.

Flanagan, Goldiamond, and Azrin (1958) were the first to investigate stuttering as an operant behavior.[3] In the "aversive period" of their ABA design, they presented bursts of loud noise (105 dB, 6000 Hz) contingent upon moments of stuttering. This procedure produced overall reductions (from the end of baseline to the end of treatment) approximating 31, 43, and 61% for their three adult subjects, and stuttering was virtually eliminated in the laboratory for one subject. Biggs and Sheehan (1969) endeavored to replicate these findings with six male adult stutterers (concurrently enrolled in treatment with the experimenter). In all three experimental conditions, subjects continually reread a passage for the duration of the baseline, 20-min experimental, and 20-min extinction conditions (ABA design). In the aversive condition (punishment), a loud noise (108 dB, 4000 Hz) was presented contingent upon every moment of stuttering. In the other two experimental conditions, noise was presented either in a negative reinforcement procedure or randomly. Each subject experienced all conditions. While the results indicated that stuttering decreased systematically from reading to reading in the aversive condition, this was true also for the other two conditions. Because all three conditions produced a similar effect, the punishment findings of Flanagan et al. were not replicated. However, the data of Biggs and Sheehan do not offer a significant challenge to those findings either, since experimental control of stuttering was not demonstrated in any of the conditions (decreases in stuttering did not reverse as would be expected with the removal of the independent variable in final extinction conditions).

Martin and Siegel (1966a) reported the first investigation of the effects of contingently presented shock on various stuttering behaviors. In care-

---

[3] Three early studies that demonstrated somewhat variable stuttering reductions (Fahmy, 1950; Sheehan, 1951; Wingate, 1959) could be interpreted as examples of combined TO and punishment by contingent presentation, but were not intended as such by their authors.

fully controlled within-subject experimental designs with three adult stutterers, they showed that either specific stuttering behaviors or "moments of stuttering" could be substantially reduced during RC shock conditions. Their results were impressive and unambiguous. But in a much later study with five adult stutterers, Martin and colleagues (Martin, St. Louis, Haroldson, & Hasbrouck, 1975) reported much less impressive and somewhat ambiguous results from a comparison between punishment and negative reinforcement using shock. Their experimental design may have been limited by the absence of replicated conditions, but the data showed that RC shock produced clear reductions in stuttering for only two of five subjects.

Other ambiguous results have emerged from group studies on the effects of RC shock. Daly and Cooper (1967) found that shock presented following or during every moment of stuttering did not produce a significantly greater decrement in stuttering frequency across five readings of a passage than a nonshock control condition, but the competition between adaptation and response-contingent stimulation for the reduction of stuttering may have seriously confounded this study (and too many others). Williams and R. B. Martin (1974), however, were able to demonstrate a significant ($p < .01$) punishment effect when stuttering reduction for 12 adults during adaptation readings, in the absence of shock, was compared to readings in which shock was presented either immediately following each moment of stuttering or as a delayed contingency (at the end of each sentence).

More contradictory data are presented for oral reading of five adult subjects by Hegde (1971) and for four adults by Janssen and Brutten (1973). These authors reported that "stuttering" (Hegde, 1971) and oral prolongations (Janssen & Brutten, 1973) not only did not reduce, but increased in some cases, under conditions of RC shock. But the credibility of these studies is problematic. For example, Hegde's data are not accompanied by reliability measures and only report number of stuttered words in shock and nonshock conditions, independent of the number of words read in each condition. Janssen and Brutten's findings are presented in difficult-to-read cumulative records and rely on baseline conditions that did not always allow behavior to stabilize before punishment was introduced. Further, some of the reliability coefficients reported were as low as .53.

Generally, RC studies using unconditioned aversive stimuli have shown somewhat ambiguous but basically supportive findings regarding the predicted effects of punishment on stuttering, especially considering the absence of carefully quantified and undoubtedly varying stimulus intensities among the shock studies. Further clarification of these issues is unlikely in view of present day restraints on the use of these kinds of stimuli with human subjects and the evidence that many other stimuli reliably modify stuttering in RC conditions.

Myriads of other presumably aversive stimuli have been presented as consequences for stuttering in experimental studies. Goldiamond (1962; 1965) presented brief periods of delayed auditory feedback (DAF) contingent upon the stutterings of three adults and found this stimulus to reliably reduce stuttering. Quist and Martin (1967), in a within-subject ABA design with three adults, showed that RC presentation of tape-recorded "wrong" also produced reliable reductions in moments of stuttering as well as for specific stuttering behaviors. Martin and Haroldson (1979) included the same stimulus in a study that compared five different treatments known to reduce stuttering frequency (described previously). Contingent *wrong* produced an average 60% reduction in stuttering and was an effective punisher for 60% of the 20 subjects, thus suggesting it to be a mild and somewhat inconsistent punishing stimulus.

Brutten (1980) also applied RC *wrong*, to prolongations only, and reported that they increased significantly in the "B" condition of one 54-minute session; however, such prolongations also displayed ABA increases in the four control sessions as well, although not to a statistically significant level.[4] Brutten suggests that different topographies of stuttering behave differently under punishment contingencies so that findings such as those reported in the preceding review may be attributed to reductions of only some forms of stuttering. The demonstration by Costello and Hurst (1981) that different topographies of stuttering covary in a response class relationship refutes Brutten's claim.

A different verbal RC stimulus was used by Reed and Godden (1977), whose subjects were two preschool children (male, age 5;10; female, age 2;9). Their stuttering was effectively eliminated during conversation with an experimenter by RC presentations of "slow down, " but it is debatable whether this result was due to punishment or instruction ("slow down" acting as an S^D), since the speech rate measures reported were not sufficiently sensitive to assess this possibility. In short, stuttering may have diminished because subjects spoke more slowly or because the verbal stimulus punished stuttering, or both.

One further RC study utilized moderately loud noise stimuli. Murray (1969) investigated the function of white noise masking in five condi-

---

[4] These within-subject data are not appropriately analyzed by the selected Wilcoxon-T test because it assumes "that sampling is random and pairs are independent" (Marascuilo & McSweeney, 1977, p. 334).

tions during the reading of 300-word passages by 30 adult stutterers, each subject reading in each condition. The frequency of stuttering during a control reading was compared with stuttering when masking was continuous, when 1-sec bursts of masking noise were presented randomly, and when RC 1-sec bursts were activated by the subject in one condition and by the experimenter in another. The latter two conditions produced stuttering frequencies that were similar to one another and that were lower than the control condition, but they were not significantly lower. In fact, they produced the least reduction in stuttering of any of the experimental conditions. Furthermore, randomly presented noise bursts produced a group mean that was lower than that of either of these RC conditions, a finding reported in no other study utilizing random stimulus presentations. The largest decrease in stuttering occurred under the continuous masking condition, which apparently preceded both the random and the RC conditions for all subjects. There are a number of factors in Murray's study that might explain these unexpected results for RC noise. These factors include the unreported accuracy with which RC stimuli were applied, the brevity of RC conditions, and the order of condition presentations. If the conditions occurred in a fixed sequence, then it is possible that the results may be peculiar to the sequence of masking and random stimulation conditions that preceded the RC conditions in this study. Another study that also appears to contain an order effect was reported by Lanyon and Barocas (1973). In Experiment II, experimenter-presented random signals were shown to produce insignificant increases in stuttering frequency (for a single subject) until they were paired with stimuli known to produce decreases in stuttering frequency, after which their random presentation produced a significant ($p < .05$) stuttering decrease, as though they had become S^- stimuli.

Another view of "punishment" effects. The literature reporting the stuttering-contingent presentation of a wide variety of assumedly aversive stimuli has been relatively consistent in demonstrating reduction of stuttering under those conditions. The findings have been so frequent, and the stimuli of such varying nature, that some writers have been led to speculate on the possibility that essentially *any* stimulus presented immediately contingent upon stuttering would produce its decrease. Two studies tested this supposition. Cooper, Cady, and Robbins (1970) investigated the effects of assumed positive, negative, and neutral RC verbal stimuli (*wrong, right,* and *tree*) on the stutterings and disfluencies of two groups of 14 adult stutterers and nonstutterers. Daly and Kimbarow (1978) replicated this study with two groups of 18 child stutterers and nonstutterers matched for age (8–18), sex, and grade. In both studies every subject participated in three experimental conditions, each requiring one session of reading under ABA conditions. During "A" conditions, no contingencies were presented. During "B" conditions, one of the three verbal stimuli was presented contingent upon every stuttering or disfluency. The data from both studies were consistent for the stutterers: Stutterings were significantly reduced under all "B" conditions, although the absence of data on word output is problematic. On the basis of these data, Cooper et al. suggest that it is possible that past researchers "simply have called the speaker's attention to the disfluencies. Perhaps the conceptualization that 'stimulus–response learning' has occurred when the speaker's disfluencies decrease after the introduction of a disfluency contingent response has been more confusing than helpful" (p. 243). And Daly and Kimbarow further speculate that "the operant model seems insufficient to explain such stuttering reductions at this time" (p. 596).

Not surprisingly, these studies generated a spirited exchange among researchers in the area (Bloodstein, 1979; Daly & Kimbarow, 1979a, 1979b; Hegde, 1979; Wingate, 1980). Hegde (1979) claimed that the results were simply consistent with stuttering behaving as an operant:

> Results obtained by Daly and Kimbarow clearly show that the three verbal stimuli *right, wrong,* and *tree* acted as punishers for disfluencies....The conclusion is inescapable that disfluencies of stuttering children were clearly affected by their consequent stimuli and therefore they belong to the operant response class. (p. 667)

Although the relative merits of *a priori* and *a posteriori* definitions of stimuli are arguable (Starkweather, 1974), it is clearly puzzling when a stimulus that appears to have no inherent valence (*tree*), or is usually a positive reinforcer for other behaviors (*right*), suddenly changes valence and acts as a punisher. Is there a plausible operant-based explanation of these findings? One good place to look is in the writings and research of Siegel. Based primarily upon his studies of the control of disfluencies of nonstuttering subjects (Siegel & Martin 1965a, 1965b, 1966, 1967, 1968; Martin & Siegel, 1969), Siegel (1970) posed a "highlighting hypothesis":

> The unique feature of disfluencies appears to be that virtually any event that highlights or brings these responses to the speaker's attention will cause their reduction. (p. 689)

> It may be that disfluencies of normal adult speakers are potential "carriers of their own punishment," such that increasing the subject's attention to the response evokes the punishing property. (p. 691)

If this characterization of disfluencies extends to stutterings, then perhaps the view of stuttering as operant behavior can be supported.

It is conceivable that moments of stuttering, and their attendant tactile, proprioceptive, and auditory feedback, could acquire negative properties via classical conditioning (Pavlov, 1927) through pairings with varieties of negative environmental events purported to surround occasions of stuttering. Siegel (1970) suggests (p. 693–694) that such response-produced punishers may be only mild conditioned aversive stimuli that might not be activated on all talking occasions because a talker's preoccupation with formulating messages and abiding by the rules of conversation overshadow awareness of and attention to moments of stuttering. However, Siegel suggests, attaching signals of any kind to moments of stuttering might serve to draw a talker's attention to (i.e., to highlight) those stutterings and thereby heighten their aversive properties. Further, once a stutterer becomes aware of occurrences of stuttering, his or her own (covert) negative evaluation of those behaviors could serve to punish their occurrence. This view, then, suggests that an operant concept of punishment, albeit in a (self-punishment) covert form, is still worth consideration as an explanation of the decelerating effect of seemingly neutral stimuli attached to stutterings.

Evidence regarding a highlighting hypothesis

The effects of response contingent neutral stimuli. Siegel verified the decelerating effects of assumedly neutral consequent stimuli on disfluencies of nonstuttering subjects (Martin & Siegel, 1969; Siegel, 1973; Siegel & Hanson, 1972; Siegel & Martin, 1966), sometimes bolstering such effects by instructions directing subjects' attention to their disfluencies. A few studies have examined the effect of ostensibly neutral stimuli on stutterings as well. Wingate's (1959) study included one condition in which stutterers were "reminded" of moments of stuttering by the RC activation of an electronic counter during repeated oral readings. Although this study is somewhat problem bound (see Martin & Ingham, 1973), the reductions in stuttering that occurred during this condition suggest that a relatively neutral stimulus may have served to control the stuttering. As one of several treatments attempted with an adult stutterer by Poppen, Nunn, and Hook (1977), a clinician raised a finger to signal the subject each time he stuttered. This seemingly neutral procedure was reported to produce a mild transient reduction in stuttering.[5] Corcoran's (1980) study, on the other hand, failed to produce significant reductions in stuttering with eight subjects when

[5] Poppen, Nunn, and Hook's (1977) first description of this procedure seemed to describe TO; however, a later description of the procedure described it as RC presentation of a neutral stimulus.

a presumably neutral light flash plus counter advance followed their stutterings.

A previously described study by James (1981c) is also pertinent to this issue. In part of this study, two groups of nine adult stutterers spoke in monologue and, following baseline, received either a 10-sec 290-Hz 60-dB tone contingent upon each moment of stuttering or a randomly presented 10-sec tone. Neither procedure produced a significant reduction in either group's stuttering. Inspection of the findings for individual subjects, however, revealed that five subjects in the contingent tone group reduced their stuttering by between 20 and 29% and 70 and 79%; but only one subject showed stuttering reduction during the random tone condition. This suggests that for some subjects, following moments of stuttering with a seemingly neutral stimulus served to reduce their frequency. This finding is all the more impressive since it is likely that many stutterings were not immediately followed by this neutral stimulus because subjects could continue to talk (and stutter) during the 10-sec tone interval.

Other findings pertinent to this issue have been reported by Haroldson et al. (1968) and Patty and Quarrington (1974). In their previously described TO study, Haroldson et al. informally reported that the red light that served as a TO signal had no systematic RC effect on stuttering frequency when it was presented alone. On the other hand, Patty and Quarrington found a stuttering contingent light flash to have no effect on any form of stuttering behavior except visible struggle, which increased.

In summary, it appears that there is evidence to suggest that presumably neutral RC stimuli sometimes reduce stuttering frequency, but these effects also appear to be more fragile and less widespread across subjects than stimuli carrying more negative connotations.

The effects of self-monitoring. It might be assumed that calling attention to stuttering through self-monitoring or self-counting procedures would be another way of releasing the hypothesized aversive properties associated with moments of stuttering, thereby offering further (indirect) evidence pertinent to a highlighting hypothesis. Self-monitoring of behaviors other than stuttering has often been reported to modify a behavior's frequency of occurrence (Nelson & Hayes, 1981). There is also a growing body of literature on the effects of subjects' self-monitoring of stutterings. It began with La Croix's (1973) study in which two male adolescent stutterers pressed a hand-held counter for each disfluency. Large, clinically significant reductions in "percent words disfluent" were observed, although knowledge of their disfluency counts and the presence of the experimenter may have contributed to the self-counting effect. Similar findings under similar conditions were replicated in informal clinical probes (ABAB) by Costello (1975).

There appear to be only two studies in the literature that provide a relatively "pure" test of the highlighting hypothesis by having subjects monitor their stutterings without provision of external feedback, and their findings disagree on the effects of such procedures on stuttering. Goldiamond's original work (1962, 1965) was all conducted having subjects record their own stutterings. He tested the reactivity of this measure and reported that "subject definition" (p. 64) did not influence the frequency of stuttering for three subjects and had only a transitory decelerating effect for one subject. In contrast, Hanson's (1978) study was designed to develop a procedure to enhance stutterers' attention to their stuttering and, hence, increase the potency of self-recording. However, simply requiring two female subjects to press a handswitch whenever they stuttered produced such clear decreases in stuttering that the experimental enhancement condition was redundant.

Further experimentation with regard to self-monitoring effects on stuttering has incorporated differing degrees of feedback. Ingham, Adams, and Reynolds' (1978) subjects were required, at various times, to speak in monologue without self-monitoring, to press a button every time they heard themselves stutter, or to press a button every time they said the word *the*, a control for the role of generalized attention to speaking. Subjects received feedback regarding their frequency counts via an electronic counter. The results illustrated the variability across subjects for which stutterers are so notorious: One (of three) subject's stuttering was reduced while one showed reliable increases. James (1981a) investigated the effects of self-administered TO in a multiple baseline across settings design with one subject and showed it to be a viable decelerater of stuttering frequency, even in settings beyond the clinic.

The accuracy of self-monitoring. Further analysis of James' (1981a) data revealed that the subject's identification and self-punishment of moments of stuttering had been less than 50% accurate, so a second experiment was undertaken to increase the accuracy of self-initiated TO and to observe its relationship to stuttering reductions. The accuracy of TO delivery was increased to 77% and stuttering was concomitantly further reduced (to less than 1% SS).

The observation of a positive relationship between accuracy of self-monitoring and amount of stuttering reduction was not upheld, however, in a subsequent study by James (1981b). In this study 33 adult stutterers signaled their own moments of stuttering by pressing a handswitch that produced a tone. It turned out that self-monitoring accuracy and reductions in stuttering frequency were significantly but *negatively* related. That is, when the subjects were grouped according to accuracy, only the low-accurate self-monitors ($\bar{x}$ = 26% accuracy) produced significant ($p<.01$) stuttering changes ($\bar{x}$ = 41% reduction). The thrust of these findings is supported by all of the self-monitoring studies that have reported the accuracy of subjects' self-counts of stutterings (Costello, 1975; Goldiamond, 1965; Hanson, 1978; Ingham et al., 1978; James, 1981a; La Croix, 1973). First, stuttering is not typically counted accurately by subjects, and second, the most affected subjects often appear to be the least accurate counters. Such inaccuracy may bear testimony to the efficacy of intermittent RC stimulation and is complemented by Adams and Popelka's (1971) and James's (1976, 1981c) reports that even experimenters may fail to deliver consequences after every stuttering, yet RC effects still occur. On the other hand, it is conceivable that subjects in these studies were counting accurately but were counting *something different* from the experimenters; perhaps they were counting "real" stutterings, and it was the experimenters' counts that were inaccurate. Perkins' recent (1983) comments regarding the observation that many stutterers perceive the feeling of a momentary involuntary loss of motor control to be the essence of their moments of stuttering, a "behavior" that might not be readily observable to an observer, would support this view.

Antecedent stimulus control and stuttering

The development of discriminative stimuli is well known in the operant conditioning literature and has been demonstrated clearly in laboratory studies with stuttering subjects. For example, Martin and Siegel (1966a, 1966b) demonstrated that a nylon strap placed on the subject's wrist or illumination of a blue light was sufficient to reduce stuttering, provided that these stimuli had been previously present during stuttering-contingent punishment. Reed and Lingwall (1980) verified this effect when they made a demonstrably neutral stimulus, continuous presence of a woman's face on a video screen, into an S^- by pairing it with stuttering-contingent female laughter. In one condition of Martin and Haroldson's (1971) previously described study, subjects' infrequent presentations of TO contingencies were ineffective in reducing each other's stuttering. However, following a period of effective experimenter-presented TO, subject-presented TO did decrease stuttering, although their accuracy of TO delivery did not improve. It was suggested that stuttering decreased because the presence of the TO paraphernalia had become S^D's for reduced stuttering during the intervening experimenter-controlled punishment condition.

Another kind of stimulus control exerted by antecedent stimuli is evident when a subject's behavior is modified by observing a model's behavior (Bandura, 1969). For example, Martin and Haroldson (1977) showed that after 20 stutterers viewed a videotape of a stutterer responding appropriately to TO treatment, 19 displayed less stuttering following the videotape than preceding it. Martin and Haroldson suggest that these findings are "consonant with the notion that stuttering is an operant behavior" (p. 25).

Verbal instructions may also function as conditioned discriminative stimuli that modify operant behaviors. Oelschlaeger and Brutten (1976) attempted to demonstrate that instructions to reduce particular kinds of speech interruptions would be functional for interjections, but not for repetitions. Statistical analyses supported this contention, but the actual ABA data were not presented for readers' scrutiny (see Footnote 4). Further, Costello and Hurst (1981) and Costello and Felsenfeld (an unpublished study described below) used instructional control to produce reductions of various forms of stuttering that Brutten and Oelschlaeger would hypothesize to be in different response classes. Martin and Siegel (1966b) demonstrated that instructions to speak fluently produced a moderate, but transient, reduction in stuttering frequency for two adult subjects, while Martin and Haroldson's (1979) similar instructions failed to produce evidence of stimulus control. In the earlier study, fluency instructions were first paired with effective contingencies for stuttering and fluency, which might account for their positive influence. Many studies reported herein have included some form of instructional control, apparently in an effort to facilitate the effects of the contingency manipulations (Corcoran, 1980; James, 1976; Lanyon & Barocas, 1973, 1975; Manning, Trutna, & Shaw, 1976; Martin & Haroldson, 1979, 1982; Patty & Quarrington, 1974; Shaw & Shrum, 1972; Williams & R. B. Martin, 1974; Wingate, 1959), although determining the differential effects of these two variables becomes impossible under these conditions. Nonetheless, behaviors that are controlled by their consequences and by conditioned discriminative stimuli are typically considered to be operant behaviors. There is evidence that stuttering fulfills these criteria.

Negative reinforcement (reinforcement by contingent withdrawal)

Now we turn to the study of the effects on stuttering of operant principles designed to increase response rates. Since increasing stuttering has relatively little clinical value, it is not surprising that little research has been conducted along these lines. However, if stuttering is conceptualized as an operant, then it would follow that environmental contingencies should increase as well as decrease stuttering.

Negative reinforcement was first investigated by Flanagan et al. (1958) in an ABA design with three adult stutterers. In an escape (negative reinforcement) period, a continuous 6000-Hz 105-dB tone was terminated for 5 sec contingent on each moment of stuttering. The resulting data trends are ambiguous in the case of two subjects because of the use of cumulative records in this report, but rough calculations indicate that stuttering increased approximately 30% from the end of baseline to the end of the escape period for all three subjects. This trend was reversed by the withdrawal of the contingencies for two subjects, while a third subject continued to produce increased stuttering (to 49% above baseline). Biggs and Sheehan's (1969) previously described replication of this study failed because none of their experimental conditions demonstrated control over stuttering—an apparent failure of experimental design rather than a failure of stuttering to respond to negative reinforcement.

Another study described previously (Martin et al., 1975), also attempted to replicate Flanagan et al.'s findings. Using ongoing shock as the aversive stimulus, and alternating negative reinforcement and punishment conditions, Martin and his colleagues produced ambiguous increases in stuttering during negative reinforcement for only one of five adult subjects, although there was an initial, transient increase in "shock-off time" for all subjects. In another study cited earlier, Goldiamond (1962; 1965) used DAF as an aversive stimulus in a negative reinforcement paradigm with two adult male subjects. In the experimental portion of an ABA design, DAF was shut off for 10 sec following each moment of stuttering. After two such sessions, stuttering in one subject had substantially increased (from a maximum of about 37% words stuttered [%WS] in baseline to about 55% WS during negative reinforcement). For the second subject, a small and immediate increase in stuttering occurred.[6]

---

[6] The most important clinical finding to come out of these studies, however, was the effect of extended periods of DAF on the speech of stutterers. Eventually the subjects reacted to DAF not by increasing stuttering and thus avoiding DAF, but by slowing their rate of speech through prolongation, thus apparently better matching bone- and air-conducted auditory feedback and (fortuitously) essentially eliminating stuttering. This finding led directly to the development of one of the most frequently used stuttering therapy procedures (Ingham, 1984, chap. 10). It is interesting to note, however, that these and other procedures are made more effective when RC consequences are added (e.g., Ingham & Andrews, 1973a; Ingham & Packman, 1977) and that the positive effects on stuttering of RC consequences alone cannot be accounted for by subject's use of prolonged speech or other fluency inducing techniques (Andrews, Howie, Dozsa, & Guitar, 1982.)

Generally, the research on negative reinforcement and stuttering only mildly supports the prediction that stuttering should increase under these kinds of reinforcement contingencies. Many of the findings in these studies, however, are blemished by order effects (Goldiamond, 1962, 1965; Martin et al., 1975), by lack of overall experimental control (Biggs & Sheehan, 1969), or by ambiguous presentations of the data (Flanagan et al., 1958). It would appear that the effect of negative reinforcement on stuttering has yet to be unequivocally determined.

Positive reinforcement (reinforcement by contingent presentation)

Several studies have investigated the effects of this kind of reinforcement on stuttering, although their effects are anything but congruent. A pivotal study by Cooper et al. (1970) and its replication by Daly and Kimbarow (1978) were discussed above. In one of their three conditions, RC *right* considerably reduced stuttering for essentially all stutterers. As noted earlier, a highlighting hypothesis would suggest that *right* served to call the stutterers' attention to stutterings and their inherent punishing properties, and that these aversive qualities overpowered whatever reinforcing characteristics *right* may have had. Presumably, this effect would be less powerful for the normal (thereby, less aversive) disfluencies of nonstuttering subjects, which was the case in both studies. Lanyon and Barocas (1975) also called upon a highlighting effect to explain why stuttering-contingent monetary gain (typically 5¢ per stutter) and monetary loss both produced reduced stuttering. They suggested that such small monetary gains might have had very little reinforcing power "in comparison with the aversive effect of self-awareness or public acknowledgment of each nonfluency" (p. 792).

Patty and Quarrington's (1974) findings do not support a highlighting hypothesis, even though they also showed 5¢ per stutter to produce decreases in stuttering whether the award of 5¢ was signaled at the time of each stutter or simply awarded at the end of the session.[7] Only visible struggle behaviors were reduced by this variable, but they actually increased when a neutral RC signal was presented alone. Oelschlaeger and Brutten (1975) upped the ante to 10¢ per stutter (this time for part-word repetitions only), but the Wilcoxon-T analysis revealed no significant frequency changes (see Footnote 4). Again, no data were included for direct inspection. Starkweather and Lucker (1978) reported that they also found presumed RC reinforcers (tokens worth 1¢ backed up by toys and candies) to decrease stuttering frequency for three of

---

[7] The latter condition is mistakenly referred to as Noncontingent Reward, although the reward was clearly contingent, only delayed.

four children (aged 10–12). However, the data for two subjects are confounded by similar reductions also occurring in the control conditions. The fourth subject increased stuttering frequency but was reported to have done so by "faked" stutterings.

Another indecisive result emerged from Corcoran's (1980) study on the effects of presumed positive (5¢) and neutral (light flash and advancement of a counter) stimuli on the stuttering frequency of eight adult stutterers. Statistical analysis of the data indicated that stuttering did not increase under either RC condition, nor did it decrease. Corcoran suggests that these findings may not have replicated the stuttering decrements found under similar conditions in other studies because experimenter expectations were controlled in this study. It certainly could be said that for much of the literature reviewed in this chapter—on both sides of the ideological fence—results could be rather reliably predicted by knowledge of the researchers' philosophical leanings. This might indicate the existence of some powerful, yet-to-be-isolated, independent variables active in RC investigations of stuttering. (See Rosenthal [1966] for an extensive account of experimenter bias.)

Two other studies provide somewhat incidental, but supportive, findings for the accelerating effects of positive stimuli on stuttering frequency. Both Shaw and Shrum (1972) and Manning et al. (1976) studied reinforcement of nonstuttered utterances in child stutterers (ages 9–10 and 6–9, respectively). Both studies utilized ABAB reversal designs (Hersen & Barlow, 1976; McReynolds & Kearns, 1983) wherein the second A condition required application of the experimental reinforcing stimulus to stutterings and disfluencies. In both studies two of the three subjects displayed stuttering rates above the original baseline levels during these reinforcement conditions.

In summarizing his recent review of all of these studies, Ingham (1984) stated:

> The findings from the "reinforcement of stuttering" studies present a fairly confusing picture. There is certainly ample evidence that some findings are contrary to those expected if stuttering is regarded as operant behavior. But there are other ways of explaining these confusing data. To begin with, in none of these studies did the subject actually fail to receive payment for speaking during the experimental conditions; thus, regardless of any performance, they were "rewarded." Consequently, the "punishing" effects of highlighted stuttering may have been greater than the reinforcement of "more money." ...A final consideration is the value of the presumed reinforcer. It may be hazardous to predict the reinforcing properties of the stimulus before an event, but this writer would be prepared to wager that markedly different data trends might have appeared in many of these studies if the contingency had been, say, $10 per stuttering instead of 10¢. (p. 229)

If a highlighting effect does exist, it might be especially confounded for adult subjects under positive reinforcement conditions. A stimulus that at once signals the occurrence of a noxious event (a moment of stuttering) and offers approval of that event (*right*, tokens, monetary gain) might logically produce ambiguous behavior changes. It might be expected, however, that the contradictions inherent in this paradigm would be lessened in younger subjects for whom stuttering might not yet have acquired aversiveness. (Three of the four studies that showed stuttering to increase under RC positive stimulation involved subjects aged 12 years or less.)

Following these assumptions, Costello & Felsenfeld (unpublished)[8] studied positive (token) reinforcement of stuttering in two female preschool stutterers, aged 4.5 and 6 years. Elaborate procedures were used to ensure that token and backup reinforcers were likely to be functional, but tokens were demonstrated preexperimentally to be functional positive reinforcers for only one subject who subsequently displayed unambiguous ABABA increases in %WS (in the range of a 30% increase). For the second subject, token reinforcers were pre-experimentally demonstrated to be nonfunctional; and they likewise did not produce changes in stuttering (i.e., neither reinforcement nor highlighting effects), although increases were reliably obtained through instructional stimulus control. These findings offer some support for the position that stuttering can be increased via positive reinforcement contingencies if the possible interference of the stutterer's negative reactions to a heightened awareness of stuttering is controlled through the use of preschool-aged (primary) stutterers who may not yet have acquired such reactions.

CONCLUSIONS

Issues regarding the onset of stuttering from the perspective of stuttering as an operant behavior have not been tackled in this chapter, primarily because there is not experimental evidence available to address this topic. Inferences can be drawn from clinical experience that indicate that behavioral treatment of stuttering in young children is highly successful (e.g., Costello, 1983; chapter 18, this volume), and from reviews of the spontaneous recovery literature that indicate some percentage of "spontaneously recovered" stutterers may have actually experienced operant-like stuttering treatment from their families (e.g., Ingham, 1983);

[8] The original version of this study is an unpublished master's thesis by Susan Felsenfeld titled *Stuttering: Operant or not?* University of California, Santa Barbara, 1979.

but no direct evidence regarding variables that are instrumental to the genesis of stuttering has been contributed to the literature, and more speculation and theorizing does not seem beneficial.[9] Moreover, issues concerning the *cause* of stuttering and issues concerning the *nature* of stuttering can be independent issues, although they seem to have become inextricably related in much writing on stuttering. That is, if stuttering is operant behavior, it does not necessarily follow that stuttering is a learned disorder. As has been stated elsewhere,

> Just as tongue protrusion might be interfered with in an apraxic or dysarthric patient, or reaching movements might be distorted in a cerebral-palsied person, tongue protrusion and reaching are still operant behaviors subject to the principles of operant learning—they are just motorically *impaired* operant behaviors. So, too, might stuttering be. (Costello & Hurst, 1983, p. 158)

An interesting complication occurs when one attempts to study experimentally the nature of stuttering as an operant behavior. That the dependent variable is an operant is assumed in most operant research. Therefore, when manipulations of consequences do not predictably affect the response, one can "blame" the consequent stimulus and then set about conducting a systematic search for stimuli that do bear a functional relationship to the dependent variable. This is the essence of the experimental analysis of behavior (and too infrequently practiced in our published research). However, when stuttering is the dependent variable and the consequent stimuli do not produce predicted effects, some researchers have "blamed" stuttering by concluding that stuttering must not be an operant. A considerable amount of information on that front is now available (and is reviewed herein), and one might conclude from these findings that *stuttering acts like operant behavior* most of the time. When it fails to, then perhaps dubious research designs—for example, the use of exactly the same stimuli for all subjects and for prescribed periods of time—have been at fault, rather than the behavior under study. It would seem that continued and extended efforts at devising experiments that utilize the flexibility and hypothesis-testing functions of the classic unfolding experiment (Platt, 1964; Sidman, 1960;

---

[9] In this context it is noteworthy that the operant procedure of extinction has been virtually ignored in the experimental literature (although it has been discussed by Wingate, [1966], and Brookshire, [1967a], and one study [Rousey, 1958] could be considered to be an indirect test of it). To effect extinction experimentally, one must (1) know what stimuli reinforce stuttering and (2) be able to control their occurrence. Where stuttering is concerned, there is no evidence that stimuli that occur in the natural environment reinforce stuttering (although speculations in this regard have been made by Daly & Cooper, [1967]; Shames & Sherrick, [1963]; Sheehan, [1951]; Siegel, [1970]; Silverman, [1976]; Wischner, [1950]; among others). So, until (1) is known, it is impossible to investigate the effects of (2). Little headway has been made in this direction.

Skinner, 1956) provide the best path to eventually tracking down the critical variables that reliably modify stuttering.

REFERENCES

Adams, M. R., & Popelka, G. The influence of "time-out" on stutterers and their dysfluency. *Behavior Therapy,* 1971, *2,* 334–339.

Andrews, G., Howie, P. M., Dozsa, M., & Guitar, B. E. Stuttering: Speech pattern characteristics under fluency-inducing conditions. *Journal of Speech and Hearing Research,* 1982, *25,* 208–216.

Azrin, N. H., & Holz, W. C. Punishment. In W. K. Honig (Ed.), *Operant behavior: Areas of research and application.* New York: Appleton–Century–Crofts, 1966.

Bandura, A. *Principles of behavior modification.* New York: Holt, Rinehart, & Winston, 1969.

Biggs, B., & Sheehan, J. G. Punishment or distraction? Operant stuttering revisited. *Journal of Abnormal Psychology, 1969, 74,* 256–262.

Bloodstein, O. The anticipatory struggle hypothesis: Implications of research on the variability of stuttering. *Journal of Speech and Hearing Research,* 1972, *15,* 487–499.

Bloodstein, O. The operant model of stuttering. *Journal of Speech and Hearing Research,* 1979, *22,* 665–666.

Bloodstein, O. *A handbook on stuttering.* Chicago: The National Easter Seal Society, 1981.

Brookshire, R. H. Comments on: "Stuttering adaptation and learning." *Journal of Speech and Hearing Disorders,* 1967, *32,* 195–198. (a)

Brookshire, R. H. Speech pathology and the experimental analysis of behavior. *Journal of Speech and Hearing Disorders,* 1967, *32,* 215–227. (b)

Brutten, G. J. Stuttering: Topography, assessment and behavior-change strategies. In J. Eisenson (Ed.), *Stuttering: A second symposium.* New York: Harper & Row, 1975.

Brutten, G. J. The effect of punishment on a Factor 1 stuttering behavior. *Journal of Fluency Disorders,* 1980, *5,* 77–85.

Brutten, G. J., & Shoemaker, D. J. *The modification of stuttering.* Englewood Cliffs, NJ: Prentice–Hall, 1967.

Cooper, E. B., Cady, B. B., & Robbins, C. J. The effect of the verbal stimulus words, "wrong," "right," and "tree" on the disfluency rates of stutterers and nonstutterers. *Journal of Speech and Hearing Research,* 1970, *13,* 239–244.

Corcoran, J. A. Effects of neutral and positive stimuli on stuttering: "Calling attention to stuttering" revisited. *Journal of Fluency Disorders,* 1980, *5,* 99–114.

Costello, J. M. The establishment of fluency with time-out procedures: Three case studies. *Journal of Speech and Hearing Disorders,* 1975, *40,* 216–231.

Costello, J. M. Operant conditioning and the treatment of stuttering. In W. H. Perkins (Ed.), *Strategies in stuttering therapy. Seminars in Speech, Language and Hearing,* 1. New York: Decker, 1980.

Costello J. M. Techniques of therapy based on operant theory. In W. H. Perkins (Ed.), *Current therapy of communication disorders.* New York: Decker, 1982.

Costello, J. M. Current behavioral treatments for children. In D. Prins & R. J. Ingham (Eds.), *Treatment of stuttering in early childhood: Methods and issues.* San Diego: College–Hill Press, 1983.

Costello, J. M., & Felsenfeld, S. *The positive reinforcement of stuttering in two preschool stutterers.* Unpublished manuscript, 1981.

Costello, J. M., & Hurst, M. R. An analysis of the relationship among stuttering behaviors. *Journal of Speech and Hearing Research,* 1981, *24,* 247–256.

Costello, J. M., & Hurst, M. R. A reply to Brutten. *Journal of Speech and Hearing Research,* 1983, *26,* 156–159.

Daly, D. A., & Cooper, E. B. Rate of stuttering adaptation under two electroshock conditions. *Behaviour Research and Therapy,* 1967, *5,* 49–54.

Daly, D. A., & Kimbarow, M. L. Stuttering as operant behavior: Effects of the verbal stimuli *wrong, right,* and *tree* on the disfluency rates of school-age stutterers and nonstutterers. *Journal of Speech and Hearing Research,* 1978, *21,* 589–597.

Daly, D. A., & Kimbarow, M. L. The operant model of stuttering: A reply to Bloodstein. *Journal of Speech and Hearing Research,* 1979, *22,* 166. (a)

Daly, D. A., & Kimbarow, M. L. Stuttering as operant behavior: A reply to Hegde. *Journal of Speech and Hearing Research,* 1979, *22,* 669–670. (b)

Egolf, D. B., Shames, G. H., & Seltzer, H. N. The effects of time-out on the fluency of stutterers in group therapy. *Journal of Communication Disorders,* 1971, *4,* 111–118.

Fahmy, M. The theory of habit control and negative practice as a curative method in the treatment of stammering. *Speech,* 1950, *14,* 24–30.

Ferster, C. B., & Appel, J. B. Punishment of S^{Δ} responding in matching to sample by time-out from positive reinforcement. *Journal of Experimental Analysis of Behavior,* 1961, *4,* 45–56.

Flanagan, B., Goldiamond, I., & Azrin, N. Operant stuttering: The control of stuttering behavior through response-contingent consequences. *Journal of the Experimental Analysis of Behavior,* 1958, *1,* 173–177.

Goldiamond, I. The maintenance of ongoing fluent behavior and stuttering. *Journal of Mathetics,* 1962, *1,* 57–95.

Goldiamond, I. Stuttering and fluency as manipulatable response classes. In L. Krasner & L. P. Ullman (Eds.), *Research in behavior modification.* New York: Holt, Rinehart & Winston, 1965.

Halvorson, J. The effects on stuttering frequency of pairing punishment (response cost) with reinforcement. *Journal of Speech and Hearing Research,* 1971, *14,* 356–364.

Hanson, B. R. The effects of contingent light-flash on stuttering and attention to stuttering. *Journal of Communication Disorders,* 1978, *11,* 451–458.

Haroldson, S. K., Martin, R. R., & Starr, C. D. Time-out as a punishment for stuttering. *Journal of Speech and Hearing Research,* 1968, *11,* 560–566.

Hegde, M. N. The effect of shock on stuttering. *Journal of the All India Institute of Speech and Hearing,* 1971, *2,* 104–110.

Hegde, M. N. Stuttering as operant behavior. *Journal of Speech and Hearing Research,* 1979, *22,* 667–669.

Hegde, M. N. Assessment and treatment of fluency disorders: State of the art. In J. M. Costello (Ed.), *Speech disorders in adults: Recent advances.* San Diego: College-Hill Press, 1984.

Hersen, M., & Barlow, D. H. *Single case experimental designs: Strategies for studying behavior change.* New York: Pergamon, 1976.

Holland, A. L. Some applications of behavioral principles to clinical speech problems. *Journal of Speech and Hearing Disorders,* 1967, *32,* 11–18.

Holland, J. G., & Skinner, B. F. *The analysis of behavior: A program for self-instruction.* New York: McGraw-Hill, 1961.

Honig, W. K. *Operant behavior: Areas of research and application.* New York: Appleton-Century-Crofts, 1966.

Ingham, R. J. Operant methodology in stuttering therapy. In J. Eisenson (Ed.), *Stuttering: A second symposium.* New York: Harper & Row, 1975.

Ingham, R. J. Spontaneous remission of stuttering: When will the emperor realize he has no clothes on? In D. Prins & R. J. Ingham (Eds.), *Treatment of stuttering in early childhood: Methods and issues.* San Diego: College-Hill Press, 1983.

Ingham, R. J. *Stuttering and behavior therapy: Current status and experimental foundations.* San Diego: College-Hill Press, 1984.

Ingham, R. J., Adams, S., & Reynolds, G. The effects on stuttering of self-recording the frequency of stuttering or the word "the." *Journal of Speech and Hearing Research,* 1978, *21,* 459–469.

Ingham, R. J., & Andrews, G. An analysis of a token economy in stuttering therapy. *Journal of Applied Behavior Analysis,* 1973, *6,* 219–229. (a)

Ingham, R. J., & Andrews, G. Behavior therapy and stuttering: A review. *Journal of Speech and Hearing Disorders,* 1973, *38,* 405–441. (b)

Ingham, R. J., & Packman, A. Treatment and generalization in an experimental treatment for a stutterer using contingency management and speech rate control. *Journal of Speech and Hearing Disorders,* 1977, *42,* 394–407.

James, J. E. The influence of duration on the effects of time-out from speaking. *Journal of Speech and Hearing Research,* 1976, *19,* 206–215.

James, J. E. Self-monitoring of stuttering: Reactivity and accuracy. *Behaviour Research and Therapy,* 1981, *19,* 291–296. (b)

James, J. E. Behavioral self-control of stuttering using time-out from speaking. *Journal of Applied Behavior Analysis,* 1981, *14,* 25–37. (a)

James, J. E. Punishment of stuttering: Contingency and stimulus parameters. *Journal of Communication Disorders,* 1981, *14,* 375–386. (c)

James, J. E., & Ingham, R. J. The influence of stutterers' expectancies of improvement upon response to time-out. *Journal of Speech and Hearing Research,* 1974, *17,* 86–93.

Janssen, P., & Brutten, G. J. The differential effects of punishment of oral prolongations. In Y. Lebrun & R. Hoops (Eds.), *Neurolinguistic approaches to stuttering.* The Hague: Mouton, 1973.

Johnson, W. *The onset of stuttering.* Minneapolis: University of Minnesota, 1959.

Kazdin, A. E. *History of behavior modification: Experimental foundations of contemporary research.* Baltimore, MD: University Park Press, 1978.

La Croix, Z. E. Management of disfluent speech through self-recording procedures. *Journal of Speech and Hearing Disorders,* 1973, *38,* 272–274.

Lanyon, R. I., & Barocas, V. S. Effects of contingent stimuli on stuttering. *Proceedings 81st Annual Convention American Psychological Association,* 1973, 539–540.

Lanyon, R. I., & Barocas, V. S. Effects of contingent events on stuttering and fluency. *Journal of Consulting and Clinical Psychology,* 1975, *43,* 786–793.

Leitenberg, H. Is time-out from positive reinforcement an aversive event? *Psychological Bulletin,* 1965, *64,* 428–441.

Manning, W. H., Trutna, P. A., & Shaw, C. K. Verbal versus tangible reward for children who stutter. *Journal of Speech and Hearing Disorders,* 1976, *41,* 52–62.

Marascuilo, L. A., & McSweeney, M. *Nonparametric and distribution free methods for the social sciences.* Monterey, CA: Brooks/Cole, 1977.

Martin, R. R., & Berndt, L. A. The effects of time-out on stuttering in a 12 year old boy. *Exceptional Children,* 1970, *36,* 303–304.

Martin, R. R., & Haroldson, S. K. The effects of two treatment procedures on stuttering. *Journal of Communication Disorders,* 1969, *2,* 115–125.

Martin, R. R., & Haroldson, S. K. Time-out as a punishment for stuttering during conversation. *Journal of Communication Disorders,* 1971, *4,* 15–19.

Martin, R. R., & Haroldson, S. K. Effect of vicarious punishment on stuttering frequency. *Journal of Speech and Hearing Research,* 1977, *20,* 21–26.

Martin, R. R., & Haroldson, S. K. Effects of five experimental treatments on stuttering. *Journal of Speech and Hearing Research,* 1979, *22,* 132–146.

Martin, R. R., & Haroldson, S. K. Contingent self-stimulation for stuttering. *Journal of Speech and Hearing Disorders,* 1982, *47,* 407–413.

Martin, R. R., & Ingham, R. J. Stuttering. In B. Lahey (Ed.), *The modification of language behavior.* Springfield, IL: Thomas, 1973.

Martin, R. R., Kuhl, P., & Haroldson, S. K. An experimental treatment with two preschool stuttering children. *Journal of Speech and Hearing Research*, 1972, *15*, 743-752.

Martin, R. R., & Siegel, G. M. The effects of response contingent shock on stuttering. *Journal of Speech and Hearing Research*, 1966, *9*, 340-352. (a)

Martin, R. R., & Siegel, G. M. The effects of simultaneously punishing stuttering and rewarding fluency. *Journal of Speech and Hearing Research*, 1966, *9*, 466-475. (b)

Martin, R. R., & Siegel, G. M. The effects of a neutral stimulus (buzzer) on motor responses and disfluencies in normal speakers. *Journal of Speech and Hearing Research*, 1969, *12*, 179-184.

Martin, R. R., St. Louis, K., Haroldson, S. K., & Hasbrouck, J. Punishment and negative reinforcement of stuttering using electric shock. *Journal of Speech and Hearing Research*, 1975, *18*, 478-490.

McReynolds, L. V. Contingencies and consequences in speech therapy. *Journal of Speech and Hearing Disorders*, 1970, *35*, 12-24.

McReynolds, L. V., & Kearns, K. P. *Single-subject experimental designs in communicative disorders.* Baltimore, MD: University Park Press, 1983.

Miller, L. K. *Principles of everyday behavior.* Belmont, CA: Brooks/Cole, 1982.

Murray, F. P. An investigation of variably induced white noise upon moments of stuttering. *Journal of Communication Disorders*, 1969, *2*, 109-114.

Nelson, R. O., & Hayes, S. C. Theoretical explanations for reactivity in self-monitoring. *Behavior Modification*, 1981, *5*, 3-14.

Oelschlaeger, M. L., & Brutten, G. J. Response-contingent positive stimulation of the part-word repetitions displayed by four stutterers. *Journal of Fluency Disorders*, 1975, *2*, 10-17.

Oelschlaeger, M. L., & Brutten, G. J. The effect of instructional stimulation on the frequency of repetitions, interjections, and words spoken during the spontaneous speech of four stutterers. *Behavior Therapy*, 1976, *7*, 37-46.

Patty, J., & Quarrington, B. The effects of reward on types of stuttering. *Journal of Communication Disorders*, 1974, *7*, 65-77.

Pavlov, I. P. *Conditioned reflexes.* London: Oxford University Press, 1927.

Perkins, W. H. The problem of definition: Commentary on "stuttering." *Journal of Speech and Hearing Disorders*, 1983, *48*, 246-249.

Poppen, R., Nunn, R. G., & Hook, S. Effects of several therapies on stuttering in a single case. *Journal of Fluency Disorders*, 1977, *2*, 35-44.

Platt, J. R. Strong inference. *Science*, 1964, *146*, 347-353.

Quist, R. W., & Martin, R. R. The effect of response contingent verbal punishment. *Journal of Speech and Hearing Research*, 1967, *10*, 795-800.

Reed, C. G., & Godden, A. L. An experimental treatment using verbal punishment with two preschool stutterers. *Journal of Fluency Disorders*, 1977, *2*, 225-233.

Reed, C. G., & Lingwall, J. B. Conditioned stimulus effects on stuttering and GSRs. *Journal of Speech and Hearing Research*, 1980, *23*, 336-343.

Rosenthal, R. *Experimental effects in behavioral research.* New York: Appleton-Century-Crofts, 1966.

Rousey, C. L. Stuttering severity during prolonged spontaneous speech. *Journal of Speech and Hearing Research*, 1958, *1*, 40-47.

Ryan, B. P. *Programmed therapy for stuttering in children and adults.* Springfield, IL: Thomas, 1974.

Ryan, B. P. Stuttering therapy in a framework of operant conditioning and programmed learning. In H. H. Gregory (Ed.), *Controversies about stuttering therapy.* Baltimore, MD: University Park Press, 1979.

Shames, G. H. Operant conditioning and stuttering. In J. Eisenson (Ed.), *Stuttering: A second symposium.* New York: Harper & Row, 1975.

Shames, G., & Sherrick, C. E. A discussion of nonfluency and stuttering as operant behavior. *Journal of Speech and Hearing Disorders,* 1963, *28,* 3–18.

Shaw, C. K., & Shrum, W. F. The effects of response-contingent reward on the connected speech of children who stutter. *Journal of Speech and Hearing Disorders,* 1972, *37,* 75–88.

Sheehan, J. G. The modification of stuttering through non-reinforcement. *Journal of Abnormal Psychology,* 1951, *46,* 51–63.

Sheehan, J. G. Conflict theory and avoidance-reduction therapy. In J. Eisenson (Ed.), *Stuttering: A second symposium.* New York: Harper & Row, 1975.

Sidman, M. *Tactics of scientific research: Evaluating experimental data in psychology.* New York: Basic Books, 1960.

Siegel, G. M. Punishment, stuttering and disfluency. *Journal of Speech and Hearing Research,* 1970, *13,* 677–714.

Siegel, G. M. Studies in speech fluency. *Journal of Communication Disorders,* 1973, *6,* 259–271.

Siegel, G. M., & Hanson, B. The effect of response-contingent neutral stimuli on normal speech disfluency. *Journal of Speech and Hearing Research,* 1972, *15,* 123–133.

Siegel, G. M., & Martin, R. R. Experimental modification of disfluency in normal speakers. *Journal of Speech and Hearing Research,* 1965, *8,* 235–244. (a)

Siegel, G. M., & Martin, R. R. Verbal punishment of disfluencies in normal speakers. *Journal of Speech and Hearing Research,* 1965, *8,* 245–251. (b)

Siegel, G. M., & Martin, R. R. Punishment of disfluencies in normal speakers. *Journal of Speech and Hearing Research,* 1966, *9,* 208–218.

Siegel, G. M., & Martin, R. R. Verbal punishment of disfluencies during spontaneous speech. *Language and Speech,* 1967, *10,* 244–251.

Siegel, G. M., & Martin, R. R. The effects of verbal stimuli on disfluencies during spontaneous speech. *Journal of Speech and Hearing Research,* 1968, *11,* 358–364.

Silverman, F. H. Communication success: A reinforcer of stuttering? *Perceptual and Motor Skills,* 1976, *42,* 398.

Skinner, B. F. A case history in scientific method. *American Psychologist,* 1956, *11,* 221–233.

Starkweather, C. W. Analysis of a controversy in stuttering. *Journal of Fluency Disorders,* 1974, *1,* 10–21.

Starkweather, C. W., & Lucker, J. Tokens for stuttering. *Journal of Fluency Disorders,* 1978, *3,* 167–180.

Williams, J. D., & Martin, R. B. Immediate versus delayed consequences of stuttering responses. *Journal of Speech and Hearing Research,* 1974, *17,* 569–575.

Wingate, M. E. Calling attention to stuttering. *Journal of Speech and Hearing Research,* 1959, *2,* 326–335.

Wingate, M. E. Stuttering adaptation and learning I. The relevance of adaptation studies to stuttering as learned behavior. *Journal of Speech and Hearing Disorders,* 1966, *31,* 148–156.

Wingate, M. E. On the Hegde–Daly and Kimbarow exchange. *Journal of Speech and Hearing Research,* 1980, *23,* 217–219.

Wischner, G. J. Stuttering behavior and learning: A preliminary theoretical formulation. *Journal of Speech and Hearing Disorders,* 1950, *15,* 324–335.

Chapter 11

Stuttering as a Prosodic Disorder

Marcel Wingate

INTRODUCTION

Although this chapter appears in a section devoted to theories of stuttering, I disclaim that what is presented here is offered as a theory of stuttering. First of all, I believe, for various reasons, that there is no existent statement about stuttering which merits designation as a theory, unless one is using the word "theory" in the vernacular sense, in which it means little more than "speculation." Stuttering has been plagued by theories which have served mainly to create devoted followers and, at the same time, obstruct understanding. As Hughlings Jackson once said, "A study of the causes of things must be preceded by a study of the things caused." In stuttering there is still much need for study of the things caused. Second, while I believe that prosodic factors are central to an understanding of stuttering, it should be obvious that prosody is not an isolated function; on one hand it is an integral part of the complex processes of language expression; on the other hand it is, at base, the reflection of a certain range of physiological functions. A theory of stuttering should be able to interrelate these, and other, matters through a set of hypotheses.

I will say, however, that pursuing investigation of stuttering in reference to prosodic features seems to me the most direct avenue to a coherent understanding of the disorder, simply because so much of the reliable speech-specific data about stuttering indicates prosodic involvement.

PROSODY: A BRIEF GENERAL STATEMENT

Prosody is not easy to define, especially in a technical sense. There is no unanimity of agreement among knowledgeable persons regarding what should be included under the rubric of prosody; in fact, it is generally acknowledged that discussions of prosody contain a certain degree of vagueness. However, such imprecision as exists need not obscure an appreciation of the essential nature of prosody nor confound an understanding of the dimensions regularly considered in discussions of it.

Prosody refers to the temporal patterns of undulation in tone, tempo, and loudness which constitute the "tune" of a spoken message. Etymologically, prosody—from the Greek *pros* "to" and *ode*, "song"—has a correspondence to the word "melody," a more familiar term which has often been used to refer to the prosodic dimensions of speech. The character of prosodic features is well reflected in the more technical term "suprasegmental," a word which is used more-or-less synonymously with prosody. Suprasegmental states a specific distinction to other features of the speech signal—the segments, or phones. *Supra*segmental is intended to refer to aspects of the speech signal which are above and beyond segmental features; they are above in the sense of being in addition to the individual phones, and beyond in the sense that they may extend over many sequential segments.

The essential suprasegmental parameters, as perceived, are pitch, loudness, and duration. In connected speech these variables participate in dimensions of the speech stream identified as stress, intonation, and, for want of a better term, speech rhythm.

It should be evident that prosodic or suprasegmental features are an integral part of language expression and comprehension. However, in spite of the fact that the study of prosody is perhaps one of the oldest pursuits in the scientific analysis of language, prosody has received less attention than have other foci of linguistic inquiry, such as phonetics, semantics, or grammar. The relative inattention to prosodic features is well reflected in our ordinary—and professional—systems for transcribing oral language. Standard English orthography includes relatively few markers, such as the comma, period, and question mark, for coding the wide range of suprasegmental variations. The situation is not much better in widely accepted professional systems for representing speech graphically; symbols for specifying segmental variations outnumber symbols for indicating prosodic features.

The evident priority given to grammatical, semantic, and phonetic aspects of language are undoubtedly due in large part to the fact that they carry the burden of meaning in communication; yet prosodic features share regularly in carrying meaning, often qualifying the information contained in the segmental, word, and phrase sequences and sometimes negating or inverting the meaning conveyed in the semantic features. Prosodic features are an important part of the speech code.

PROSODIC INVOLVEMENT IN STUTTERING
Direct evidence

Information which can be considered to bear directly on prosodic involvement in stuttering centers in the prosodic dimension of linguistic stress. There is substantial evidence that linguistic stress is intimately involved in stuttering. The first experimental evidence indicating a significant relationship between stuttering and stress appeared in a series of studies authored primarily by Spencer F. Brown between 1935 and 1945 (Brown, 1937, 1938a, 1938b, 1938c, 1943, 1945; Brown & Moren, 1942; Johnson & Brown, 1935, 1939). It is of some interest that this series, which turned out to be a sequence of analyses of certain language variables related to stuttering, was initiated as an effort to identify sounds that might be particularly difficult for stutterers. The search for difficult sounds was disappointing. In the studies of speech sounds per se (Johnson & Brown, 1935, 1939) it was found that all stutterers did not have difficulty with (stutter on) the same sounds. Furthermore, the data did not reveal a special group of sounds which stood out clearly from the rest as being notably difficult. However, the frequency with which the various sounds were stuttered could be arranged in rank order, and from this ranking, those sounds whose rank order value was above the average were identified, for computational purposes, as "difficult." This procedure resulted in a criterion that words beginning with a vowel or one of four "easy" consonants were less frequently associated with stuttering than were words beginning with the other consonants.[1]

Thus, the first language-related variable which Brown reported to be related to stuttering was:

(1) Words beginning with a consonant other than /w, hw, h, t, ð/ were stuttered more often than words beginning with other sounds. Further analysis of his data revealed certain other variables which were regularly associated with stuttering.

(2) Words from the grammatical classes of nouns, verbs, adjectives, and adverbs (identified in the writings of subsequent authors as content words) were stuttered much more often than such word classes as articles, prepositions, and conjunctions (classes identified in later writings as function words).

(3) Long words, those having five letters or more, were stuttered more often than short words.

(4) Words occurring early in a sentence—among the first three—were stuttered more often than later words in a sentence.

(5) Stuttering appeared most often with the first sound of a word.

(6) Stuttering almost always occurred in relation to a stressed syllable.

It is pertinent to note that the fifth variable was not newly revealed in Brown's work. The marked tendency for stuttering to apparently involve the initial sound of a word had been reported informally many times before. It has also been reported formally and informally many times since; in fact, this concurrence has been so widely known that it has the status of a given. It is also pertinent to note that the variable of word-initial sound actually encompasses the first variable in the list, for it is in respect to word-initial sounds that the matter of difficult sounds has relevance. That is, when a stutterer claims to have difficult sounds (in some writings, feared sounds) he is referring to those sounds when they occupy word-initial position only.[2]

Actually, Brown developed his discussions in respect to the first four variables, and presented the data to show that stuttering was progressively more likely to occur on words in proportion to which they possessed the characteristics identified in these four variables.

Brown's theoretical bias oriented him to apply to these findings a psychological interpretation which centered on the assumption that a stutterer is intensely preoccupied with his speech performance and overly concerned with doing well. Brown was therefore predisposed to explain his findings in terms that would reflect this assumed preoccupation of stutterers. He explained all of the variables listed above as having, in one way or another, a psychological "prominence" for the stutterer.[3]

Overall, Brown focused most of his attention on the variable listed here as 2—the grammatical factor. He did so partly because the data regarding the relationship between stuttering and the grammatical class of words was more stable and consistent than for the other three variables he discussed, and partly because this variable was particularly amenable to a psychological explanation centering around a presumed concern about communicating adequately. Brown contended that, because nouns, verbs, adjectives, and adverbs have more inherent meaning than the other classes of words, they are more important to the meaning of a sentence. Therefore, the stutterer is more concerned about speaking them well, and therefore he is more likely to stutter on them.

The findings constituting the core of Brown's discussions have been investigated, generally corroborated, and in some sense expanded by a considerable amount of subsequent research. Two publications by Hahn (1942a, 1942b) appeared within a short time of Brown's own publications; however, a lengthy hiatus then followed. Twenty years later a recurrence of interest in this line of research was reflected in publications by Conway and Quarrington (1963), Lanyon (1968, 1969), Quarrington (1965), Quarrington, Conway, and Siegel (1962), Schlesinger, Forte, Fried, & Melkman (1965), Soderberg (1962, 1966, 1967), and Taylor (1966a, 1966b). Most of this research was addressed to some combination of the four variables which occupied Brown's attention, and there was particularly heavy emphasis on the variable which appealed most to him—the grammatical factor. All of these publications corroborated Brown's findings in some way; again, especially in regard to the relationship of stuttering to grammatical class.

For present purposes our interest in the subsequent research is more with the fact, rather than the details, of the corroboration it yielded. It is important to know that the kind of findings reported by Brown are repeatable, and therefore reliable. In particular, repeated consistent findings of a substantial relationship between stuttering and grammatical class are especially valuable in view of the fact that this apparent effect of grammatical class is better explained as an expression of prosodic function. We will return to this shortly.

First, let us comment on the remaining variable, 6, in the list presented earlier. This variable, reflecting linguistic stress, was compromised by Brown's interpretation of it as due to psychological prominence. He likened the role of stress to the role he conjectured for early sentence position, and therefore the identity and unique contribution of stress were lost in his general discussions, which centered on meaning.[4] Probably in consequence, stress was also largely ignored in the subsequent research, which followed Brown's line of analysis and discussion.

Failure to adequately consider stress was an omission having grand proportions. In the first place, among the "new" findings which emerged from Brown's data, stress was by far the most impressive: It could be shown to have a stronger relationship to stuttering occurrence than any of the other variables except word-initial position (to which it is closely related). Moreover, the variable of grammatical class can be incorporated easily within the variable of linguistic stress.

The key to explaining grammatical class as an expression of stress lies in the matter of the rules for stress assignment in English. The significance of these rules for understanding the apparent grammatical factor in stuttering was not discussed in the literature until fairly recently (Wingate, 1979); the essence of this account is as follows. In English, words of certain grammatical classes are typically, and most often, spoken only with certain levels of stress relative to other word classes. The classes of words which have been found to be frequently associated

TABLE 11-1. Frequency of Stuttering Associated with Various Grammatical Classes Grouped According to Eight Conventional Parts of Speech.[a]

Distinction Made by Brown[b]	Grammatical Class	Median Percent Stuttering
"High" Stuttering Frequency	Adjectives	8.2
	Nouns	7.65
	Adverbs	6.5
	Verbs	3.75
"Low" Stuttering Frequency	Pronouns	2.45
	Conjunctions	2.0
	Prepositions	1.75
	Articles	0.6

[a]After Brown, 1937.

[b]And accepted in subsequent research.

with stuttering are those word classes that typically receive heavy stress. In contrast, the grammatical classes of words *in*frequently stuttered are the word classes which typically receive weak stress or are unstressed.

Brown's separation of the grammatical classes into two categories, one with high stuttering and the other with low stuttering, turned out to be partially, but quite importantly, incorrect. Table 11-1 (from Brown, 1937) presents the data on which Brown divided the "eight conventional parts of speech" into two categories, as indicated on the left. Note that among the rank values of the top four classes (high stuttering frequency) the value for verbs is not as close to the values of the three higher classes as one should expect if these four classes function as equivalent expressions of the same influence (which is then assumed to differentiate these four classes, as a category, from the remaining four classes). In fact, the difference between adverbs and verbs (2.75) is over twice as great as the difference (1.30) between verbs and the next ranked class on the list, pronouns. Furthermore, the difference between adverbs and verbs is greater than the difference between verbs and each of the following

TABLE 11-2. Frequency of Stuttering Associated with Various Grammatical Classes: Refined Classification[a]

Grammatical Class	Median Percent Stuttering
Participial adjectives	14.1
Proper nouns	9.6
Gerunds	8.05
Adjectives	8.0
Adverbs	6.95
Nouns	6.6
Root verbs (in verb phrase)	5.25
Simple verbs	4.7
Subordinating conjunctions	3.8
Relative pronouns	3.15
Personal pronouns	2.55
Infinitives	2.1
Coordinating conjunctions	2.0
Prepositions	1.9
Auxiliary verbs	1.6
Possessive pronouns	1.2
Articles	0.6
Prepositions linked to verbs	0.0

[a] After Brown, 1937.

three classes in the list. Consequently, there is more justification for separating nouns, adjectives, and adverbs as one group and verbs, pronouns, prepositions, conjunctions, and articles as the other. The significance of the comparisons we have just made becomes clear if we look carefully at the analysis of concurrence between stuttering and a more refined grammatical classification.

Table 11-2, also from Brown (1937), presents the rank order for incidence of stuttering of a refined list of grammatical classes. The rank sequence of classes in this list reveals the error in combining all forms of verbs and conjunctions, among others, into composite classes, as in Table 11-1. In Table 11-2, various forms of the several grammatical classes are found dispersed throughout the list; they do not follow the sequence indicated in Table 11-1. Clearly, some classes of function words are stuttered more frequently than certain types of content words. Stuttering is not, then, related directly to grammatical class.

The differential incidence of stuttering revealed in Table 11-2 *is* directly related, however, to the level of stress which words of the various classes are likely to receive when spoken. According to the rules of English stress assignment, nouns, gerunds, adjectives, and adverbs are word classes that receive heavy stress. So are root verbs and main verbs; but, in contrast, auxiliary verbs and infinitives are most likely to be unstressed. Similarly, possessive pronouns are typically unstressed; personal pronouns are much more likely to be stressed. Also, coordinating conjunctions are much less likely to receive stress than are subordinating conjunctions. And articles and prepositions are almost always spoken without stress.

The foregoing analysis provides very substantial grounds for seriously doubting that there is a "grammatical factor," as such, in stuttering. Evidently the observed relationship of grammatical classes to stuttering incidence is simply an artifact of a classification system which, although useful for other purposes, in this instance obscures the critical variable.

All of the research cited so far has dealt with data derived from speech samples obtained through oral readings of prose material. Hejna (1955) obtained comparable data from spontaneous speech samples of stutterers and applied the same analyses reported in the Brown series. The spontaneous speech samples were obtained by having individual stutterers talk about various subjects as suggested by topic headings printed separately on small cards and made available to each individual to select as needed. Although this speaking situation is not equivalent to ordinary conversational circumstances, it did require individual subjects to produce connected speech generated independently at the moment. Also, other aspects of the experimental situation were contrived to approximate many facets of ordinary speaking circumstances.

Hejna found that, in spontaneous speech also, stuttering is associated with the same variables revealed in Brown's work. However, while his findings were generally consistent with Brown's data, Hejna's findings regarding the grammatical class of words, word length, early words in sentences, and kind of initial consonant were somewhat different from previous findings based on samples of oral reading. On the other hand, his data relative to the association of stuttering with word-initial position and with stressed syllables fully corroborated the similar findings from other research.

We have noted before that word-initial position and word stress are closely related in English. Table 11-3 presents data which reflect this close relationship. The percentage figures in the right-hand section of

TABLE 11-3. Distribution of the Stressed Syllable in Polysyllabic Words

Source	Number of words	Percent stressed on syllable				
		1	2	3	4	5
Brown	3276	78	—	—	—	—
Hejna	5976	78	—	—	—	—
Voelker	510	63	31	5	1	0
Berger	543	72	25	2	1	0

the table identify the distribution of the stressed syllable in polysyllabic words. The first two sets of entries in the table are from Brown (1938b) and Hejna (1955). Both authors identified only the total number of polysyllabic words and the number of these words which bore initial syllable stress. The number of words in the Brown study represents the number of polysyllabic words spoken by each subject. The number of words from the Hejna study is a random sample of all words spoken by all subjects and constitutes approximately 12.5% of the total corpus (this sample was used as a reference for various comparisons made in his analyses). The second two entries are data from word lists compiled in two studies of frequency of word usage (Berger, 1967; Voelker, 1942). They are included here to show that when word stress falls on other than the first syllable of a polysyllabic word it will most likely fall on the second syllable. In other words, for most polysyllabic words, stress occurs very early in the word.

In the research reviewed so far the analyses relating to stress were limited to polysyllabic words, evidently because one can tell, even for polysyllabic words in isolation, where the stress will occur. In ordinary connected speech, stress frequently falls on certain single-syllable words as well as on the normally accented syllable of polysyllabic words. It is important to know if the reported relationship between stuttering and stressed syllables applies to single-syllable words, too. One would expect that it should; the relationship of stuttering and stress should be independent of word length in connected speech. A test of this supposition was made in a study reported by the present author (Wingate, 1984a).

In connected speech the assignment of stress to certain words is determined by the role played by those words in relationship to other words in the utterance (sentence, phrase). There is a certain latitude regarding how the stress pattern of any particular utterance will be expressed, with variation affected by several sources of influence. At the same time, there is, for any utterance, a kind of "citation reference, " an idealized pattern for the utterance, which represents the way in which one would expect the vast majority of native speakers to say it, assuming that all speakers had a common intention in mind. The citation, or criterion, pattern of an utterance can be reproduced, intuitively, by a native speaker of the language. However, a more objective basis for identifying criterion form would be to have an expert linguist select the criterion example from actual samples of the utterance. The latter method was used in this study investigating concurrence of stuttering and stress in connected speech.

The objective in this study was to compare a representative sample of stutters occurring in connected speech with the stress pattern occurring in a normally spoken sample of the same sequence. Such comparison required that both data sets be obtained from an oral reading of the same material. Data for the stress pattern were derived from the criterion sample, which was obtained as follows. Individual tape recordings of 10 normal speakers reading the test material were played for a linguist known for his expertise in prosodics, who, by paired-comparison technique, selected the sample which most closely approximated citation form for an ordinary expression of the material. The tape recording of this criterion sample was then played through a Graphic Level recorder, an instrument which gives a permanent record of variation in intensity (loudness) of the speech signal. Peaks in intensity were accepted as representatives of points of stress.

The data set for stutter occurrences was obtained from 35 stutterers who read the passage individually. The syllables on which each stutter occurred were recorded for each individual, and the frequency of stuttering at each locus was summed for all subjects.

The correspondence of the two sets of data is presented in Figure 11-1. The comparison utterance is: "From within the small ship the passengers felt the movement of the heavy swells, though now the ship was riding well. On through the stormy night it had struggled over huge waves, in constant danger of swamping. " The thin vertical lines mark the correspondence of each syllable with the appropriate peak on the Graphic Level recorder tracing, which is the lower of the two curves in the figure. The upper curve is a smoothed plot of the frequency of stutters occurring at the various syllables in the utterance.

As expected, there is a clear concurrence of stuttering frequency with intensity variation, regardless of word length. Many stutters occur on

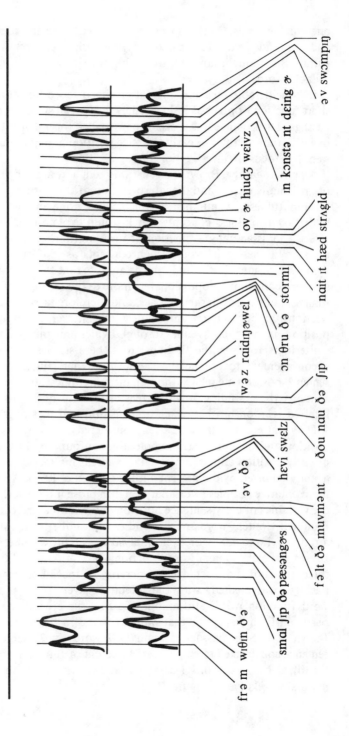

FIGURE 11-1. Concurrence of stutter frequencies (upper curve) and intensity peaks (lower curve) on sequential syllables of the test material. Stutter frequencies were obtained from 35 subjects. The intensity display is a Graphic Level recorder tracing of a criterion talker speaking the material (see text).

one-syllable words, which happen to be stressed. Note also that stuttering and amplitude peaks concur frequently on certain function words (from, within, the, though, now, on, through), most of which are also single-syllable words.

In considerable measure, this latter concurrence (of stuttering and short function words) was influenced by the special structure of the *Ship* passage. This passage was specially constructed for use in another study in which the variables of early sentence position and grammatical class were the focus of investigation (Wingate, 1979).

As noted earlier, Brown's discussions centered around the variable of grammatical class and the interpretation of this variable in terms of meaningfulness. A number of the studies done in the 1960s were undertaken to assess concepts which would explain that the position effect, too, is actually a function of meaningfulness. In those studies it was hypothesized, through such concepts as "information load, " "gradient of meaning, " and "uncertainty, " that the early words in a sentence contribute proportionately more to the meaning of a sentence than do later words in the sentence, and therefore (assuming a positive relationship between meaningfulness and stuttering) early sentence position is another avenue through which meaningfulness elicits stuttering. However, the findings from these studies did not provide encouragement to pursue the supposition that stuttering and early sentence position are related through meaningfulness. In fact, data from some of these studies provided reason to raise questions about the inferred relationship between word position and meaningfulness.

One matter that had not been considered in the studies of word position and meaning was the potential confounding of the variables of early position and grammatical class. This matter was addressed in a study reported by the present author (Wingate, 1979). Analysis of 10 representative samples of ordinary English prose indicated that, indeed, the variables of early sentence position and grammatical class are confounded: Content words were found to outnumber function words by a ratio of 1.6 to 1.0. Moreover, analysis of the prose material used by Brown yielded a content word/function word ratio of 2.2:1.0 in the first three words of those sentences. Therefore, a special passage, the *Ship* passage, was created, with the intent to invert the typical content word/function word ratio among the first three words of sentences, particularly in respect to that ratio as found in the material used by Brown. The *Ship* passage contains 362 words in 21 sentences, each sentence constructed to emphasize placement of function words among the first three positions (see the first two sentences above, in the discussion relative to Figure 11-2).

Data to compute stuttering frequency on words of the *Ship* passage were obtained from 35 stutterers who read the passage individually. Table 11-4 presents a summary of the distribution of content words and function words in positions as one of the first three words of a sentence or in some other sentence position, and the frequency with which words of these two categories were stuttered in those positions.

Overall, stuttering occurred much more frequently with content words than function words (7.1 to 2.8). This result is consistent with previous research and was to be expected since most of the words (299) are in their ordinary relationship to each other in a prose sequence. However, the content word/function word ratio of stuttering is reversed relative to early sentence position: Function words, usually not found as frequently in early sentence positions (and also not as often stuttered, and not stressed) were stuttered much more frequently when intentionally placed in early sentence positions. At the same time, in contrast to what had been found before, the relative amount of stuttering on the first three words is actually *less* than on words occurring in later sentence positions. Both of these results are contrary to expectation based on the previous research, and its interpretation.

These results indicate that grammatical class and early sentence position are not separate factors in their influence on stuttering. Although both variables appear to have an effect on stuttering which is independent of the other, the influence of grammatical class evidently is qualified by position, and the influence of position apparently is affected by grammatical class. The seeming contradiction, or at least bemusing complexity, posed by these findings are readily resolved, again, by explanation in terms of linguistic stress.

Earlier we noted that, in its apparent relationship to stuttering, the effect of grammatical class can be resolved as being simply an artifactual reflection of linguistic stress. The effect of position can also be accounted for within an explanation centered in linguistic stress. Stress occurs regularly in the early portion of sentences and at the beginning of clauses within sentences. Research reported by Lieberman (1967) shows that the intonation pattern of the typical declarative sentence, or a constituent of a derived phrase marker of a sentence, is characterized by an initial surge of physiological activity which underlies what is perceived as stress.

The expression of stress in the effects of both grammatical class and position is reflected in the rank order, in Table 11-2, of subclasses of pronouns and conjunctions. Relative pronouns and subordinating conjunctions typically occur at the beginning of clauses, and frequently as early words in sentences; it is because of such position occurrences that they are stressed more often than possessive pronouns and

TABLE 11-4. Influence of Early Sentence Position on the Content Word/Function Word Ratio of Stuttering

Position	Content Words	Function Words	All Classes
First three			
words	17	46	63
stutters	64	237	301
ratio	3.7	5.1	4.8
Other			
words	189	110	299
stutters	1393	198	1591
ratio	7.4	1.8	5.3
Total			
words	206	156	362
stutters	1457	435	1892
ratio	7.1	2.8	5.2

coordinating conjunctions, which are stuttered much less often. In this respect, it is pertinent to note that Bloodstein and Gantwerk (1967) found a tendency for stuttering to occur unusually often on pronouns and conjunctions in the speech of stuttering youngsters, an effect which evidently was due largely to the high frequency of stuttering on the first word of sentences. Data reported by Conway and Quarrington (1963) and by Soderberg (1967) indicated a *within* sentence position effect on stuttering which seemed to reflect the beginning of a clause. In fact, Soderberg noted that the unusually high proportion of stuttering on function words in his data appeared to reflect the fact that such words frequently occurred in early positions in clauses.

The important role of stress in stuttering was also reflected in a study of stuttering and word length. In an effort to isolate the effect of word length per se the present author (Wingate, 1967) constructed two lists of words, one made up of 30 two-syllable words and the other consisting of 30 pairs of single-syllable words. The two lists were matched phonemically: each pair of the single-syllable words was phonemically equivalent to one of the words in the two-syllable list, although all words differed in standard English spelling. Examples of the two lists are as follows:

fan sea	fancy
row stir	roaster
bay bee	baby
not whole	knothole

Through use of an apparatus specially constructed for the purpose, the list of one-syllable word pairs was presented, one pair at a time, to each of the stutterer subjects in a manner such that the subject said the words of each pair in rapid succession (but, of course, as separate words (syllables)). The list of two-syllable words was presented in a comparable manner, that is, one word at a time. The method of presentation had the expected effect: fluent utterances of the two-syllable words were unremarkable (that is, quite ordinary) and fluent utterances of word pairs sounded like their two-syllable counterparts being spoken with equal stress on both syllables.

The results were quite impressive: 73 stutters occurred on the 60 single-syllable words (a ratio of 1.2:1.0); 93 stutters occurred on the 30 two-syllable words (a ratio of 3.1:1.0). The difference is highly significant.

Note that the absolute amount of stuttering on the two-syllable words is greater than on single-syllable words even though there were only half as many two-syllable words. The ratio of stuttering on the two-syllable words is 2.5 times greater than on single-syllable words.

Stutters occurred in word-initial position for all words of both lists, a finding which has significance relative to matters of both initial position and difficult sounds. Since the initial phone in words of the two-syllable list were the same initial phone in at least half of the words of the single-syllable list, one would expect at least the same frequency of stuttering in both lists if a phonetic factor is important in stuttering. However, there was (absolutely) more stuttering on the two-syllable (shorter) list. This result is also of significance relative to the matter of word-initial position: the single-syllable list had twice as many word-initial positions, yet elicited fewer stutters, than the two-syllable list. This finding suggests that, although it is certainly notable that stuttering occurs so frequently in word-initial position, other influences evidently contribute materially to precipitating stuttering at those points. The findings of this study show clearly that factors associated with word length are a substantial part of this contribution. In this study the major dimension of the word length difference was that the long words had a prosodic pattern, marked basically by variation in stress over the two syllables. In contrast, the single-syllable words were spoken as separate syllabic units. (One is reminded here of the fact that stutterers can speak quite fluently to a pattern of one syllable per beat.) These findings provide evidence that prosodic factors influence stuttering occurrence even at the level of individual words.

There are obvious differences between speaking isolated words and speaking words in sequence—that is, connected speech. For present purposes we will limit discussion to such differences as they relate to oral reading, which we can accept as a modified analog of spontaneous speech.

A major dimension of the difference between the oral reading of isolated words and of connected prose is that the latter has a prosodic pattern with much more variation than the reading of even polysyllabic words. Interestingly, one of Brown's findings (Brown, 1938) was that his subjects stuttered markedly less when they read the words of the passages as a list of words than when reading the actual passages. Similar evidence comes from other sources (for example, Eisenson & Horowitz, 1945). The two differences might well be related; that is, the much higher frequency of stuttering in connected speech might, again, reflect the fact that prosodic features are a major dimension of connected speech.

A study designed to test this hypothesis was reported by the present author (Wingate, 1966). The objective in that study was to determine if the frequency of stuttering would be sensitive to prosodic changes in connected speech. The stuttering adaptation procedure seemed to offer the most suitable vehicle for isolating and measuring the effect of prosodic change. In the standard adaptation procedure, subjects speak (read aloud) the same material several times in succession, and the frequency of stuttering decreases progressively over the successive readings. For this study, designed to assess the effect of prosodic change, a special passage was constructed which would permit various changes in punctuation yet leave the sequence of words unchanged. It was thus possible to create several different versions of the passage, each having identical word order but differing punctuation. These variations in punctuation called for, and could be expected to produce, different prosodic patterns.

Comparisons were made of the frequency of stuttering when subjects read one version of the passage five times in succession (the standard procedure) with the frequency of stuttering occurrence when the same subjects read five differently punctuated versions of the passage one after the other. The results of the study are presented in Figure 11-2. The broken line, plotted for stuttering frequency in repeated reading of the same version of the passage, describes a curve typical for the

FIGURE 11-2. Stuttering adaptation with five successive oral readings of the same passage (A) compared to adaptation with sequential oral reading of five altered versions of the same passage (B).

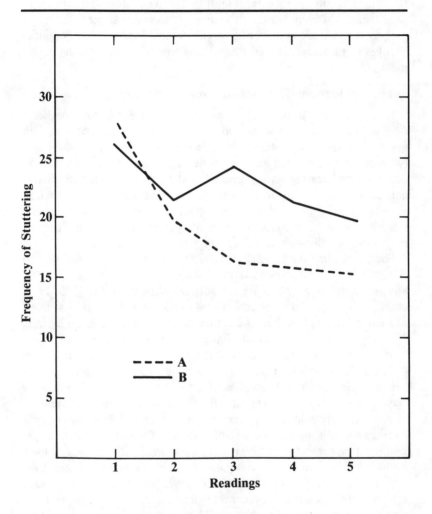

standard stuttering adaptation sequence, in which stuttering decreases progressively with successive readings. The solid line shows the frequency of stuttering under the condition of prosodic change, when the subjects read a slightly different version of the passage in each successive reading.

It was expected that the two curves would have the same level at origin, as they do. Also, it was expected that both curves would show a comparable decrease for the second reading; this is a routine finding in stuttering adaptation studies, including those using changing material, and appears to reflect a true adaptation (to the overall circumstances). In contrast, the points representing the last three readings are significantly different for the two curves. It seems clear that the typical progressive decrease in stuttering was obstructed by the (actually minor) changes in prosody required in speaking the differing versions of the passage.[5]

Indirect evidence: The ameliorative conditions

It has been known for a long time that stuttering can be very markedly reduced if the stutterer speaks under certain circumstances or in certain manners. These circumstances include singing, speaking rhythmically (with or without various accompaniments), choral speaking, speaking under reduced hearing acuity, speaking under delayed auditory feedback, and a few other circumstances.[6] An adequate discussion of these circumstances would require much more space than is available here; the interested reader is referred to the sources cited below. For the present purposes the following brief summary must suffice.

For a long time the beneficial influences of the various ameliorative circumstances were explained in multiple ways. Recently, however, analyses developed by the present author (Wingate, 1969, 1970, 1976, chap. 7, 8) support the deduction of a unified explanation: that in all of these circumstances there is a common core of influences. In essence, the common core consists of change in manner of speaking which involves, in substantial measure, changes of a prosodic nature.

The expression of prosody is a complex function which, at the peripheral level, evidently involves the entire speech mechanism in some way. At the same time, the laryngeal voice source is a major dimension of prosodic formation. By extension, then, laryngeal function is implicated as a significant element in stutter events. The implication of laryngeal function suggested by the analyses mentioned above (Wingate, 1969, 1970) led to a number of investigations of voicing and laryngeal function in stutterers. From many different angles this research has yielded evidence of irregularities in vocal control and anomalous laryngeal function among stutterers. Freeman (1979) has reviewed a number of these studies published by that date. It should be noted that certain earlier sources had also reported evidence of similar anomalies in stutterers (for example, Chevrie-Muller, 1963; Henrickson, 1936; Travis, 1926). This evidence is highly consistent with the findings, reviewed here, which indicate the salience of linguistic stress in stuttering.

One should keep in mind, however, that stress is not exclusively a laryngeal function. Some years ago Ohman's work (Ohman, 1967) led him to hypothesize that in the expression of stress all muscle systems participating in the speech act receive an increment of innervation which is expressed as increases in what may be called "effort." Subsequent research bearing on this area of speech physiology has lent support to Ohman's hypothesis. When the physiology of prosodic variation is better understood we shall be better able to understand a major dimension of stuttering. At the same time, study of the prosodic involvement in stuttering may contribute to an understanding of the processes of speech expression.

One last note, of a practical nature: Most current—including the supposedly "new"—methods of stuttering therapy, and many of the old methods too, incorporate techniques which involve prosodic manipulation (see Wingate, 1976; 1984b).

NOTES

[1]The report by Johnson and Brown that words beginning with vowels are less often stuttered than words beginning with consonants was evidently the first time this finding was reported as part of a formal experimental study. However, it had been noted previously in other kinds of reports. It also has been reported many times since.

[2]This remarkably reliable finding itself seriously qualifies the notion of "difficult" or "feared" sounds.

[3]The explanation of "psychological prominence" may be plausible in regard to grammatical class, word-initial position, early sentence position, and even word length. However, it seems heavily strained as an explanation regarding stress. Most speakers are only dimly aware, if aware at all, of where stress is to fall in words or lengthier utterances, even though, as native speakers, they intuitively stress properly when speaking.

[4]Although there is a close relationship between stress and meaning, Brown's discussion of meaning was limited to its semantic aspect.

[5]Since all versions of the passage contained (a) exactly the same words in (b) exactly the same sequence, there would be no reason to expect other than the usual adaptation curve if stuttering is really a "response" to "stimuli" which are somehow incorporated in the words. (The latter explanation is the classic, and standard, explanation of adaptation data.)

[6]Some of these circumstances are not as potent in their influence but deserve consideration in an overall account of ameliorative effects. See Wingate, 1976, chap. 8.

REFERENCES

Berger, K. The most common words used in conversation. *Journal of Communication Disorders*, 1967, *1*, 201–214.

Bloodstein, O., & Gantwerk, B. F. Grammatical function in relation to stuttering in young children. *Journal of Speech and Hearing Research*, 1967, *10*, 786–789.

Brown, S. F. The influence of grammatical function on the incidence of stuttering. *Journal of Speech Disorders,* 1937, *2,* 207–215.

Brown, S. F. A further study of stuttering in relation to various speech sounds. *Quarterly Journal of Speech,* 1938, *24,* 390–397. (a)

Brown, S. F. Stuttering in relation to word accent and word position. *Journal of Abnormal and Social Psychology,* 1938, *33,* 112–120. (b)

Brown, S. F. The theoretical importance of certain factors influencing the incidence of stuttering. *Journal of Speech Disorders,* 1938, *3,* 223–230. (c)

Brown, S. F. An analysis of certain data concerning loci of 'stutterings' from the viewpoint of general semantics. Papers from the *Second American Congress of General Semantics,* 1943, *2,* 194–199.

Brown, S. F. The loci of stutterings in the speech sequence. *Journal of Speech Disorders,* 1945, *10,* 181–192.

Brown, S. F., & Moren, A. The frequency of stuttering in relation to word length during oral reading. *Journal of Speech Disorders,* 1942, *7,* 153–159.

Chevrie-Muller, C. A study of laryngeal function in stutterers by the glottographic method. *Proceedings, VII Congres de la Societe de medicine de la voix et de la parole.* Paris, October 1963.

Conway, J., & Quarrington, B. Positional effects in the stuttering of contextually organized verbal material. *Journal of Abnormal and Social Psychology,* 1963, *67,* 299–303.

Eisenson, J., & Horowitz, E. The influence of propositionality on stuttering. *Journal of Speech Disorders,* 1945, *10,* 193–197.

Freeman, F. J. Phonation in stuttering: A review of current research. *Journal of Fluency Disorders,* 1979, *4,* 79–89.

Hahn, E. F. A study of the relationship between stuttering occurrence and grammatical factors in oral reading. *Journal of Speech Disorders,* 1942, *7,* 329–335. (a)

Hahn, E. F. A study of the relationship between stuttering occurrence and phonetic factors in oral reading. *Journal of Speech Disorders,* 1942, *7,* 143–151. (b)

Hejna, R. F. *A study of the loci of stuttering in spontaneous speech.* Doctoral dissertation, Northwestern University, 1955.

Henrickson, E. H. Simultaneously recorded breathing and vocal disturbances of stutterers. *Archives of Speech,* 1936, *1,* 133–149.

Johnson, W., & Brown, S. F. Stuttering in relation to various speech sounds. *Quarterly Journal of Speech,* 1935, *21,* 481–496.

Johnson, W., & Brown, S. F. Stuttering in relation to various speech sounds: A correction. *Quarterly Journal of Speech,* 1939, *25,* 20–22.

Lanyon, R. I. Some characteristics of nonfluency in normal speakers and stutterers. *Journal of Abnormal Psychology,* 1968, *73,* 550–555.

Lanyon, R. I. Speech: Relation of nonfluency to information value. *Science,* 1969, *164,* 451–452.

Lieberman, P. *Intonation, perception, and language.* Cambridge, MA: MIT Press, 1967.

Ohman, S. E. G. Word and sentence intonation: A quantitative model. Stockholm: *Quarterly Program Status Report,* Speech Transmission Laboratory, Royal Institute Technology, 1967, *2–3,* 20–54.

Quarrington, B. Stuttering as a function of the information value and sentence position of words. *Journal of Abnormal Psychology,* 1965, *70,* 221–224.

Quarrington, B., Conway, J., & Siegel, N. An experimental study of some properties of stuttered words. *Journal of Speech and Hearing Research,* 1962, *5,* 387–394.

Schlesinger, I. M., Forte, M., Fried, B., & Melkman, R. Stuttering, information load and response strength. *Journal of Speech and Hearing Disorders,* 1965, *30,* 32–36.

Soderberg, G. A. Phonetic influences upon stuttering. *Journal of Speech and Hearing Research,* 1962, *5,* 315-320.

Soderberg, G. A. The relations of stuttering to word length and word frequency. *Journal of Speech and Hearing Research,* 1966, *9,* 584-589.

Soderberg, George A. Linguistic factors in stuttering. *Journal of Speech and Hearing Research,* 1967, *10,* 801-810.

Taylor, I. K. The properties of stuttered words. *Journal of Verbal Learning and Verbal Behavior,* 1966, *5,* 112-118. (a)

Taylor, I. K. What words are stuttered? *Psychological Bulletin,* 1966, *65,* 233-242. (b)

Travis, L. E. A phono-photographic study of the stutterer's voice and speech. *Psychological Monographs,* 1926, *36,* 109-140.

Voelker, C. H. The one thousand most frequent spoken words. *Quarterly Journal of Speech,* 1942, *28,* 189-197.

Wingate, M. E. Prosody in stuttering adaptation. *Journal of Speech and Hearing Research,* 1966, *9,* 550-556.

Wingate, M. E. Stuttering and word length. *Journal of Speech and Hearing Research,* 1967, *10,* 146-152.

Wingate, M. E. Sound and pattern in "artificial" fluency. *Journal of Speech and Hearing Research,* 1969, *12,* 677-686.

Wingate, M. E. Effect on stuttering of changes in audition. *Journal of Speech and Hearing Research,* 1970, *13,* 861-873.

Wingate, M. E. Concurrence of stuttering instances and stress loci. *Journal of Fluency Disorders,* 1984, in press. (a)

Wingate, M. E. A rational management of stuttering. In M. Peins (Ed.), *New approaches in stuttering therapy.* Boston: Little, Brown & Co. In press, 1984. (b)

Wingate, M. E. *Stuttering: Theory and treatment.* New York: Irvington/Wiley, 1976.

Wingate, M. E. The first three words. *Journal of Speech and Hearing Research,* 1979, *22,* 604-612.

Chapter 12

Stuttering as a Cognitive–Linguistic Disorder

Curt E. Hamre

HISTORICAL PERSPECTIVE

Higher mental functions have been implicated in stuttering for more than two centuries. In the early 1700s, for example, Mendlessohn blamed a "collision between ideas"; in the middle 1700s Rullier felt that speed of thinking was out of phase with the capacity of speech organs to carry out instructions; and, in the early 1800s Magendie suggested that "organic" intelligence underlying speech was deficient in stutterers. In the mid-to-late 1800s speculation concerning the neural correlates of "thought" processes was stimulated by the discoveries of Broca and Wernicke in aphasia, and stuttering was seen by Chevrin, Marshall, Thomé, Hammond, Sankow, Rouma, and others as symptomatic of impaired function of motor or speech centers in the brain (Klingbeil, 1939).

That thought-language disruption is revealed by (or "causes") stuttered speech is a notion held by both lay people and experts. For example, this was a frequent explanation of childhood stuttering offered by parents in Johnson's (1959, pp. 164-167) study. More formal speculation of cognitive-linguistic malfunction as a source of stuttering includes (a) Bluemel's (1957, p. 40) speech disorganization view that in "stammering. . .mental speech is *quenched*, and thus there is a period of mutism in which oral speech becomes impossible"; (b) Sheehan's (1975) approach–avoidance conflict version of Mendlessohn's "collision between ideas"; and (c) Bloodstein's (1975) idea that *belief* (that speech is difficult) explains the origin of the disorder and "the moment of stuttering. " In addition, Eisenson's (1975) interpretation specifies both cognitive (perseveration) and linguistic (propositionality) sources of stutterings. Wingate (1976) has interpreted stuttering phenomenology within a language-speech ("vocalization") framework with an emphasis on prosodic and phonetic variables. Fransella (1972) described a regimen of therapy with major emphasis on reconstructing stutterers' thoughts and beliefs. And Stocker (1976) and Ryan (1974) have proposed therapy approaches which, they feel, control relevant language requirements.

In short, several variants of cognitive-linguistic paradigms of stuttering continue to be attractive to many students of stuttering. In fact, it is common to hear proponents of various "theories" of stuttering comment that "stuttering is a language disorder." For example, in Wyatt's (1969) book, stuttering is described as one of the *language and learning disorders in children* caused by a developmental crisis in mother-child relationships. And it is legitimate for her to use this "language" orientation to stuttering, because it derives from Freud's model of the link between unconscious thought and language function.

To examine stuttering as a cognitive-linguistic disorder, it is advisable to consider each domain (cognition, language) as well as the hyphen that joins/separates them. Bates, Benigni, Bretherton, Camaioni, and Volterra (1977, p. 280) described a rigorous examination of five positions on the interdependence among these domains plus a third, social development—no mean task. They pointed out that consideration of the possible permutations yields "something in the vicinity of 32,768 models for the interdependencies that hold among language, thought, and social development." (It should not be surprising, then, that there are an adequate number of models to accommodate whatever speculation might appear on stuttering as a cognitive-linguistic disorder.) Later, Bates (1979, p. 5) said that "proponents can be found for just about every one of these positions. . . and . . .the field would be in less of a muddle if researchers clarified their stand on what is, after all, nothing other than the classical debate on the relationship between language and thought."

The "field" to which Bates referred was language development. This chapter is concerned with only one dimension of this field, the development of normally fluent speech versus the development of stuttered speech. Our major goal is to clarify the main features of each of the 11 conceptual models of language in Table 12-1 and to render the field in "less of a muddle" by considering how each model has influenced explanatory models of stuttering. Relevant research and clinical principles will be included in discussion of each model.

The reader may also refer to the Appendix which provides a reference for each Table 12-1 perspective, in most cases an early major proponent of that particular view of language. The "stuttering derivation"

TABLE 12-1. Conceptual Models of Language and Stuttering:
Definitions

MODEL	LANGUAGE DEFINITION	STUTTERING DEFINITION
Sociological	Language is a code used by all connected by speech based on consensual validation.	Stuttering is a concept agreed upon by certain cultures.
Anthropological	Language is a mold for thinking—it determines thought.	Stuttering represents a distorted mental category for events which can be behaviorally described.
General Semantic	Language provides only abstractions from reality, a means of forming inferences.	Stuttering occurs as a response to inferences that speech will be difficult.
Psychoanalytic	Language is a tool for organizing and revealing amorphous unconscious thought.	Stuttering reveals nature of unconscious presentations.
Statistical	Language is highly variable information.	Stuttering is tied to implicit calculations of symbol redundancy.
Cybernetic	Language production is a self-regulated act.	Stuttering represents a disruption in speech feedback mechanisms.
Behavioral	Language is behavior and adheres to behavioral laws such as the law of effect.	Stuttering is classically and/or instrumentally conditioned behavior.
Pragmatic	Language involves a match between the available code and communicative circumstances.	Stuttering varies with communicative features.
Cognitive	Language is an "overlaid function"; it attaches to basic concepts.	Stuttering reflects malfunctioning conceptual processes.
Linguistic	Language is a system which can be described by logical rules of semantics, syntax, and phonology.	Stuttering involves restricted application of phonologic and prosodic rules.
Neurological	Language is a complex set of neural processing operations.	Stuttering represents an occasional inability to process language formulation and/or execution requirements.

references identify experiments or position papers based on assumptions of the language model while the "concept" column identifies a word that captures a distinctive feature for each model.

SOCIOLOGICAL MODEL

The first three models embody separate aspects of the most influential language perspective on stuttering, the "evaluational" (or "semantogenic" or "diagnosogenic") theory championed by Wendell Johnson. What we have labeled a *sociological* model is credited to de Saussure in 1915 (1959) who, according to Ogden and Richards (1945, p. 4), was "regarded by perhaps a majority of French and Swiss students as having for the first time placed linguistics upon a scientific basis. " He distinguished between language ("la langue") and speech ("la parole"); the former referring to the common word images and grammatical system in the brains of all users of a particular language ("consensual validation"), the latter representing an individual's use of language. Consistent with this view, Johnson's (1944) theory proposed that the absence of a word for stuttering in a culture meant the absence of the concept, so "so-called stutterings" (normal disfluencies) would be coded appropriately as rather uninteresting characteristics of normal speech. One clinical implication was that the members of one language community—the family of a stuttering child—should delete "stuttering" and the word image from their code. And many clinicians have lent consensual validation to such recoding; it is common to see "rhythm" or "disfluency" used in lieu of "stuttering" in their diagnostic reports, referrals, and publications.

ANTHROPOLOGICAL MODEL

The second model is termed *anthropological* because its core argument asserts that use of a particular language determines a particular way of thinking which is peculiar to that culture (Sapir, 1921; Whorf, 1956). This is a "strong" version of the hypothesis; a "weak" version is that verbal labels aid recall on some perceptual tasks, evidently by providing attentional focus for coded details (Brown, 1958, pp. 229–233; Carmichael, Hogan, & Walter, 1932; Lenneberg & Roberts, 1956; Osgood & Sebeok, 1954, pp. 192–203). In short, the evidence has vitiated the strong version and provided support for the weak version. Williams (1957) employed the strong and weak version positions in discussing how language molds stutterers' thoughts.[1] He pointed out that stutterers become accustomed to making statements, such as "I stuttered, " which foster an animistic belief that something beyond their control "just happened. " This exemplifies the strong position and, like the model from which it is drawn, is without experimental support. It seems likely that stutterings do, in fact, "just happen," and that this is another example of language ("I stuttered") revealing thought rather than determining thought. Thus, clinicians may lose credibility by suggesting otherwise to some older stutterers who "know it just happens"—those who are at Piaget's "formal operations" stage, approximately 12 years and older (Flavell, 1963, pp. 204–211).

Williams' (1957, 1971) appeal to the weak version is consonant with Johnson's (1955) "static analysis" procedure and can claim support from evidence (cited above) that verbal labels facilitate attentional focus. He provided a variety of descriptive examples and analogies which stutterers can cognitively attach (or "code") to modifiable portions of stuttering patterns and which may facilitate an understanding of the talking process.

GENERAL SEMANTIC MODEL

The *general semantic* philosophy can be viewed as an applied form of linguistic determinism (Johnson, 1946; Korzybski, 1933), but it is treated separately because its definitional cornerstone (Table 12-1) emphasizes that *all* observations are only inferences drawn from what is real and that all language (including first-order description) requires further inference. A so-called "fact," then, is only an abstraction, "an expurgated version, so to speak, of something concerning which we can only conjecture" (Johnson, 1946, p. 94).

Johnson's "evaluation" theory of stuttering development has been reiterated most regularly by Bloodstein (1961, 1975),[2] whose explanation of stuttering (cause and definition) (1975) appears to be derived explicitly from both of the aforementioned principles of the general semantic model: (a) Language is inference from what is observed, and (b) observations are only abstracts of the true state of affairs (facts). In his view, stuttering is caused by "virtually anything" which leads the child to *infer* that speech is difficult. In addition, stuttering cannot be defined "since no observations can be made to determine whether a definition is 'correct'." Without a definitional possibility, then, "the 'initial' symptoms, or 'onset', of stuttering" cannot be observed—"In the most basic sense they are concepts, not facts."

Johnson's theory of the onset and development of stuttering continues as a dominant force in the field. A recent survey (St. Louis & Lass, 1981) revealed that the majority of 1,902 speech pathology and audiology students from 33 states who participated in the survey prefer this explanation.[3]

PSYCHOANALYTIC MODEL

Considering the extent of Freud's contributions to neural correlates of language, his *psychoanalytic* model only represents his focus on one major *function* of language (Table 12-1). Travis' (1940) interpretation is a rather direct view of stuttering as a linguistic artifact that is revelatory of unconscious thought. And Wyatt's (1969) "language" theory, noted earlier, explains stuttering in accord with this model.

STATISTICAL MODEL

The *statistical* model is rooted in probability (the basis of information theory) and has achieved prominence[4] primarily because language is highly variable and "must be studied statistically" (Miller, 1951, pp. 8–9).[5] A basic assumption is that quantitative measures can clarify the nature of human language, and three measures which emanate from the model have been applied to stuttering: (a) Some words are used more frequently than others; (b) some are longer; and (c) in a string of six words, for example, some words are more predictable—more likely than others to be used in fifth (or any other) position; this is a "transitional probability" measure. Well-known findings for older (12 years +) stutterers (reviewed by Bloodstein, 1981 and St. Louis, 1979) show that stutterings occur more often on infrequent, long, and unlikely, words in an utterance. Goldman-Eisler (1958) also found that normal speakers' frequency and duration of pauses increased on "low probability" compared to "high probability" phrases. Similarly, a widely used aphasia battery (Goodglass & Kaplan, 1972) compares patients' performance on "low probability" and "high probability" phrases, and several aphasia batteries require patients to say words of increasing length, a difficult task for many patients with apraxia of speech (Hamre & Harn, 1979).

The statistical model, then, has produced measures which evidently tap lexical retrieval processes and aspects of speech production facility. In the language model taxonomy presented here, such issues are best pursued with reference to "cognitive" or "neurological" operations (discussed later), although they are often cited as "linguistic factors" (e.g., St. Louis, 1979). In fact, this model was rather short-lived as a linguistic theory, because it explains language in terms of linear "finite state processes," but language is hierarchical; "English is not a finite state language" (Chomsky, 1964, p. 21).[6]

It should also be noted that such measures would be inappropriate for studying young children in the process of acquiring fluent or stuttered speech. It appears that the question, "Which words or word combinations are most familiar to this child?" would have to consider individual differences (Nelson, 1981) rather than population norms.

CYBERNETIC MODEL

The *cybernetic* model of language, as proposed by Fairbanks (1954), was a *speech* model that emphasized continuous sensory influences. "Cybernetics" dates to Weiner's 1948 book by that name and refers to systems (e.g., thermostats) that automatically regulate themselves by comparing feedback (e.g., temperature of room) to output; such systems are "servosystems," and the Fairbanks thesis is that speech is guided similarly by feedback obtained from tactile and proprioceptive receptors in the vocal tract, and by auditory feedback.

One should remember that Weiner (1948) intended cybernetics as a model for cognitive, as well as motor, processes to appreciate its use as a conceptual model of language. Schuell, Jenkins, and Jiménez-Pabón (1964, pp. 118–133), for example, suggested cybernetics as an analog to a language system and referred to Hebb's (1949) reverberatory circuits ("cell assemblies") as a potential neural correlate of central feedback loops. More recently, one of Schuell's coauthors, Jenkins (with Shaw, 1975) argued for a model that recognizes the "all-of-a-pieceness" of speech–language–communication interdependence.[7]

One cybernetic interpretation of stuttering as a cognitive–linguistic disorder was provided by Mysak (1960, 1966). Because the feedback loop is the building block in cybernetics, we can summarize Mysak's model by suggesting that he created feedback loops for constructs discussed earlier—stutterers' (and listeners') misevaluations (Johnson), conflicts (Sheehan), and unconscious feelings (Freud). Although it is difficult to imagine empirical means of testing Mysak's thesis, the role of feedback in motor *speech* automaticity has been actively pursued. Because such studies represent one interpretation of peripheral activity during stutterings, they will be considered in later discussion of a neurological model.

BEHAVIORAL MODEL

The search for a mental *motif force* underlying a variety of human acts ("mentalism") was misdirected energy, according to Skinner (1938), and should be supplanted by a descriptive focus on what can be observed. He is responsible for (a) encouraging acceptance of the notion, "response," attached to simple and complex acts (e.g., rat bar-pressing for food, person defining "beauty"); (b) the assumption that many complex "responses" (operants) are lawfully tied to unobservable stimuli; and (c) the idea that response-contingent stimulation ("reinforcement") which is followed by altered frequency of a target "response" (law of effect) verifies the lawfulness of the stimulus–response link.

This position became a language model with the publication of Skinner's *Verbal Behavior* in 1957, the same year in which Osgood described an alternative behavioral model of language which he felt accounted for facts ignored (purposely) by Skinner. Osgood said, for example, that the ability to recognize a face from partial exposure required that we acknowledge links between "mediated" stimuli and responses (within the brain). Also, while Skinner said that an explanation of "meaning" was beyond the purview of psychology, Osgood employed "representational" mediated responses and stimuli to explain how "assigns" (words) become meaningful through association with other signs.

Skinner's model (of *language*) was thoroughly criticized in a now classic paper by Chomsky (1959), and several behaviorists (Jenkins, Palermo, Reese) in the 1970s acknowledged deficiencies of stimulus-response and mediation principles in accounting for language (Muma, 1978, pp. 32-33). We will not catalog those deficiencies here, but the reader may wish to compare this literature to Wingate's (1962, 1966b, 1966c, 1976) thorough analysis of learning theory explanations of stuttering. Such a study will reveal why research of the last decade in language and stuttering has focused on processes within the central nervous system—the "black box" from which Skinner had hoped to escape. This paradigm shift seems to have been occasioned by evidence that instrumental and classical conditioning offer inadequate explanations of stuttering (and language) onset and development.

The study by Flanagan, Goldiamond, and Azrin (1958) was the first to show that frequency of stuttering could be controlled using a 105-dB tone (and relief from it); stutterers stuttered less when the tone followed each stuttering, and more when that was required to turn the tone off. A spate of similar reports appeared in the 1960s and 1970s (cf. Bloodstein's review, 1981), including two of particular interest here. Cooper, Cady, and Robbins (1970) found that stuttering contingent presentations of "right," "wrong," and "tree" were equally effective in reducing stutterings; Daly and Kimbarow (1978) verified this finding with school-aged children using the same procedure. If one is not satisfied with the Skinnerian position that these words were all "punishment" because "response" frequency decreased, what accounts for reduced stuttering? A simpler explanation was suggested by Wingate's (1959) interpretation that subjects reduced stuttering frequency (when signaled electronically for each instance), because these signals drew their attention to speech.

Learning theorists have suggested how one might focus on external stimuli ("reinforcement"), even though events within a stutterers' brain, which are unobservable, may be required to explain stuttering. Shames (1975), for example, suggested that clinicians could offer approval (reinforcement) for positive *content* in stutterers' statements to alter their *beliefs*. He expressed the hope that "operant technology" would enjoy wider application (Shames, 1975, p. 315), but the foregoing review suggests that stutterers' attention, interpretation, and belief (internal and unobservable cognitive functions) are important variables. If such internal functions are essential ingredients of an adequate explanation, then the "death of behavior modification" (Krasner, 1976) may spur interest in a cognitive technology.[8] For example, rather than attacking the problem of delivering reinforcement on time—before a fluent syllable or two follow an instance of stuttering (M. Adams & Popelka, 1971)—perhaps we should acknowledge that stutterers interpret reinforcement (negative or positive) as information and that they may benefit from better "knowledge-of-results" (J. Adams, 1978).

PRAGMATIC MODEL

In recent years, there has been a major paradigm shift toward a "synergistic" (holistic, gestalt) orientation to language development with pragmatics at the core (Prutting & Elliot, 1979). Bates (1976) argued that "all language is pragmatic to begin with" and later developed propositions on a thought–communication synergy that is basic to the emergence of symbolic abilities (Bates, 1979).

A unique feature of pragmatics is its thorough analysis of communication variables. Methodology derived from this model would be the approach of choice for clinical and experimental research on stuttering as a "communication" disorder. Tough (1977) and Wells (1981), for example, have described options open to speakers in "modes" of conversation (e.g., description, narration, explanation, and emoting). Various studies revealing that stutterings typically occur at the beginnings of utterances may, in fact, only reveal that initiation is a factor for certain conversational modes.

Prutting and Kirchner (1983) have described an assessment procedure that is elaborated from "speech act" (Searle, 1969) theory. It would be interesting to know how stutterings are distributed within certain subtypes of propositional, illocutionary, and perlocutionary acts. This orientation may also be useful for individual assessment and as one baseline for evaluations of progress. For example, some speech act requirements may present more difficulty than others, for some stutterers, in terms of establishing and maintaining fluency.

We have observed clinically that some young stutterers (2–5 years of age) are more responsive to a "modeling" strategy than others. That is, if a clinician or parent converses with slow, prolonged speech, some young stutterers adopt similar speech, and this seems to transfer readily to extraclinical circumstances. We recently became aware of research by Street (1983) on "convergence"—the manner in which some parameters (tempo, pauses) of the speech of one speaker are adopted by a second speaker in a dialogue. In short, it appears that some stuttering children may "converge" more readily than others, and it seems likely that research on this and other pragmatic variables can provide insight on the nature and treatment of stuttering.

COGNITIVE MODEL

The major thrust of a cognitive orientation to language is that there are concepts and operations underlying language comprehension and production. Piaget's "mental schemas" are prerequisite to language development and his studies of cognitive growth represent the most extensive work on this perspective. Bates (1979), Bruner (1981), and Searle (1983) provide strong arguments that cognitive and pragmatic functions make joint and equal contribution to the earliest acquisition of "intentions," the source of symbolic ability.

There are findings which suggest that research on cognitive variables may also be fruitful for understanding aspects of stuttering. It is interesting to consider, from a cognitive perspective, evidence cited by Eisenson (1975) in support of "rigidity" or "preservation" in stutterers. The tasks used, such as quickly printing, alternating between upper and lower case letters, are similar to Piagetian tasks that are used to explore reversibility and other dimensions of operational thought. Wingate's findings that stutterers performed poorly on slurvian translation (1967) and on phonetic anagrams and backward speech tasks (1971) support the inference that aspects of operational thought may not be as "fluent" as necessary for fluent speech.

Sigel and Cocking (1977) detailed a hierarchy of processes which comprise a "cognitive distance" construct—the ability to symbolically represent events removed from immediate experience. They identified types and degrees of "distancing" strategies revealed in utterances, and a closer examination of this construct may reveal a relationship to spoken fluency. For example, there are fewer pauses in speech when material is *predictable* (Goldman-Eisler, 1958), and it seems that more stutterings occur when material is *propositional* (Eisenson & Horowitz, 1945). Both predictability and propositionality are evanescent constructs, but they probably involve cognitive processes which affect the efficiency of speech formulation. Cognitive distancing may be an operation common to both constructs; and the relationship between Sigel and Cocking's distancing strategies and frequency of stuttering is an empirical question. Of course, it is clinically useful to identify variables related to stuttering frequency, because such variables can often be controlled, in part, by the clinician. For example, it is our experience that fewer stutterings occur during picture description (less cognitive distance?) than when attempting to explain how to play a game, such as soccer (more cognitive distance?).

The research on "expectancy" by Milisen (1938) and several others (Bloodstein, 1981) has revealed that some stutterers are rather good at predicting words in a paragraph on which they will stutter; others are not. It is reasonable to offer a cognitive interpretation of this finding, namely, that some stutterers have more reliable personal knowledge of their stuttering than others. It may be that those who are good at predicting offer a better prognosis for improvement because they bring this insight to the clinical endeavor.

Stuttering therapy involves the client's cognitive participation (Wingate, 1976, p. 263). A common clinical principle recurs in the literature regarding the merits of having a stutterer assume responsibility for his or her therapy. While no one advocates pursuit of this goal with, say, a 4-year-old child, it is pertinent to ask at what stage of cognitive growth can a child be expected to play a role in therapy planning, implementation, evaluation.

Finally, we would recommend replacing an emphasis on reinforcement types and schedules with exploration of the type of information, or knowledge of results most useful to clients at various stages of cognitive growth. Williams (1971), for example, has provided clinicians with examples of information which seem to help stuttering children understand talking. Likewise, Guitar (1975) found that explicit knowledge of results on the status of muscle tension through EMG was helpful to stutterers.

LINGUISTIC MODEL

The stuttering definition derived from a linguistic model (Table 12-1) addresses only two linguistic systems (phonology and prosody) because stutterings, by definition, violate rules for those systems (cf. chap. 11, this volume). It may seem odd that stuttering researchers interested in "language factors" have not exploited linguistic methods of study, but there has been a substantial shift in emphasis within linguistics during the past two decades. In the main, this has been a shift from a focus on structure to a focus on language functions and individual differences in acquisition and use (Muma, 1978, p. 306).

A succinct statement of language from a linguistic view was provided by Jakobson (1941/1968, pp. 72–76; 1972) who said that speech requires two operations—*selection* of units (morphemes, phonemes, etc.) and their *combination*. A listing of the units on which stuttering frequently occurs represents the state of the art of much "linguistic" research on stuttering. For example, a review of Brown's (1938, 1945) so-called "linguistic factors" (St. Louis, 1979) shows that stutterings *tend to occur on* (a) sentence initiation, (b) longer more so than shorter words, (c) certain parts of speech more so than others, (d) consonants more so than vowels, and (e) stressed rather than unstressed syllables. In the main, these findings have been replicated by numerous investigators (see reviews by Bloodstein, 1981, and St. Louis, 1979).

A linguist, of course, would ask, "Are all sentence–initial, long, content words beginning with consonants stuttered?" The complete answer is more than "no"; that is, one should add that "the majority of them are not stuttered." The linguist might next inquire, "Have you examined the contexts—syntactic, semantic, phonological, and prosodic—of stutterings?" To which one might respond, "No...well, MacKay and Soderberg (1970a, 1970b) and Soderberg (1972) found that some phonetic environments are particularly conducive to stuttering." At which point the linguist might comment, "If that could be verified in a representative sample of spontaneous speech, then one should be able to describe phonologic rules for stuttering loci. However, once stutterings have been identified in a sample, then you would also want to determine if there are co-occurring syntactic structures, semantic functions and relations, and prosodic features."

Such an exchange points out that Brown's factors are not "linguistic" unless one adopts a taxonomic view of linguistics which was popular earlier in this century (Muma, 1978, p. 31). For whatever target one might be interested in (articulation error, stuttering, etc.), linguists would recommend that a traditional "parts of speech" notion be discarded in favor of constituent analyses—that target loci be examined for co-occurring verbals, nominals, adverbials, and adjectivals. Adopting a linguistic orientation involves the study of the *contexts* of stutterings rather than the unit (phoneme, part of speech, etc.) that stutterings occur *on*.

If stutterings conform to a linguistic pattern, or reliably co-occur with certain cognitive or pragmatic variables, then we would expect to find individual differences in such patterning. Such research would be most useful with young stutterers, since individual differences abound in acquisition of all linguistic systems (Nelson, 1981). General patterns predictive of stutterings may emerge; we now know that certain aspects of (nonphonetic) context appear to predict misarticulations from studies by Paul and Shriberg (1982) and Campbell and Shriberg (1982).

The clinical "pay-off" for contextual analyses of a child's own language corpus is more immediate. With a knowledge of contexts which co-occur with stutterings, a clinician can prepare materials (controlled syllable strings, speech act opportunities, etc.) that range from easy to difficult. And such analyses may provide a baseline for later comparison that is more informative and relevant than typical measures such as stuttering frequency, speech rate, and the like.

NEUROLOGIC MODEL

There is compelling evidence that the human brain is uniquely designed for linguistic operations (Lenneberg, 1967; Milner, 1976; Pribram, 1971). Table 12-1 identifies language and stuttering definitions which conform to a "neurolinguistic" perspective.

Some of the neurolinguistic research is of particular interest for stuttering. It has been known for some time that cortical and subcortical electrical stimulation produces speech arrest (tonic stuttering?) and syllabic repetitions (clonic stuttering?) in some patients (Penfield & Roberts, 1966; Ojemann, 1976). It is interesting that, even with precise electrode placement in the ventrolateral thalamus, Ojemann (1976) found that the disfluencies noted above occurred in a small percentage of patients and that they occurred only intermittently. Obviously, there are individual differences in neural speech processes, and their disruption is clearly conditional—dependent on contexts which are unknown but probably include ongoing phonetic and prosodic activity.[9]

Such observations may suggest neurophysiological processes which are involved in spoken fluency, but the reverberations produced by electrode stimulation of speech circuits undoubtedly differ grossly from the electrochemical fluctuations that occur naturally in the course of conversational speech. Apparent aberrancies in neural speech processes *do* occur in both fluent and stuttered utterances of stutterers (Agnello, 1975; Conture, Brewer, & McCall, 1977; Di Simoni, 1974; Freeman & Ushijima, 1978; Shapiro, 1980; Zimmerman, 1980a, 1980b, 1980c). While measures of peripheral neuromuscular activity, especially those of laryngeal structures (Starkweather, 1982), have been of prominent interest in recent years, several investigations have also provided compelling evidence that higher level, more central, speech–language programming deficits may underlie stutterings in conversational speech (Cooper & Allen, 1977; Hand & Haynes, 1983; Wingate, 1966a, 1967, 1971).

Zimmerman (1980a) favored a peripheral feedback interpretation of stuttering based on his finding that six adult stutterers demonstrated aberrant lower lip and jaw movement patterns, but he also pointed out that "the timing relationships and the kinematic parameters underlying them may be slaves to a superordinate spatial coordinate system." There are cognitive–linguistic inputs to such a "superordinate spatial coordinate system" (Kent, Netsell, & Abbs, 1979), and some inputs may be abnormal in persons who stutter. Coarticulatory disturbances also appear to be a central feature of stuttering (Agnello, 1975; Stromsta, 1965), and the *fact* of coarticulation demonstrates that preplanning (above a peripheral, "feedback" level) is required for normal speech (Buckingham & Hollien, 1978).

Buckingham and Hollien (1978) pointed out that "unquestionably, the initiation of the utterance is a particularly difficult event to understand." They offered a top-down ("open-loop") explanation of probable processes involved in utterance initiation, and it seems likely that stutterings may result from disruption of these processes; many stutterings occur on attempts to initiate an utterance, and it is illogical to propose that these occur because of *auditory feedback* anomalies (Wingate, 1970).[10] There is also growing evidence to support the hypothesis that motor speech is preplanned in sizable phonetic strings (Anderson, 1981; Flege, 1983). From this perspective, stuttering may involve a cognitive–linguistic disorder affecting preplanning (feedforward) rather than feedback processing. Empirical evidence supporting this view includes: (a) Word-finding appears to be difficult for many stutterers (Boomsliter & Solomon, 1963; Boysen & Cullinan, 1971; Telser, 1970; Weuffen, 1961); (b) central phonetic coding deficits are prominent in stutterers (Wingate, 1967, 1971); (c) durational inconsistencies of repeated utterances are pathognomic of stuttering; (d) lateralized hemispheric function appears to differ in stutterers (Hand & Haynes, 1983); and (e) coarticulation abnormalities (cited above) are a component of stutterers' speech.

One of the most intriguing questions facing the profession is the extent to which speech is regulated in a top-down ("open-loop") and/or bottom-up ("closed-loop") manner. Adams (1976, 1978) has marshaled evidence to support a closed-loop interpretation, but adds that "motor behavior is draped with more cognitive activity than most are willing to admit" (Adams, 1976). In the main, he reviewed evidence that the rate of firing and distribution of tongue muscle spindles is adequate to support the hypothesis of virtually immediate feedback in speech regulation. Likewise, Zimmerman (1980a, 1980b, 1980c) has postulated that stutterings may occur because brainstem reflexes are bombarded with highly irregular feedback from stutterers' variable articulatory movements.

While our view is that the weight of evidence favors the interpretation that stuttering is characterized by intermittent language—speech formulation irregularities, future research may support Zimmerman's hypothesis that impaired motor (kinematic) feedback accounts best for stuttering phenomenology. Progress toward an understanding of the neural bases of stuttering will probably be evolutionary rather than revolutionary, and research addressed to all aspects of neurolinguistic processing is needed. Ultimately, we seek a parsimonious explanation of why stutterings occur where they do in spontaneous speech.

NATURE OF THE SEARCH

It is wise to know what one is looking for before preparing the search, and Perkins and Curlee (1969) provided clear guidelines for framing questions. It is perhaps obvious that posing relevant questions concerning stuttering is more important than finding solutions to irrelevant, trivial questions. For students of language acquisition, Bates (1979, pp. 14-19) has delineated four types of questions pertinent to "cause" which she derived from an Aristotelian framework: *Efficient, material, final,* and *formal.* The fourth view ("formal") may be the wisest referent when one is considering a search of the "cause of stuttering." Bates said that "formal" causality refers to "the principles or laws that govern the range of possible outcomes in a given situation."

For a language perspective on stuttering, the "outcomes" of first-order interest are stuttered and nonstuttered utterances *and* their contexts (or "given situation"). What, then, are the "principles or laws that govern" utterances? While one might select principles derived from a myriad of models, the foregoing discussion should reveal our bias, namely, that principles supported by research on pragmatic, cognitive, linguistic, and neurological bases of utterances are the best candidates for revealing stuttering regularities—or "formal" causes.

Finally, *using principles of these four models,* a new direction for stuttering research emerges which requires development of hypotheses in the following domains:

1. *Descriptive:* To refine our understanding of topographies of stuttered and nonstuttered utterances;

2. *Developmental:* To identify characteristics of early (prelinguistic) utterances which may emerge later as stuttering, and to identify the principles which appear to govern acquisition of stuttered and nonstuttered utterances;

3. *Comparative:* To clarify commonalities between stuttered utterances and other errors of utterance production (for example, apraxia of speech, misarticulations of various types, "speech errors");

4. *Clinical:* To specify utterance variables that will be most germane to assessment, therapy, and measures of change during and following therapy.

NOTES

[1] This is an expanded version of one aspect of "a general interaction hypothesis" contained in a report (Johnson, 1959, pp. 236-264) to which Williams contributed.

[2] Bloodstein (1975, p. 52) has argued that his "continuity hypothesis" provides a clear divergence from Johnson's theory because Johnson "could not or did not choose to free himself from the notion that something could only be either stuttering or normal." Actually (and conservatively), that claim would appear to misrepresent Johnson's non-Aristotelian efforts.

[3] Wingate's (1962, 1976) examination of the relevant evidence suggests that it would be wise to pursue other explanations of stuttering.

[4] Perhaps the best known product of this model is the outline of a communication system (Source-Transmitter-Channel-Receiver-Destination) in the seminal publication by Shannon and Weaver (1949, p. 5).

[5] The interested student should see Carroll (1964, pp. 52-61), Lounsbury (in Osgood & Sebeok, 1954, pp. 93-94), Miller (1951, pp. 41-42), and Wilson (in Osgood & Sebeok, 1954, pp. 35-44) for excellent introductions to these issues.

[6] Difficulties in applying this model to language behavior are reviewed by Wilson and Carroll (in Osgood & Sebeok, 1954, pp. 44-47, 103-110). Chomsky's *Syntactic Structures* (1964) revolutionized linguistic theory, in part, by demonstrating the limitations of a linear view.

[7] This "synergistic" (Prutting & Elliot, 1979) orientation represents the current Zeitgeist for cognitive-linguistic-pragmatic models essentially unlinked to neurological constructs (Bates, 1979; Bruner, 1981). These models will be discussed later, but it is relevant to note here that the neurologically based cybernetic philosophy provided a good deal of the impetus for the favored focus on the "one-ness" of interactive systems.

[8] Note that Bloodstein (1981, chap. 5) continues to interpret stuttering as "behavior"—a "response" to a variety of "stimuli." He argues that the lawful relationship between stimuli and response (stuttering) is demonstrated best by the "consistency effect." The reader is encouraged to consider Wingate's (1966b, 1966c) examination of learning theory and the evidence that the "consistency effect" may be a misnomer (Hamre & Wingate, 1973).

[9] Milner's (1976) excellent review of postnatal CNS development reveals that individual differences also characterize findings from research on structural, histological, and EEG measures.

[10] Perkins (1983) is the most recent among many authors who have proposed auditory feedback disruption as a source of stutterings. However, some other malfunction must produce utterance-initial, silent, tonic stutterings which occur without so much as a glottal pulse.

REFERENCES

Adams, J. Issues for a closed-loop theory of motor learning. In G. Stelmach (Ed.), *Motor control: Issues and trends.* New York: Academic Press, 1976.

Adams, J. Theoretical issues for knowledge of results. In G. Stelmach (Ed.), *Information processing in motor control and learning.* New York: Academic Press, 1978.

Adams, M., & Popelka, G. The influence of "time-out" on stutterers and their dysfluency. *Behavior Therapy,* 1971, *2,* 334-339.

Agnello, J. Laryngeal and articulatory dynamics of dysfluency interpreted within a vocal tract model. In L. Webster & L. Furst (Eds.), *Vocal tract dynamics and dysfluency.* New York: Speech and Hearing Institute, 1975.

Anderson, S. Vowel timing and linguistic organization of articulatory sequences in jargonaphasia. In J. Brown (Ed.), *Jargonaphasia.* New York: Academic Press, 1981.

Bates, E. Pragmatics and sociolinguistics in child language. In D. Morehead & A. Morehead (Eds.), *Normal and deficient child language.* Baltimore: University Park Press, 1976.

Bates, E. The ontogenesis of symbols: Cognition and communication in infancy. New York: Academic Press, 1979.

Bates, E., Benigni, L., Bretherton, I., Camaioni, L., & Volterra, V. From gesture to the first word: On cognitive and social prerequisites. In M. Lewis & L. Rosenblum (Eds.), *Interaction, conversation, and the development of language.* New York: Wiley, 1977.

Bloodstein, O. The development of stuttering: III. Theoretical and clinical implications. *Journal of Speech and Hearing Disorders,* 1961, *26,* 67–82.

Bloodstein, O. Stuttering as tension and fragmentation. In J. Eisenson (Ed.), *Stuttering: A second symposium.* New York: Harper & Row, 1975.

Bloodstein, O. *A handbook on stuttering.* Chicago: National Easter Seal Society, 1981.

Bluemel, C. *The riddle of stuttering.* Danville, IL: Interstate, 1957.

Boomsliter, P. & Solomon, R. Symbolic development as a factor in stuttering. *Asha,* 1963, *5,* 781 (abstract).

Boysen, A., & Cullinan, W. Object-naming latency in stuttering and nonstuttering children. *Journal of Speech and Hearing Research,* 1971, *14,* 728–738.

Brown, R. *Words and things.* New York: Macmillan, 1958.

Brown, S. Stuttering with relation to word accent and word position. *Journal of Abnormal and Social Psychology,* 1938, *33,* 112–120.

Brown, S. The loci of stutterings in the speech sequence. *Journal of Speech Disorders,* 1945, *10,* 181–192.

Bruner, J. The social context of language acquisiton. *Language and Communication,* 1981, *1,* 155–178.

Buckingham, H., & Hollien, H. A neural model for language and speech. *Journal of Phonetics,* 1978, *6,* 283–297.

Campbell, T., & Shriberg, L. Associations among pragmatic functions, linguistic stress, and natural phonological processes in speech-delayed children. *Journal of Speech and Hearing Research,* 1982, *25,* 547–553.

Carmichael, L., Hogan, H., & Walter, A. An experimental study of the effect of language on the reproduction of visual perceived form. *Journal of Experimental Psychology,* 1932, *15,* 73–86.

Carroll, J. *Language and thought.* Englewood Cliffs, NJ: Prentice-Hall, 1964.

Chomsky, N. A review of *Verbal behavior,* by B. F. Skinner. *Language,* 1959, *35,* 26–58.

Chomsky, N. *Syntactic structures.* The Hague: Mouton, 1964.

Conture, E., Brewer, D., & McCall, L. Laryngeal behavior during stuttering. *Journal of Speech and Hearing Research,* 1977, *20,* 661–668.

Cooper, M., & Allen, G. Timing control accuracy in normal speakers and stutterers. *Journal of Speech and Hearing Research,* 1977, *20,* 55–71.

Cooper, E., Cady, B., & Robbins, C. The effect of the verbal stimulus words *wrong, right,* and *tree* on the disfluency rates of stutterers and nonstutterers. *Journal of Speech and Hearing Research,* 1970, *13,* 239–244.

Daly, D., & Kimbarow, M. Stuttering as operant behavior: Effects of the verbal stimuli *wrong, right,* and *tree* on disfluency rates of school-age stutterers and nonstutterers. *Journal of Speech and Hearing Research,* 1978, *21,* 589–597.

de Saussure, F. *Course in general linguistics (1915)*. New York: Philosophical Library, 1959.

Di Simoni, F. Preliminary study of certain timing relationships in the speech of stutterers. *Journal of the Acoustical Society of America*, 1974, *56*, 695–696.

Eisenson, J. Stuttering as perseverative behavior. In J. Eisenson (Ed.), *Stuttering: A second symposium*. New York: Harper & Row, 1975.

Eisenson, J., & Horowitz, E. The influence of propositionality on stuttering. *Journal of Speech Disorders*, 1945, *10*, 193–197.

Fairbanks, G. Systematic research in experimental phonetics, I: A theory of the speech mechanism as a servosystem. *Journal of Speech and Hearing Disorders*, 1954, *19*, 133–139.

Flanagan, B., Goldiamond, I., & Azrin, N. Operant stuttering: The control of stuttering behavior through response contingent consequences. *Journal of Experimental Analysis of Behavior*, 1958, *1*, 173–177.

Flavell, J. *The developmental psychology of Jean Piaget*. Princeton, NJ: Van Nostrand, 1963.

Flege, J. The influence of stress, position, and utterance length on the pressure characteristics of English /p/ and /b/. *Journal of Speech and Hearing Research*, 1983, *26*, 111–118.

Fransella, F. *Personal change and reconstruction*. New York: Academic Press, 1972.

Freeman, F., & Ushijima, T. Laryngeal muscle activity during stuttering. *Journal of Speech and Hearing Research*, 1978, *21*, 538–562.

Goldman-Eisler, F. The predictability of words in context and the length of pauses in speech. *Language and Speech*, 1958, *1*, 226–231.

Goodglass, H., & Kaplan, E. *The assessment of aphasia and related disorders*. Philadelphia: Lea & Febiger, 1972.

Guitar, B. Reduction of stuttering frequency using analog electromyographic feedback. *Journal of Speech and Hearing Research*, 1975, *18*, 672–685.

Hamre, C., & Harn, W. The effects of masking on apraxia: Evidence from spectrographic data. In H. Hollien & P. Hollien (Eds.), *Current issues in the phonetic sciences*. Amsterdam: Benjamins, 1979.

Hamre, C., & Wingate, M. Stuttering consistency in varied contexts. *Journal of Speech and Hearing Research*, 1973, *16*, 238–247.

Hand, C., & Haynes, W. Linguistic processing and reaction time differences in stutterers and nonstutterers. *Journal of Speech and Hearing Research*, 1983, *26*, 181–185.

Hebb, D. *The organization of behavior*. New York: Wiley, 1949.

Jakobson, R. *Kindersprache, aphasie, und allgemeine lautgeselze*. Uppala: Almqvist & Wiksell, 1941. [English trans. *Child language, aphasia, and phonological universals*.] The Hague: Mouton, 1968.

Jakobson, R. Verbal communication. *Scientific American*, 1972, *227* #3, 72–80.

Jenkins, J., & Shaw, R. On the interrelatedness of speech and language. In J. Kavanagh & J. Cutting (Eds.), *The role of speech in language*. Cambridge, MA: MIT Press, 1975.

Johnson, W. The indians have no word for it: Stuttering in children and adults. *Quarterly Journal of Speech*, 1944, *30*, 330–337, 456–465.

Johnson, W. *People in quandaries*. New York: Harper, 1946.

Johnson, W. The descriptional principle and the principle of static analysis. In W. Johnson (Ed.), *Stuttering in children and adults*. Minneapolis: University of Minnesota, 1955.

Johnson, W. *The onset of stuttering*. Minneapolis: University of Minnesota, 1959.

Kent, R., Netsell, R., & Abbs, J. Acoustic characteristics of dysarthria associated with cerebellar disease. *Journal of Speech and Hearing Research*, 1979, *22*, 627–648.

Klingbeil, G. The historical background of the modern speech clinic. *Journal of Speech Disorders,* 1939, *4,* 115-132.

Korzybski, A. *Science and sanity.* Lancaster, PA: Science Press, 1933.

Krasner, L. Psychology in action: On the death of behavior modification: Some comments from a mourner. *American Psychologist,* 1976, *31,* 387-388.

Lenneberg, E. *Biological foundations of language.* New York: Wiley, 1967.

Lenneberg, E., & Roberts, J. The language of experience: A study in methodology. *International Journal of American Linguistics,* 1956, Memoir 13.

MacKay, D., & Soderberg, G. *Action at a distance in speech production: Context-dependent stuttering.* Los Angeles: Unpublished manuscript, University of California, 1970. (a)

MacKay, D., & Soderberg, G. *The syllabic form of stuttered segments.* Los Angeles: Unpublished manuscript, University of California, 1970. (b)

Milisen, R. Frequency of stuttering with anticipation of stuttering controlled. *Journal of Speech Disorders,* 1938, *3,* 207-214.

Miller, G. A. *Language and communication.* New York: McGraw-Hill, 1951.

Milner, E. CNS maturation and language acquisition. In H. Whitaker & H. Whitaker (Eds.), *Studies in neurolinguistics* (Vol. 1). New York: Academic Press, 1976.

Muma, J. *Language handbook.* Englewood Cliffs, NJ: Prentice-Hall, 1978.

Mysak, E. Servo theory and stuttering. *Journal of Speech and Hearing Disorders,* 1960, *25,* 188-195.

Mysak, E. *Speech pathology and feedback theory.* Springfield, IL: Thomas, 1966.

Nelson, K. Individual differences in language development. Implications for development and language. *Developmental Psychology,* 1981, *17,* 170-187.

Ogden, C., & Richards, I. *The meaning of meaning.* New York: Harcourt, Brace, 1945.

Ojemann, G. Subcortical language mechanisms. In H. Whitaker & H. Whitaker (Eds.), *Studies in neurolinguistics* (Vol. 1). New York: Academic Press, 1976.

Osgood, C. Motivational dynamics of language behavior. In M. Jones (Ed.), *Nebraska symposium on motivation.* Lincoln: University of Nebraska Press, 1957.

Osgood, C., & Sebeok, T. Psycholinguistics: A survey of theory and research problems. *Journal of Abnormal and Social Psychology,* 1954, *49,* (suppl.).

Paul, R., & Shriberg, L. Associations between phonology and syntax in speech-delayed children. *Journal of Speech and Hearing Research,* 1982, *25,* 536-547.

Penfield, W., & Roberts, L. *Speech and brain mechanisms.* New York: Atheneum, 1966.

Perkins, W. Onset of stuttering: The case of the missing block. In D. Prins & R. Ingham (Eds.), *Treatment of stuttering in early childhood.* San Diego: College-Hill Press, 1983.

Perkins, W., & Curlee, R. Causality in speech pathology. *Journal of Speech and Hearing Disorders,* 1969, *34,* 231-238.

Pribram, K. *Languages of the brain.* Englewood Cliffs, NJ: Prentice-Hall, 1971.

Prutting, C., & Elliott, J. Synergy: Toward a model of language. In N. Lass (Ed.), *Speech and language: Advances in basic research and practice,* Vol. 1. New York: Academic Press, 1979.

Prutting, C., & Kirchner, D. Applied pragmatics. In C. Prutting & T. Gallagher (Eds.), *Pragmatic assessment and intervention issues in language.* San Diego: College-Hill Press, 1983.

Ryan, B. *Programmed therapy for stuttering in children and adults.* Springfield, IL: Thomas, 1974.

Sapir, E. *Language.* New York: Harcourt, Brace & World, 1921.

Schuell, H., Jenkins, J., & Jiménez-Pabón, E. *Aphasia in adults.* New York: Harper & Row, 1964.

Searle, J. *Speech acts.* New York: Cambridge University Press, 1969.

Searle, J. *Intentionality*. New York: Cambridge University Press, 1983.

Shames, G. Operant conditioning and stuttering. In J. Eisenson (Ed.), *Stuttering: A second symposium*. New York: Harper & Row, 1975.

Shannon, C., & Weaver, W. *The mathematical theory of communication*. Urbana: University of Illinois Press, 1949.

Shapiro, A. An electromyographic analysis of the fluent and dysfluent utterances of several types of stutterers. *Journal of Fluency Disorders*, 1980, *5*, 203-231.

Sheehan, J. Conflict theory and avoidance-reduction therapy. In J. Eisenson (Ed.), *Stuttering: A second symposium*. New York: Harper & Row, 1975.

Sigel, I., & Cocking, R. Cognition and communication: A dialectic paradigm for development. In M. Lewis & L. Rosenblum (Eds.), *Interaction, conversation, and the development of language*. New York: Wiley, 1977.

Skinner, B. *The behavior of organisms*. New York: Appleton-Century-Crofts, 1938.

Skinner, B. *Verbal behavior*. New York: Appleton-Century-Crofts, 1957.

Soderberg, G. The context effect: Stuttering as a function of interactions between phonetic features. *Asha*, 1972, *14*, 472 (abstract).

Starkweather, C. Stuttering and laryngeal behavior: A review. *ASHA Monographs*, 21. Rockville, MD: American Speech-Language-Hearing Association, 1982.

St. Louis, K. Linguistic and motor aspects of stuttering. In N. Lass (Ed.), *Speech and language: Advances in basic research and practice* (Vol. 1). New York: Academic Press, 1979.

St. Louis, K., & Lass, N. A survey of communicative disorders students' attitudes toward stuttering. *Journal of Fluency Disorders*, 1981, *6*, 49-80.

Stocker, B. *Stocker probe technique for diagnosis and treatment of stuttering in young children*. Tulsa: Modern Education Corp., 1976.

Street, R. Noncontent speech convergence and divergence in adult-child interactions. In R. Bostrom (Ed.), *Communications yearbook* 7. Beverly Hills, CA: Sage, 1983.

Stromsta, C. A spectrographic study of dysfluencies labeled as stuttering by parents. *De Therapia Vocis et Loquellae*, 1965, *1*, 317-320.

Telser, E. *An assessment of word finding skills in stuttering and nonstuttering children*. Doctoral dissertation, Northwestern University, 1970.

Tough, J. *The development of meaning*. London: Unwin Education Books, 1977.

Travis, L. The need for stuttering. *Journal of speech disorders*, 1940, *5*, 193-202.

Weiner, N. *Cybernetics*. New York: Wiley, 1948.

Wells, G. *Learning through interaction*. New York: Cambridge University Press, 1981.

Weuffen, M. Untersuchung der Wortfindung bei normalsprechenden und stotternden Kindern und Jugendlichen im Alter von 8 bis 16 Jahren. *Folia Phoniatrica*, 1961, *13*, 255-268.

Whorf, B. *Language, thought, and reality*. Cambridge, MA: MIT Press, 1956.

Williams, D. A point of view about stuttering. *Journal of Speech and Hearing Disorders*, 1957, *22*, 390-397.

Williams, D. Stuttering therapy for children. In L. Travis (Ed.), *Handbook of speech pathology and audiology*. New York: Appleton-Century-Crofts, 1971.

Wingate, M. Calling attention to stuttering. *Journal of Speech and Hearing Research*, 1959, *2*, 326-335.

Wingate, M. Evaluation and stuttering. *Journal of Speech and Hearing Disorders*, 1962, *27*, 106-115; 244-257; 368-377.

Wingate, M. Behavioral rigidity in stutterers. *Journal of Speech and Hearing Research*, 1966, *9*, 626-629. (a)

Wingate, M. Stuttering adaptation and learning: I. The relevance of adaptation studies to stuttering as "learned behavior." *Journal of Speech and Hearing Disorders*, 1966, *31*, 148–156. (b)

Wingate, M. Stuttering adaptation and learning: II. The adequacy of learning principles in the interpretation of stuttering. *Journal of Speech and Hearing Disorders*, 1966, *31*, 211–218. (c)

Wingate, M. Slurvian skill of stutterers. *Journal of Speech and Hearing Research*, 1967, *10*, 844–848.

Wingate, M. Effect on stuttering of changes in audition. *Journal of Speech and Hearing Research*, 1970, *13*, 861–873.

Wingate, M. Phonetic ability in stuttering. *Journal of Speech and Hearing Research*, 1971, *14*, 189–194.

Wingate, M. *Stuttering theory and treatment*. New York: Irvington, 1976.

Wyatt, G. *Language learning and communication disorders in children*. New York: Free Press, 1969.

Zimmerman, G. Articulatory dynamics of fluent utterances of stutterers and nonstutterers. *Journal of Speech and Hearing Research*, 1980, *23*, 95–107. (a)

Zimmerman, G. Articulatory behaviors associated with stuttering: A cinefluorographic analysis. *Journal of Speech and Hearing Research*, 1980, *23*, 108–121. (b)

Zimmerman, G. Stuttering: A disorder of movement. *Journal of Speech and Hearing Research*, 1980, *23*, 122–136. (c)

APPENDIX: Language Model References and Key Concept

MODEL	REFERENCE	CONCEPT	STUTTERING DERIVATION
SOCIOLOGICAL	de Saussure, F., *Course in general linguistics (1915).* New York: Philosophical Library, 1959.	CONSENSUAL VALIDATION	Johnson, W., The indians have no word for it. *QJS,* 1944, *30,* 330–337.
ANTHROPOLOGICAL	Whorf, B., *Language, thought, and reality.* Cambridge: MIT, 1956.	DETERMINISM	Williams, D. A point of view about stuttering. *JSHD,* 1957, *22,* 390–397.
GENERAL SEMANTIC	Johnson, W. *People in quandries.* New York: Harper, 1946.	INFERENCE	Bloodstein, O. The development of stuttering. *JSHD,* 1961, *26,* 67–82.
PSYCHOANALYTIC	Lafal, J. Freud's theory of language. *Psychoan. Quart.,* 1964, *33,* 157–175.	TOOL	Travis, L. The need for stuttering. *JSD,* 1940, *5,* 193–202.
STATISTICAL	Shannon, C., & Weaver, W. *The mathematical theory of communication.* Urbana: Univ. of Illinois, 1949.	INFORMATION	Quarrington, B. Stuttering as a function of information value... *J. Abn. Psychol.* 1965, *70,* 221–224.
CYBERNETIC	Fairbanks, G. Systematic research...Speech mechanism as a servosystem. *JSHD,* 1954, *19,* 133–139.	SELF-REGULATION	Mysak, E. Servo theory and stuttering. *JSHD,* 1960, *25,* 188–195.

APPENDIX: Language Model References and Key Concept—(Cont'd)

MODEL	REFERENCE	CONCEPT	STUTTERING DERIVATION
BEHAVIORAL	Skinner, B. *Verbal behavior.* New York: Appleton–Century–Crofts, 1957.	REINFORCEMENT	Flanagan, B., Goldiamond, I. & Azrin, N. Operant stuttering... *J. Exper. Anal. Beh.*, 1958, *1*, 173–177.
	HEURISTIC LANGUAGE MODELS		
PRAGMATIC	Searle, J. *Speech acts.* New York: Cambridge Univ. Press, 1970.	COMMUNICATION	Siegel, G., & Haugen, D. Audience size and variations in stuttering behavior. *JSHR*, 1964, *7*, 383–388.
COGNITIVE	Piaget, J. *The language & thought of the child.* New York: Harcourt, 1926.	CONCEPTS	Fransella, F. *Personal change and reconstruction...Treatment of Stuttering.* New York: Academic Press, 1972.
LINGUISTIC	Chomsky, N., & Halle, M. *The sound pattern of English.* New York: Harper, 1968.	SYSTEMS	Muma, J. Syntax of preschool fluent & dysfluent speech: A transformational analysis. *JSHR*, 1971, *14*, 428–441.
NEUROLOGICAL	Pribram, K. *Languages of the brain.* Englewood-Cliffs: Prentice–Hall, 1971.	PROCESSING	Eisenson, J. A perseverative theory of stuttering. In J. Eisenson (Ed.), *Stuttering: A symposium.* New York: Harper, 1958.

Chapter 13

Stuttering as a Sequencing and Timing Disorder

Donald G. MacKay and
Maryellen C. MacDonald

The present chapter takes up the problem of stuttering where Van Riper (1982) left off. Van Riper (p. 45) defined stuttering as a disruption of the simultaneous and successive programming of muscular movements required to produce a speech sound or its link to the next sound in a word. Anticipation of this programming difficulty can then cause struggle and avoidance reactions which are secondary, variable, and learned. However, the primary difficulty lies in the programming of sequence and timing, and Van Riper summarized several sources of evidence for this basic thesis. For example, asynchronies or lags have been observed in all of the speech muscles of stutterers, not only during overt instances of stuttering but also during their seemingly fluent speech (Zimmerman, 1980). The temporal coordination of voice, respiration, and articulation is apparently disrupted during fluent as well as nonfluent utterances of stutterers. Stutterers are also less able to repeat the temporal pattern of a sentence or sequence of finger taps than nonstutterers (Cooper & Allen, 1977), as if their neural clocks are less accurate or more susceptible to mistiming.

Van Riper next showed how timing disruptions might account for many of the basic phenomena observed in research on stuttering. An example is the rhythm effect, where fluency is enhanced when a stutterer speaks in time with a metronome or any other rhythmic stimulus (visual, auditory, or tactile), provided the rhythm is not abnormally fast. According to Van Riper (1982) externally generated rhythm may help facilitate the timing of motor patterns which are prone to asynchrony in stutterers. Fluency is likewise improved when stutterers sing because musical rhythm may help facilitate timing of the syllables corresponding to the notes.

Despite this evidence favoring his hypothesis (see also Perkins, Bell, Johnson, & Stocks, 1979), Van Riper concluded his book on a pessimistic note and gave three reasons for his pessimism. First, he found it "very difficult to evaluate the degree of support all of this scattered and often indirectly focused research lends to the position that stuttering involves a disruption in timing." Second, lacking a theory of how timing is achieved in fluent or unstuttered speech, Van Riper was unable to specify the nature and cause of the hypothesized timing difficulty. Finally, Van Riper was concerned that viewing stuttering as a timing disorder may be incompatible with data indicating that stuttering is related to the processing of auditory feedback.

Expressions of discontent similar to Van Riper's are rampant in recent literature. Preus (1981) calls the state of stuttering research "deplorable" (p. 13), and Bloodstein (1969) finds stuttering theories either descriptive in nature or so vague as to be unhelpful. As Bloodstein points out, to call stuttering a perseverative response, a symbolic sucking activity, or a miniature convulsion, only describes rather than explains it. Similarly, attributing stuttering to anxiety, stress, or delayed myelinization of cortical neurons is theoretically unhelpful unless a detailed causal explanation can be provided for at least one specific, real-time example of the moment of stuttering.

THE METATHEORY UNDERLYING STUTTERING RESEARCH

The present chapter addresses all of these concerns and another more general one which is relevant to virtually all research and theories of stuttering to date. It concerns the metatheory underlying past stuttering research. Under this metatheory, stuttering can be studied by itself, independent of both data and theories on how normal, error-free speech is achieved. In short, this metatheory views stuttering research as a field unto itself with its own special methodology, phenomena, and theories.

This metatheory explains why few studies of stuttering have made attempts to integrate the findings from normal speakers with those from stutterers (Garber & Siegel, 1982) and why studies of stuttering have proceeded in virtual isolation from the remainder of psychology and speech science. Moreover, this metatheory has provided a serious obstacle to our understanding of stuttering and its relationship to other speech errors. Any theory developed under this metatheory is, at best, a stab in the dark. Constructing a separate theory of stuttering is analogous to constructing a separate theory of backfires for explaining why cars sometimes emit explosive noises from their exhaust systems. To really explain backfires one must begin with an understanding of the principles of internal combustion which govern the normal functioning of an automobile engine. Similarly, to explain stuttering, one must begin with an understanding of the mechanisms underlying the production of error-free speech (see MacKay, 1969b, 1970a).

Of course there are good reasons why stuttering research has adopted a "stab-in-the-dark" metatheory and has proceeded independently of theories of normal speech production. The field has an understandable desire to provide immediate relief for stutterers, and theories of normal speech production from which to derive an explanation of stuttering, or any other class of speech errors, have been slow in coming and "woefully sketchy" (Van Riper, 1982). The reason for such sketchiness lies in the number and complexity of the processes that must be timed and sequenced in the control of fluent speech. First, there are many different levels or systems of control: the sentential system for controlling the sequencing of words in sentences; the phonologic system for controlling the sequencing of syllables and phonemes within words; and the muscle movement system for controlling and coordinating the laryngeal, respiratory, and articulatory muscles for producing speech sounds.

Moreover the processes within each of these systems are extremely complex. Considering only the lowest level speech musculature, over 100 different muscles may be involved in producing a single word, and each must get its appropriate nervous impulses at the required moment in the sequence if the word is to be spoken without disruption. At the time Van Riper (1982) wrote, both the normal events and the disruption of these events during the moment of stuttering were considered so complex as to preclude detailed theoretical description. Woeful sketchiness was inevitable.

However, recent years have seen significant advances in the understanding of processes underlying the sequencing and timing of speech, especially within the sentential and phonologic systems (see MacKay, 1982), and there is reason to believe that similar mechanisms may play a role within the muscle movement system as well. We will begin by outlining a general theory of speech production and then examine how and why the postulated mechanisms for timing and sequencing fluent speech may become disrupted during moments of stuttering. We shall focus especially on the question of where in the speech production system stuttering originates and on how this theory may account for phenomena such as the effects of adaptation and altered feedback on the occurrence of stuttering.

A GENERAL THEORY OF SPEECH PRODUCTION

The basic components underlying motor control in the theory are content nodes, each consisting of one or more neurons (MacKay, 1982).

In the case of speech production, the content nodes are organized into three independently controllable systems: the muscle movement system, the phonological system, and the sentential system. Content nodes within the muscle movement system represent muscle-specific patterns of movement involving the respiratory system, larynx, and articulatory organs such as the tongue, velum, and lips. Content nodes within the phonologic and sentential systems represent not specific muscles but cognitive units for controlling the movements making up a preprogrammed sequence such as a word or a phrase.

The motor program for words

To keep matters simple, we focus on the relatively small number of nodes making up the motor program for producing a single word. The components of a word can be represented by a hierarchy of interconnected content nodes (see MacKay, 1972, and Treiman, Salasoo, Slowiaczek, & Pisoni, 1982, for detailed evidence bearing on the organization of nodes underlying words). The highest level content node represents the concept underlying the word. By way of illustration, consider the noun, *practice*, which is represented by a single content node in the sentential sytem (see Figure 13-1). When *practice* (noun) becomes activated, its connected syllable nodes *prac* (initial stressed syllable) and *tis* (unstressed syllable) become primed or readied for activation. Unlike activation, priming varies in degree and summates over time up to some asymptotic level. Also unlike activation, priming is automatic and parallel in nature and requires no special triggering mechanism to determine when or in what sequence it occurs. However, activation must occur in a predetermined sequence if the word is to be produced without error. In the example under consideration, each node will be activated in the order shown in Figure 13-1.

Syllable nodes such as *prac* (initial stressed syllable) are part of the phonologic system and are connected to nodes representing phonologic compounds such as *pr* (initial consonant group) and *ac* (vowel group). These in turn are connected to nodes representing phonemes such as *p* (initial stop) and *r* (liquid). A phoneme node such as *p* (initial stop) is connected to distinctive feature nodes which are connected in turn to a hierarchy of muscle movement nodes representing patterns of movement for the various muscles such as the obicularis oris muscle for the lips (see Figure 13-1). The structure of connections between nodes in the muscle movement system (unlike the phonologic and sentential systems) is currently unknown.

FIGURE 13-1. The organization of selected content nodes within the sentential, phonological, and muscle movement systems for producing the noun *practice*. Numbers indicate order of activation of the units shown and the domain or sequential class of each node appears in brackets. See text for explanation.

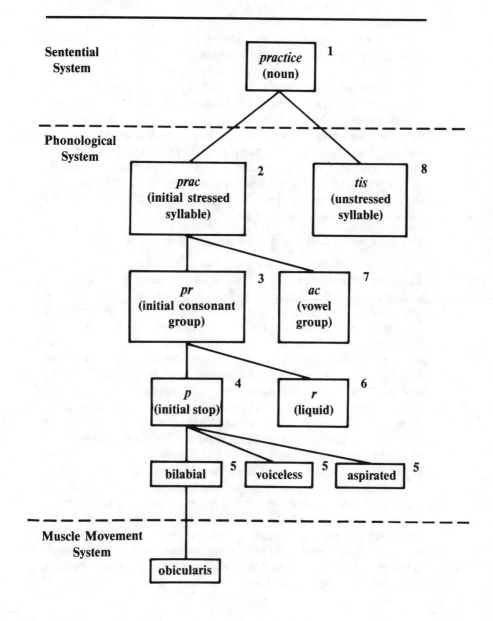

Nodes are hypothesized to share three dynamic properties which are relevant to the occurrence of stuttering and other speech errors: priming, activation, and linkage strength.

Priming. Priming is an excitatory input that active nodes pass on to nodes connected to them. The priming a node receives summates over time up to an asymptotic level, at which point a node is fully readied for activation.

Activation. Activation is the highest level of activity of a node. It is all or none in nature and is self-sustained for a specifiable period of time. Activation of the lowest level muscle movement nodes is necessary for behavior to occur, and the order and timing of activation of these nodes determines the sequence and timing of activity in the final output.

Linkage strength. Linkage strength is a long-term characteristic of the connection between nodes which determines the asymptotic level and rate at which a connection passes priming from one node to another. The main variable influencing linkage strength is practice: the frequency with which a particular connection has been activated in the past. Increased linkage strength yields lower probabilities of error for a given rate of speech (see MacKay, 1982).

The sequential activating mechanism: Sequence nodes

Activation of nodes that have been primed is achieved by a nonspecific activating mechanism which is responsible for activating an entire set or domain of nodes. Sequence nodes (capitalized in the examples to follow) are posited as a nonspecific activating mechanism for activating content nodes in proper serial order. For example, the sequence node NOUN is responsible for activating *practice* (noun) and every other node representing noun concepts. At any one time, however, a sequence node activates only one content node—the one with the greatest degree of priming. This "most-primed-wins principle" applies to the activation of every node in every system, including the sequence nodes themselves. In the case of content nodes, the node with the greatest degree of priming will normally be the one that has just been primed via its connection to an activated node which is superordinate in the hierarchy (see Figure 13-1). Sequence nodes are an independently stored set of nodes within each system, and the connections between them represent the sequential constraints for the classes of content nodes in question. For example, the sequence nodes INITIAL STOP and INITIAL LIQUID for producing the initial consonant cluster (*pr*) in *practice* are connected in such a way as to represent the fact that stops invariably precede liquids in initial clusters in English. This precedence relation among sequence nodes is achieved by an inhibitory connection. Thus, INITIAL STOP inhibits INITIAL LIQUID and dominates in degree of priming whenever these two sequence nodes are simultaneously primed by content nodes. As a consequence, INITIAL STOP can be activated first under the most-primed-wins principle as the most primed node in the domain of phonological sequence nodes.

The temporal activating mechanism: Timing nodes

Timing nodes represent the components of an internal clock which determines when the sequence nodes become activated. Timing nodes bear the same relation to sequence nodes that sequence nodes bear to content nodes. A sentence time node is connected to sequence nodes for activating the content nodes coding the components of sentences. A phonologic time node is connected to sequence nodes for activating the content nodes coding the components of syllables. And a muscle time node is connected to sequence nodes for activating the content nodes controlling muscle movements within the laryngeal, respiratory, and articulatory systems. Timing nodes, therefore, constitute the underlying basis for organization of the nodes into the three systems discussed in the introduction. Each timing node sends out pulses at specifiable intervals, but the mean pulse rate for the three timing nodes differs. For example, the phonologic time node must generate more pulses per second than the sentence time node since phonemes are produced faster than words (by a factor of about 5 on the average). However, the three timing nodes are coupled and operate in a correlated manner when simultaneously active: If the sentence time node is speeded up, the phonologic and muscle time nodes are speeded up proportionally. Whenever a timing node becomes activated it simultaneously primes the entire set of sequence nodes connected to it, and this priming summates quickly over time so that the sequence node with the greatest degree of priming reaches threshold and becomes activated.

Finally, the timing nodes for the three systems can be independently controlled. If only the sentence time node becomes activated, propositional thought without internal (phonological) speech will occur. If both the sentence and phonological time nodes become activated, internal speech will occur without overt movement of the speech musculature (even though the appropriate muscle movement nodes will have been primed). Only when all three timing nodes are simultaneously active will speech take place.

An example

To illustrate how the timing and sequence nodes interact to determine whether, when, and in what order content nodes become activated, we

FIGURE 13-2. Processes underlying activation of three content nodes in the phonological system (circles), their corresponding sequence nodes (rectangles), and timing node (triangle).

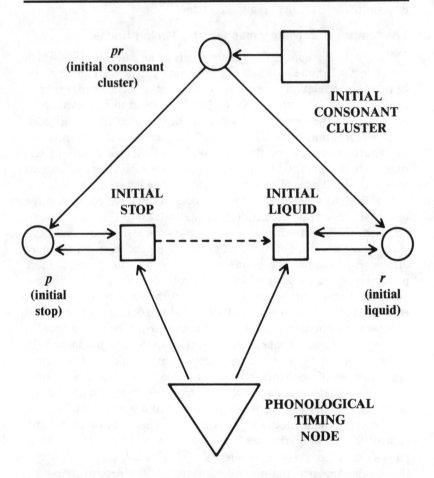

propose to focus on the first two phonemes in *practice*. Identical processes are assumed to underlie activation of nodes at every level in any system (see MacKay, 1982, for a more detailed account of these processes).

The nodes and connections between them which are relevant to this example are shown in Figure 13-2. Unbroken connections are excitatory, and the dotted connection between sequence nodes (rectangles) is inhibitory. The node representing the superordinate component *pr* (initial consonant cluster) is activated first. This simultaneously primes two subordinate content nodes: p (initial stop) and r (initial liquid) which in turn prime their corresponding sequence nodes INITIAL STOP and INITIAL LIQUID. The inhibitory link temporarily reduces the priming of INITIAL LIQUID relative to INITIAL STOP, and the latter is activated with the first pulse from the phonological time node. Once activated, INITIAL STOP strongly primes the entire domain of initial stop nodes and one of these, p (initial stop), having just been primed, has greatest priming and becomes activated under the most-primed-wins principle.

Following activation, INITIAL STOP becomes self-inhibited. This releases the inhibition on INITIAL LIQUID, which now achieves the most priming in the domain of phonologic sequence nodes and becomes activated with the next pulse from phonologic time. INITIAL LIQUID therefore strongly primes its domain of nodes, but having just been primed, r (initial liquid) achieves greatest priming, reaches threshold soonest, and becomes activated under the most-primed-wins principle.

ERRORS WITHIN THE THEORY

Error-free output occurs under this theory when an "intended-to-be-activated" content node has greater priming than any other node in its domain when the triggering mechanism is applied, that is, whenever the sequence node for the domain of content nodes is activated. The "intended-to-be-activated" node is the one that is receiving priming from a superordinate node in the output sequence, that is, the directly connected content node immediately higher in the hierarchy. This priming summates over time and eventually exceeds the priming of all other nodes in the domain, by time t_1 in Figure 13-3. At this point or any point in time thereafter, the triggering mechanism will activate the intended-to-be-activated node under the most-primed-wins principle and the output is error-free.

Errors occur whenever another node in the domain has greater priming than the intended-to-be-activated node when the triggering mechanism is applied. The fundamental cause of errors is that other, extraneous sources contribute priming which sometimes can exceed the systematically increasing priming for the intended-to-be-activated node when the triggering mechanism is applied. As a consequence, the wrong node becomes activated under the most-primed-wins principle, and an error occurs. Because of the shape of the priming function (see Figure 13-3), errors will be more likely the faster the rate of speech (i.e., the sooner the triggering mechanism is activated following onset of priming (t_0) for every node in the hierarchy).

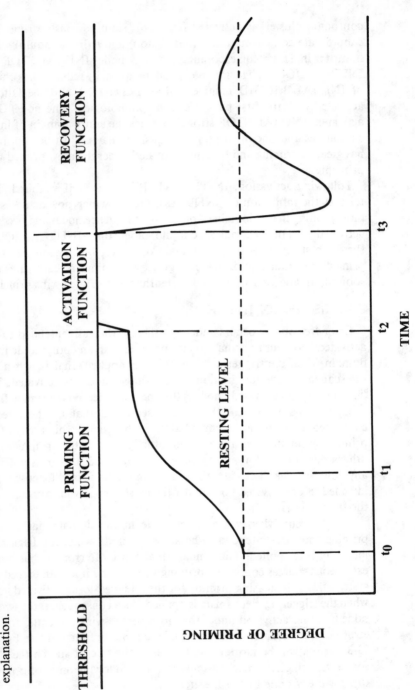

FIGURE 13-3. The priming, activation, and recovery functions for a node within a hypothetical domain of nodes. Onset of priming begins at a time t_0, onset of activation at time t_2, and onset of recovery at time t_3. See text for explanation.

Even Freudian slips are explainable in this way. Consider for example the Freudian substitution of *bottle scarred* for *battle scarred,* spoken of a general who is covertly believed to be incompetent as a result of "hitting the bottle." This covert belief independently primes the node for *bottle,* so that *bottle* (noun) has greater priming than the intended-to-be-activated node, *battle* (noun), when the triggering mechanism is applied to the domain of noun nodes. The wrong node is activated, with the resulting word substitution, because the triggering mechanism automatically activates the most primed node in its domain.

This example, of course, deals with high-level components, but errors involving lower level, phonological, and muscle movement components require a similar explanation. For all substitution errors the theory predicts that the intended and substituted components will belong to the same domain or sequential class (represented in brackets in Figure 13-1). The theory also predicts that, within limits, errors will increase as a function of rate of utterance (see MacKay, 1982).

FEEDBACK WITHIN THE THEORY

Auditory feedback is processed, according to the theory, in the same way as other speech inputs. Sensory analysis nodes constitute the first stage of processing, followed by "mental nodes," the systems of phonological and sentential nodes discussed above. This means that the same mental nodes provide the basis for both producing and perceiving cognitive units such as phrases, words, syllables, and phonemes. Top-down connections between nodes for a word are responsible for producing the word, whereas bottom-up connections are responsible for perceiving it.

Because mental nodes have both bottom-up and top-down connections, the possibility of reverberatory effects that can lead to stuttering exists at every level in every system. The reasoning can be illustrated for two hierarchically connected but otherwise arbitrary nodes: A (superordinate) and B (subordinate). During production, A becomes activated and primes B via the top-down connection. However, subsequent activation of B could lead to a reactivation of A because of the bottom-up connection required for perception involving both these same nodes. Self-inhibition following activation is hypothesized, therefore, to ensure that bottom-up priming resulting from the activation of subordinate nodes does not lead to reactivation of higher level nodes. Following self-inhibition, a normal recovery cycle with rebound from inhibition is posited in which self-priming rises above and then slowly returns to resting level (see Figure 13-3).

Self-inhibition following activation also prevents normal (undelayed) auditory feedback from causing stuttering. Feedback processed by sensory analysis nodes normally returns to and primes the same low-level mental nodes that were responsible for generating the just completed speech output. However, inputs arriving during the period of self-inhibition do not add enough priming to make self-inhibited nodes the most primed in their domain. As a consequence, just activated nodes will not become reactivated when the triggering mechanism is applied to their domain during ongoing production of the remainder of the word or sentence.

INTEGRATION OF STUTTERING INTO THE THEORY

Stuttering is similar to other errors in speech in several respects. Like all other errors, stuttering decreases with repetition or practice in producing a sentence (the adaptation effect; see Brenner, Perkins, & Soderberg, 1972) and with reduction in the rate of speech. Both these effects are readily explained under the theory outlined above (see MacKay, 1982). However, stuttering differs from other speech errors in at least three respects discussed below, which give clues to its etiology within the theory.

The surface characteristics of stuttering

Stutterers exhibit three characteristic phenomena (repetitions, prolongations, and blocks) which differ markedly from other errors in speech. Moreover, these three phenomena predominate in stuttering: Stutterers make other types of errors with no greater frequency than normal speakers.

Repetitions. Repetitions in stuttering usually involve a single consonant or consonant cluster, and only occasionally a syllable or monosyllabic word (Van Riper, 1982). In the present theoretical framework, it is as if nodes, once activated, have a tendency to be reactivated. The reason for this tendency is currently unknown but several possibilities suggest themselves from the theory. One is that the nodes of stutterers may manifest an abnormal priming and recovery cycle (illustrated in Figure 13-4). Under this hypothesis, priming summates abnormally slowly in stutterers, and rebounds abnormally sharply following self-inhibition. As a consequence, a just activated sequence node would have a high probability of being the most primed node in its domain, so that it becomes reactivated with the next pulse from the timing node. The result is, of course, a repetition such as *p-practice*, and the nodes can undergo this cycle again, resulting in a third *p*. However, the cycle cannot go on indefinitely, because reactivated nodes

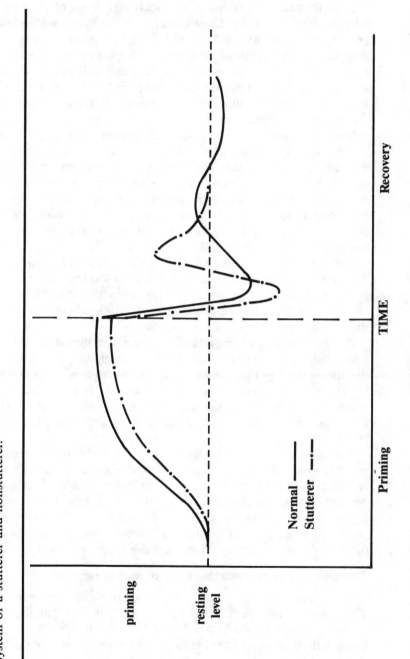

FIGURE 13-4. The hypothesized priming and recovery functions for a node within the speech muscle movement system of a stutterer and nonstutterer.

become fatigued and cannot rise to such high levels of priming on rebound from inhibition. Consequently they no longer achieve more priming than the next-to-be-activated node. Another reason why repetitions eventually stop is that priming for the next-to-be-activated nodes continues to summate during the time that malfunctioning nodes are being reactivated. Thus, the longer the period of stuttering, the more likely that the correct node will be activated with the next pulse from the triggering mechanism.

Major disfluencies occur under this account when several nodes malfunction as a group. However, minor disfluencies, undetectable by the human ear, may occur when only a few muscle movement nodes malfunction. This would explain why stutterers display slower transitions between sounds and greater asynchrony between lip and jaw movements than nonstutterers uttering the same syllables, and why utterances judged by ear to be fluent reveal abnormalities when analyzed by cine-radiography (Zimmerman, 1980).

Prolongations. Prolongations involve the unbroken lengthening of a (continuant) phoneme. A stutterer making this sort of error on *practice* might prolong the *r* to three or four times its normal duration. Descriptively, it is as if the articulators become locked in position during the production of the continuant sound.

Blocks. The most severe problem of stuttering is the inability to utter any sound at all, occurring most often at the beginning of an utterance but also at the beginning of words within an utterance. As Van Riper (1982) pointed out, blocks can be viewed as a special type of prolongation where one or more articulators (the velum, lips, or glottis) are "locked" in an obstructive position, virtually prohibiting airflow and preventing speech.

The cause of blocks and prolongations is currently unknown but the present theoretical framework suggests several possible mechanisms. One is that the nodes of stutterers sometimes fail to terminate activation because of a malfunction in the self-inhibition mechanism. It seems reasonable to suppose that malfunctions in the normal self-inhibition process may be related to the abnormal recovery cycle discussed above (see Figure 13-4), but details of this relationship remain to be worked out.

The distributional characteristics of stuttering

Stuttering occurs mainly at the beginning of words and utterances. The reason, under the theory, can be attributed to "anticipatory priming. " Note the numbers in Figure 13-1, which indicate the order in which the corresponding nodes must be activated for error-free output. Activating Node 1 simultaneously primes Nodes 2 and 8, but since 8 can only be activated after 2, 3, 4, 5, 6, and 7 have been activated, the priming of 8 constitutes "anticipatory priming" which summates during the interval that these other nodes are being activated. Anticipatory priming may, therefore, reduce the probability of stuttering by overcoming the slow buildup of priming in the intended-to-be-activated nodes of stutterers for the later components of a word or sentence (see Figure 13-4).

The level at which stuttering originates

Some stuttering theories attribute the problem to the highest level motivational and belief systems of stutterers (Sheehan, 1958; Johnson, 1938, respectively), well above the highest level (sentential) system discussed here. Others attribute the problem to lower levels, for example, the muscle movement system (Perkins et al., 1979), or even sensory systems (e.g., the stapedial reflex at the ear drum, Webster & Lubker, 1968). Still others such as Mysak (1960) contend that stuttering occurs at several levels and involves output components of many different sizes. However, there are four major reasons for believing that stuttering can be localized within the muscle movement system.

First, stutterers do not report stuttering during internal speech (J. Sheehan, personal communication).[1] Since stutterers frequently report stuttering when speaking aloud to themselves (Van Riper, 1982), reduced speaking anxiety associated with interpersonal communication cannot fully account for the absence of stuttering during internal speech. By way of contrast, other speech errors have been observed to occur with equal frequency in internal and overt speech. For example, Dell (1980) found that spoonerisms (e.g., *throat cutting* misproduced as *coat thrutting*) were equally frequent when normal subjects produced tongue twisters either aloud or to themselves. Within the present theory, this finding suggests that spoonerisms, unlike stuttering, can be localized within the phonological system rather than the muscle movement system. Secondly, the probability of stuttering increases with the number of muscle movement components that are involved. Stutterers are most fluent when they are instructed only to move their lips, less fluent when whispering, and least fluent when engaging in full-fledged articulation (Brenner et al., 1972). These findings are clearly consistent with the hypothesis that stuttering involves a disorder within the muscle movement system. Third, stutterers appear to have difficulty with the muscle movements for speech, independent of the phonological system which normally controls the overall sequencing and timing of these movements. For example, in response to a pure tone stimulus, some stutterers are slower than nonstutterers in initiating lip closure

(McFarlane & Prins, 1978) and laryngeal voicing (Cross & Luper, 1979) but not throat clearing or finger pressing (Reich, Till, & Goldsmith, 1981). Finally, stutterers show no deficits in the perception of speech. They never misperceive someone to say "ppppplease" when in fact the person said "please." This fits the hypothesis that stuttering does not originate in the sensory analysis nodes (which are specific to perception) or in the phonologic nodes (which govern both perception and production) but rather in the muscle movement nodes (which are specific to production).

The hypothesis that stuttering reflects a malfunction within the muscle movement system, of course, does not imply that higher level processes cannot contribute to the frequency of stuttering. High-level factors such as anxiety and syntactic ambiguity can affect motor control at every level and thereby influence the probability of stuttering (see MacKay, 1969a).

STUTTERING AND THE PROCESSING OF AUDITORY INPUT

So far we have been viewing stuttering as a disorder in the control of sequencing and timing. To determine whether this view is compatible with data relating stuttering to audition, we now review five observations which point to a connection between stuttering and the processing of auditory input: (1) Stuttering can be virtually eliminated for some stutterers with the flick of a switch introducing white noise within the frequency range of speech and loud enough to mask the stutterer's returning auditory feedback (Shane, 1955). (2) The stapedial reflex of the middle ear appears to differ between stutterers and nonstutterers. The stapedius muscle normally contracts 100–165 msec prior to phonation, thereby reducing the amplitude of eardrum vibration and attenuating the hearing of one's own voice. Webster and Lubker (1968) found that the stapedial reflex is less stable in stutterers than nonstutterers, and Horovitz, Johnson, Pearlman, Schaffer, and Hedin (1978) found that under conditions of anxiety, stutterers show less stapedial attenuation than nonstutterers. (3) Auditory processing of an about-to-be-produced word appears to guide and facilitate its production. For example, stutterers often release themselves from a block when someone else utters the word on which they are having difficulty (Barr & Carmel, 1970). Similarly, stuttering is ameliorated when stutterers shadow words they hear or produce words in unison with another speaker. (4) Some stutterers become more fluent when their returning auditory feedback is delayed by means of a recording and reproducing device (Huchinson & Burke, 1973; Novak, 1978; Preus, 1981; Webster, Shumacher, & Lubker, 1970). (5) Repetition errors resembling those of stutterers can be obtained in normal individuals by amplifying as well as delaying their returning auditory feedback. The effects of delayed auditory feedback have been the object of a large number of studies which we summarize briefly below. For adults, repetition errors due to delayed auditory feedback increase as a function of delay up to about .2 sec, and then decrease, with longer delays, but never disappear completely even with delays as long as .8 sec (MacKay, 1968). The peak delay producing the greatest number of repetition errors lengthens as an inverse function of age; .2 sec for adults, .375 for children aged 7–9, and approximately .75 sec for children aged 4–6 (MacKay, 1968), but not as a function of language familiarity: When bilinguals speak either their more or their less familiar language under delayed auditory feedback, their peak delay remains the same (MacKay, 1969b). Language familiarity only influences the *degree* of disruption at any given delay. Bilinguals make more repetition errors when producing their less familiar language under delayed auditory feedback (MacKay, 1970b), but practice in producing a sentence reduces the number of errors when subjects subsequently produce the sentence under delayed auditory feedback (MacKay, 1970b). The amount of disruption also diminishes with age, since practice, familiarity, and experience in producing speech increase as children grow older (MacKay, 1968). Mechanical distortions of the returning auditory feedback likewise reduce the disruptions resulting from delayed auditory feedback (Hull, 1952; see also MacKay, 1969c).

Theoretical explanation of the auditory effects

Until quite recently, feedback control theory has provided the main framework for explaining the relation between stuttering and the processing of auditory feedback (see Mysak, 1960). We begin, therefore, by outlining the nature of feedback control theory and its problems before addressing the auditory effects within the present theory. Under feedback control theory, feedback from sensory systems plays a direct role in controlling ongoing action, so that delaying this feedback results in control errors such as stuttering. Feedback control theory has never achieved a detailed explanation of instances of stuttering (Garber & Seigel, 1982), and on close inspection fails to explain many of the general effects as well. Consider delayed auditory feedback, for example. Why is there a delay that produces maximal disruption of speech? Under feedback control theory, disruption should either remain constant or increase monotonically as a function of delay. Why is it necessary to amplify the returning feedback in order to bring about articulatory errors? Why do subjects speak louder when their amplified auditory feedback is delayed? Under feedback control theory, amplified feedback should cause them to speak softer rather than louder. Why does practice or familiarity with a sentence reduce the effects of delayed auditory feedback? Under Adams' (1976) feedback control theory, practice strengthens an internal trace of the expected feedback, and successive movements are driven by the discrepancy between ongoing feedback and the expected feedback or feedback trace. This means that practice should *increase* rather than *decrease* the probability of errors for sentences produced under delayed auditory feedback. These observations suggest that articulation is not under direct feedback control (see also Siegel & Pick, 1974) and that a new explanation of the relation between stuttering and the processing of auditory input is needed.

The present theory provides such an explanation. Consider first the effects of delayed auditory feedback in normal subjects. Following activation, the nodes responsible for speech are self-inhibited and then undergo a normal cycle of recovery. This recovery cycle includes a period of hyperexcitability during which the nodes have greater than normal sensitivity, with a peak occurring approximately 200 msec following onset of activation and a return to resting level by 300 msec following onset of activation (see Figure 13-3). This explains why the delay of .2 sec produces maximal disruption of speech. When feedback arrives .2 sec after onset of activation, it delivers additional (bottom-up) priming to the just activated nodes that produced it at precisely the time when these nodes are hyperexcitable and most easily reactivated.[2] Amplification of the returning feedback adds further strength to the priming of the just activated nodes, and when these three sources of additional priming (amplification, hyperexcitability, and normal bottom-up priming) combine to exceed the top-down priming of appropriate nodes, these just activated nodes will be reactivated under the most-primed-wins principle, with an effect resembling the repetition errors of stutterers.

Errors under delayed auditory feedback decrease with slower rates of speech since slower rates enable temporal summation to augment top-down priming of nodes for an intended output. This may explain why some subjects speak slower at the most disruptive feedback delay (.2 sec) despite instructions to speak always at maximum rate: By speaking slower they can overcome the effects of the returning feedback and gain better control over the output. A similar strategy may explain why subjects also speak louder at the most disruptive delays, rather than softer, as usually occurs with amplified but undelayed feedback (see Siegel & Pick, 1974).

Consider now the relationship between pathological stuttering and the processing of auditory feedback. Under the theory, stuttering occurs whenever the just activated nodes receive greater priming than the nodes to be activated next. There are two hypotheses to account for this under the theory. One hypothesis is that the returning feedback is delayed by about .2 sec within the sensory analysis nodes of stutterers (due possibly to abnormally slow response times of these nodes) and acquires greater than normal amplitude due to a malfunction of the stapedial reflex (which normally attenuates the amplitude of self-produced feedback). As a consequence, the normal auditory feedback of these stutterers will achieve the conditions which disrupt the speech of normal speakers receiving delayed and amplified auditory feedback. The other hypothesis is that the nodes of stutterers evidence an abnormal recovery cycle, such as that illustrated in Figure 13-4. Both hypotheses predict that masking the returning auditory feedback will reduce the probability of stuttering and amplifying it will have the opposite effect. Both hypotheses predict release from stuttering when auditory input "guides" speech production. Thus stuttering is overcome when someone else utters the word on which the stutterer is blocking since the input helps prime the appropriate nodes to the level required for activation. Likewise, shadowing and choral rehearsal prevent stuttering by augmenting the priming of the appropriate or next-to-be-activated nodes. Finally, both hypotheses predict that the delay producing maximal interference with speech will be shorter for stutterers than nonstutterers. Further research is needed, especially to test the latter prediction, since systematic comparisons of the effects of different delays on stutterers' and nonstutterers' speech have never been undertaken. Studies examining stutterers under delayed auditory feedback have either used only a single feedback delay, have failed to amplify the returning feedback, or have neglected basic controls for speech rate, distraction effects, order of the delays, and possible practice effects over repeated readings of the same materials.

CONCLUSION

The present chapter began with a critique of the metatheory underlying previous theories of stuttering and then outlined a new and more promising metatheory for guiding future theories. Under this new metatheory, theories of stuttering must begin with a detailed explanation of how normal error-free speech is achieved. Only then can they explain how these normal mechanisms become disrupted during the moment of stuttering.

The chapter then describes a theory of stuttering which is consistent with this new metatheory and uses the theory to explain phenomena such as the effects of adaptation and altered feedback on the occurrence of stuttering. However, the most important contribution of the theory is that it postulates a specific hypothesis as to the level in the speech production system that stuttering arises. The theory also integrated two major approaches to stuttering which have been developing independently over the past several decades, one considering stuttering as a disorder of motor control and the other as a disorder in the processing of auditory feedback (see Garber & Seigel, 1982).

Futher research is needed to test the theory proposed here. More importantly, further theoretical work within the framework of the metatheory proposed here is needed to bridge the long-standing gap between normative psychology and stuttering research. Recent years have seen a great deal of research into errors in behavior (see for example Fromkin, 1980), and this area is likely to become a major concern of psychological models over the next decade (see Neisser, 1982). It would be unfortunate if stuttering does not become part of that larger concern since bridging the gap has benefits for both psychology and stuttering research. Under the metatheory proposed here, an understanding of the processes underlying fluent speech is necessary in order to understand its disruption in a complex speech disorder such as stuttering. But it is equally true that transient malfunctions such as stuttering need to be explained in theories of normal behavior, since a complete and adequate theory must be capable of predicting all of the ways that an output system will break down.

NOTES

[1] C. Van Riper, in a subsequent personal communication, reports that some stutterers do claim to stutter during internal speech. This unexpected difference in expert opinion suggests that this issue warrants empirical investigation in the manner illustrated in MacKay (1982, Figure 1) and Dell (1980).

[2] For purposes of exposition this explanation has been simplified by ignoring (a) the time it takes for the muscles to come into action following onset of activation of the muscle movement nodes, (b) the time it takes airborn auditory feedback to arrive at the ears, (c) the time it takes the sensory analysis nodes to process the feedback and delivery bottom-up priming to the lowest level phonologic nodes, and (d) the time it takes to pass this priming on to the just activated muscle movement nodes.

REFERENCES

Adams, J. A. Issues for a closed-loop theory of motor learning. In G. E. Stelmach (Ed.), *Motor control: Issues and trends.* New York: Academic Press, 1976.

Barr, D. F., & Carmel, N. R. Stuttering inhibition with the high frequency narrow band masking noise. *Journal of Auditory Research,* 1970, *10,* 59–61.

Bloodstein, O. *Handbook of stuttering.* Chicago: National Easter Seal Society for Crippled Children and Adults, 1969.

Brenner, N. C., Perkins, W. H., & Soderberg, G. A. The effect of rehearsal on frequency of stuttering. *Journal of Speech and Hearing Research,* 1972, *15,* 483–486.

Cooper, M. H. & Allen, G. D. Timing control accuracy in normal speakers and stutterers. *Journal of Speech and Hearing Research,* 1977, *20,* 55–71.

Cross, D. E., & Luper, H. L. Voice reaction time of stuttering and nonstuttering children. *Journal of Fluency Disorders,* 1979, *4,* 661–68.

Dell, G. *Phonological and lexical encoding in speech production: An analysis of naturally occurring and experimentally elicited speech errors.* Unpublished doctoral dissertation, University of Toronto, 1980.

Fromkin, V. A. *Errors in linguistic performance: Slips of the tongue, ear, pen, and hand.* New York: Academic Press, 1980.

Garber, S. R., & Siegel, G. M. Feedback and motor control in stuttering. In D. K. Routh (Ed.), *Learning, speech, and the complex effects of punishment.* New York: Plenum Press, 1982.

Horovitz, L. J., Johnson, S. B., Pearlman, R. C., Schaffer, E. J., & Hedin, A. K. Stapedial reflex and anxiety in fluent and disfluent speakers. *Journal of Speech and Hearing Research,* 1978, *21,* 762–767.

Huchinson, J. M., & Burke, K. M. An investigation of the effects of temporal alteration in auditory feedback upon stutterers and clutterers. *Journal of Communication Disorders,* 1973, *6,* 193–205.

Hull, F. M. *Experimental investigation of speech disturbance as a function of the frequency distortion of delayed auditory feedback.* Unpublished PhD thesis, University of Illinois, 1952.

Johnson, W. The role of evaluation in stuttering behavior. *Journal of Speech Disorders,* 1938, *3,* 85–89.

MacKay, D. G. Metamorphosis of a critical interval: Age-linked changes in the delay in auditory feedback that produces maximal disruption of speech. *Journal of the Acoustical Society of America,* 1968, *19,* 811–21.

MacKay, D. G. Effects of ambiguity on stuttering: Towards a theory of speech production at the semantic level. *Kybernetik,* 1969, *5,* 195–208. (a)

MacKay, D. G. Forward and backward masking in motor systems. *Kybernetik,* 1969, *6,* 57–64. (b)

MacKay, D. G. To speak with an accent: Effects of nasal distortion on stuttering under delayed auditory feedback. *Perception and Psychophysics,* 1969, *5,* 183–88. (c)

MacKay, D. G. Context-dependent stuttering. *Kybernetik,* 1970, *7,* 1–9. (a)

MacKay, D. G. How does language familiarity influence stuttering under delayed auditory feedback? *Perceptual and Motor Skills,* 1970, *30,* 655–69. (b)

MacKay, D. G. The structure of words and syllables: Evidence from errors in speech. *Cognitive Psychology,* 1972, *3,* 210–27.

MacKay, D. G. The problems of flexibility, fluency, and speed–accuracy trade-off in skilled behavior. *Psychological Review,* 1982, *89,* 483–506.

McFarlane, S. J., & Prins, D. Neural response time of stutterers and nonstutterers. *Journal of Speech and Hearing Research,* 1978, *21,* 768–78.

Mysak, E. Servo theory and stuttering. *Journal of Speech and Hearing Disorders,* 1960, *25,* 188–195.

Novak, A. The influence of delayed auditory feedback on stutterers. *Folia Phoniatrica,* 1978, *30,* 278–85.

Neisser, U. Understanding psychological man. *Psychology Today,* 1982, *16,* 40.

Perkins, W. H., Bell, J., Johnson, L, & Stocks, J. Phone rate and the effective planning time hypothesis of stuttering. *Journal of Speech and Hearing Research,* 1979, *22,* 747–55.

Preus, A. *Identifying subgroups of stutterers.* Oslo: University of Oslo Press, 1981.

Reich, A., Till, J., & Goldsmith, H. Laryngeal and manual reaction times of stuttering and nonstuttering adults. *Journal of Speech and Hearing Research,* 1981, *24,* 192–196.

Shane, M. L. S. Effect on stuttering of alteration of auditory feedback. In W. Johnson (Ed.), *Stuttering in children and adults.* Minneapolis: University of Minnesota Press, 1955.

Shane, M. L. S. Effect on stuttering of alternation in auditory feedback. In W. Johnson & R. R. Levitenneger (Eds.), *Stuttering in children and adults.* Minneapolis: University of Minnesota Press, 1955.

Sheehan, J. G. Conflict theory of stuttering. In J. Eisenson (Ed.), *Stuttering: A symposium.* New York: Harper & Row, 1958.

Siegel, G. M., & Pick, H. L. Auditory feedback in the regulation of voice. *Journal of the Acoustical Society of America,* 1974, *56,* 1618–1624.

Treiman, R., Salasoo, A., Slowiaczek, L., & Pisoni, D. Effects of syllable structure on adults' phoneme monitoring performance. *Research on Speech Perception Progress Report* 8. Bloomington: Indiana University, 1982.

Van Riper, C. *The nature of stuttering.* Englewood Cliffs, NJ: Prentice–Hall, 1982.

Webster, R., & Lubker, R. B. Interrelationships among fluency producing variables in stuttered speech. *Journal of Speech and Hearing Research,* 1968, *11,* 219–23.

Webster, R. L., Schumacher, S. J., & Lubker, R. B. Changes in stuttering frequency as a function of various intervals of delayed auditory feedback. *Journal of Abnormal Psychology,* 1970, *75,* 45–49.

Zimmerman, G. N. Articulatory behavior associated with stuttering: A cineradiographic analysis. *Journal of Speech and Hearing Disorders,* 1980, *23,* 108–21.

Chapter 14

Stuttering as a Temporal Programming Disorder

Ray D. Kent

INTRODUCTION

This chapter is based on a commentary (Kent, 1983) written in response to a paper by Andrews, Craig, Feyer, Hoddinott, Howie, and Neilson (1983). The primary purpose of the Andrews et al. paper was to assert the major replicated facts about stuttering; the intent of the commentary was to evaluate the theoretical interpretation given to these facts by Andrews et al. and to suggest an alternate interpretation. I hesitate to call this alternate interpretation a theory. It might be more correctly called a theoretical perspective. However, it does have some of the attributes of a theory, one of which is that it leads to testable predictions about stuttering. However, as the reader will notice, this theoretical interpretation is not so fully developed as a theory ought to be.

The crux of this interpretation is that a primary difference between stutterers and nonstutterers lies in their capacity to generate temporal programs, or time structures of action. By temporal program I do not mean the extreme version of program described in the motor control literature that speaks of preplanned movements which are executed in the desired sequence without any reliance on feedback (Keele, 1968). Rather, the temporal program envisaged here is essentially a time plan or pattern useful for both perceptual processing of sequential patterns and for the regulation of motor sequences. The temporal program is not a means to motor regulation in the absence of feedback. Quite the contrary, it is a means to the effective use of feedback by giving specifications for the timing and nature of feedback information most suited to accomplish motor objectives. In like manner, Sternberg, Monsell, Knoll, and Wright (1978) proposed that sequence control can involve both advance planning and feedback. One possible role of feedback is to function as a cue to trigger onsets of subunits in a sequence. The operation of the temporal program in speech production may involve sensory and motor components so inextricably meshed, from the very beginning of movement control, that the sensory–motor distinction loses its traditional meaning (cf. Reed, 1982).

In their careful review of the literature on stuttering, Andrews et al. (1983) described several characteristics of stutterers. There is not space in this chapter to consider these characteristics in detail, but I want to draw attention to some that may relate to an hypothesized deficiency in the establishment and maintenance of temporal patterns used for the processing of auditory stimuli and the motor regulation of speech. This discussion will emphasize some points of long standing in the literature on stuttering, in particular, sex differences, anomalous hemispheric asymmetry, perceptual–motor deficits, and fluency inducing conditions.

Andrews et al. note that as a group stutterers "differ in IQ-distribution, are late and poor talkers, have difficulties in stimulus recognition/recall in complex auditory tasks, and lag in tests of sensory-motor response. " The salient presenting symptom of stuttering is an impairment in the rhythm or fluency of speech. As Andrews et al. remark, "there is a consensus that repetitions and prolongations are necessary and sufficient for the diagnosis of stuttering to be made. " Of course, a diagnosis is rarely made apart from a consideration of history; otherwise the distinctions between verbal apraxia and stuttering would be even more troublesome than they are (Rosenbek, 1980). Repetitions and prolongations are not unique to stuttering, and this point becomes important when we consider the general issue of speech motor control in the face of some kind of obstacle to communication, whether it be internal (such as neurologic disorder) or external (such as anxiety-producing social situations). Obviously, we must distinguish between stuttering as a symptom (and not uniquely associated with the diagnostic category of "stutterer") and stuttering as a diagnosis.

Andrews et al. tell us some other characteristics about the stutterer: He (a deliberate departure from nonsexist writing given that male stutterers outnumber females by about 3 to 1) probably has a genetic predisposition to stutter. One can defend the proposition that boys, whether they stutter or not, "are late and poor talkers, have difficulties in stimulus recognition/recall in complex auditory tasks, and lag in tests of sensory–motor response.[1] That is, boys differ from girls in ways that stutterers typically differ from nonstutterers.

ANOMALOUS HEMISPHERIC ASYMMETRIES

The possibility of anomalous hemispheric dominance in stutterers is an idea of long standing. Andrews et al. consider possible differences in lateralization from Moore and Haynes' (1980) perspective that "stuttering occurs because right hemisphere processing which is claimed not to be a segmental processor, has a reduced capacity to handle the temporal segmental relationships necessary to the production of individual phrases or utterances. " Andrews et al. suggest that this proposal needs further evidence to show that the right hemisphere processes verbal material *independent* of the time dimension. However, this is a very narrow and perhaps misleading view of a large and complicated literature on hemispheric differences. I believe that a more accurate perspective is that both hemispheres are capable of processing in the time domain but differ in their preferred temporal ranges. Clinical and experimental evidence (reviewed by Hammond, 1982, and Kent, 1984) and cytoarchitectonic asymmetries of the auditory cortices (Seldon, 1981a, 1981b) indicate that the left hemisphere is capable of finer temporal resolution than the right. Evidence mounts that the nondominant hemisphere may contribute primarily to the processing of information distributed over relatively long intervals, such as linguistic context (Dwyer & Rinn, 1981), affective and prosodic content (Ross, Harney, de Lacoste-Utamsing, & Purdy, 1981), speaker recognition (Van Lancker & Canter, 1982) and various other complex linguistic functions (Wapner, Hamby, & Gardner, 1981; Delis, Wapner, Gardner, & Moses, 1983). Thus, the left and right hemispheres may process simultaneously different temporal ranges of input (or output) information. If so, a central processor is charged with the role of integrating these two lines of temporal processing.

Attention frequently has been drawn to similarities between stuttering and certain neurologic speech disorders. Some investigators have gone so far as to propose that stuttering is a form of apraxia. Caplan (1972) concluded from a comparison of stutterers with persons having a predominantly expressive aphasia with coexisting anomia and apraxia, that the mutual patterns of difficulty included: difficulty with initiation, with longer words, with consonants more than with vowels, and generally with intricate patterns of motor coordination.[2] Caplan concluded, as did Shtremel (1963), that stuttering is a form of apraxia. These studies are not cited to argue that stuttering is an apraxic syndrome, but rather to indicate how closely stuttering can resemble some types of neurologic disorder. The resemblances have been quite compelling to the ears of some investigators (Johns & Darley, 1970; Trost, 1971). A reasonable conclusion on the matter is that "stuttering is a frequent speech response to a number of different abnormalities in the neural substrates serving speech–language function" (Rosenbek, 1980, p. 247).

Acquired stuttering presents a particularly interesting disorder in the consideration of neurobehavioral risk factors for communicative disorders. A recent article by Mazzucchi, Moretti, Carpeggiani, & Parma (1981) described 16 cases of acquired stuttering in adults and reviewed other cases discussed in the literature. Some of the conclusions reached by the authors are as follows. First, acquired stuttering always has been associated with organic lesions. Second, acquired stuttering often is accompanied by aphasic signs. Third, psychogenic factors have not been identified. Fourth, complete right-hand dominance usually is observed (although more direct evidence of left hemisphere dominance is not available). Finally, the disorder is largely prevalent in males (by a ratio as high as 15:1).

Mazzucchi et al. drew other conclusions from their data, some of which are not in complete accord with previous reports. One of these is of special interest here: "in our experience, the signs indicating clinical–pathologic correlations point invariably to the left hemisphere, when lesions are unilateral" (p. 29). This conclusion is consistent with Flor-Henry's (1978) proposal that males are particularly vulnerable to dominant hemisphere dysfunction.[3] Thus, acquired stuttering may be grouped with other dominant hemisphere disorders as a characteristically male syndrome.

The results reported by Mazzucchi et al. pointed to certain similarities between adult acquired stuttering and developmental stuttering. First, no significant phonological differences were observed between the two types of stuttering. Second, they reported some cases of "acquired" stuttering which actually were "a worsening of a previous mild developmental stuttering, or a relapse of developmental stuttering following a neurologic episode" (p. 29).

Although the evidence is inconclusive regarding anomalous hemispheric asymmetry for speech production in stutterers, evidence favors the proposition that stutterers differ from nonstutterers on tests of central auditory function. Some writers have concluded that a neurological central dysfunction is an etiological factor in stuttering. But a different perspective is cast on this issue by a recent experiment reported by Wynne and Boehmler (1982). They administered a test of central auditory function to two groups of nonstutterers, a relatively fluent group and a relatively disfluent group. The two groups differed significantly, with the disfluent group performing more poorly. One interpretation of this study is that differences in central auditory function occur within the general population, and that impaired central auditory function is a predisposing or contributing factor to the etiology of stuttering. Studies of central auditory function show a general pattern of contrast across three group comparisons: Nonstutterers outperform stutterers; fluent nonstutterers outperform less fluent nonstutterers; and girls outperform boys over the age range of at least 7–15 years (Mirabile, Porter, Hughes, & Berlin, 1978). *Thus, it appears that temporal processing ability for auditory signals is correlated with verbal fluency.*

Timing breakdowns of a sort that may be similar to stuttering have been observed in tasks in which one limb taps a rhythm while another limb simultaneously taps a regular beat (Ibbotson & Morton, 1981). Performance on this task was easy when the right hand tapped the rhythm but was disrupted severely when the left hand tapped the rhythm. Breakdowns in the nonpreferred condition usually took one of two forms: (1) a partial or complete reversal of the streams (for example, both hands tapping the rhythm), or (2) inability to initiate movement. These experiments demonstrate the susceptibility to breakdown of a motor control system faced with the task of maintaining simultaneous temporal patterns. Speech also may be composed of simultaneous temporal patterns, such as temporal patterns for segmental articulation and those for prosody (analyses of sequencing errors committed by normal talkers show that prosodic and segmental features are readily disassociated; Fromkin, 1971). In this sense, the timing breakdowns in limb-tapping experiments may be *evidence of a critical vulnerability of central mechanisms that generate or maintain the temporal structure of action.*

Using a dual-task paradigm, Sussman (1982) examined interference effects for concurrent tasks of language output (reading or counting) and tapping with either the right or left hand. Left-handed subjects and right-handed stutterers showed symmetric interference effects, whereas right-handed nonstutterers showed interference effects consistent with a left hemisphere lateralization for both language and motor control of the contralateral hand. Of the three groups studied, the stutterers had the largest absolute levels of interference for dual language/tapping tasks but, interestingly, the lowest absolute levels of disruption for a dual task of object chimera and hand tapping. Thus, the stutterers were highly vulnerable to disruption of language but resistant to disruption of visual imagery.

Evidence of inaccurate timing control in stutterers has been presented by Cooper and Allen (1977). They concluded that "stutterers as a group appear to have less accurate clocks than do normal speakers, as evidenced by the consistently poorer average ranks of their RV (relative variance) scores for all tasks" (p. 65). The tasks included repeated sentences, paragraphs, nursery rhymes, and finger tapping (intended as a control condition). A particularly interesting outcome was that relative to normal speakers, the stutterers performed most poorly on the nursery rhyme task. Cooper and Allen (1977) concluded that the stutterers were not able to capitalize on the intrinsic rhythmic structure of the speech material. A similar interpretation, based on the thesis of this chapter, is that the stutterers could not generate reliable temporal programs appropriate to the structure of the speech materials.

SPECULATIONS ON GENETIC FACTORS

The possibility of a left hemisphere focus of a neurological disorder underlying stuttering is particularly interesting in view of recent proposals that certain speech and language disorders, such as dyslexia and stuttering, and certain autoimmune diseases are more likely to occur in left-handers than right-handers. Norman Geschwind (whose views are summarized by Marx, 1982) proposed that the basis of these speech and language disorders in left-handed individuals is an excess production of, or hypersensitivity to, testosterone in the fetus. Testosterone is secreted in large amounts by the fetal testes, and there is evidence that this hormone can influence brain development, particularly, in Geschwind's opinion, by slowing growth of the left hemisphere. Thus, males are more likely than females to be left-handed and to have dyslexia or stuttering. (It is pertinent here that a majority of young stutterers have concomitant disorders, such as emotional disturbance, neurologic impairment, and disorders of articulation, language, or voice; Blood & Seider, 1981). Interestingly, the sex ratio for dyslexia in school populations is about 3 to 1 (males to females), which is about the same ratio as that for male stutterers to female stutterers. It is also interesting that reading ability is correlated with *auditory blending* (Lexier, 1979) and *auditory comprehension* (Jarvis, 1974; Jackson & McClelland, 1979) whereas little evidence exists that reading ability is correlated with visual speech, visual memory, or visual–auditory pattern integration (McGuinness, 1981).[4]

The vulnerability of the developing brain to damage or to inhibition of growth is poorly understood. Some insights might be gained by examining maturational differences for different parts of the brain. That is, different parts of the brain have different rates of growth. From the data of Blinkov and Glezer (1968), it appears that between the second trimester and birth, the cortical surface area increases by about 140% for the frontal association region, about 330% for the inferior parietal association region, and about 460% for the temporal association region. Cortical regions with higher rates of growth may be more susceptible to damage or growth-retarding effects. Differential vulnerability related to growth could extend well into postnatal life. As Whitaker, Bub, & Leventer (1981) observed, "the surfaces of these neocortical zones associated with higher mental processes show a far greater degree of enlargement over their birth measurements (about 9 times) than do those of the primary motor and sensory areas (about 5 times) and those of the phylogenetically older insular and limbic regions (about 4 times)" (p. 60).

A major factor in explaining differential vulnerability between the left and right cerebral hemispheres is that the left has a lesser circulation (Flor-Henry, 1978). Better irrigation of the right hemisphere should help protect it against damage. Supporting evidence has been reported by Paolozzi (1970), who examined 20,256 EEG records for neurological patients. When only the cases with space-occupying intracerebral lesions were considered, Paolozzi observed an increase in left-sided pathology. Such an increase was not seen when only extracerebral lesions were considered. Thus, intracerebral lesions are more likely to occur on the left side. Furthermore, evidence of the vulnerability of the male brain is shown by a 30-year clinical study in which males outnumbered females by a ratio of 3:1 in the occurrence of intracranial abscesses (McClelland, Craig, & Crockard, 1978). The incidence of abscesses varied widely across lobes: frontal (25%), temporal (29%), parietal (10%), cerebellar (6%), and occipital (3%). Thus, the frontal and temporal lobes were more susceptible to damage or disease. These figures may reflect a relationship between etiology and the inherent susceptibility of a lobe to disease. The major etiology was chronic otitis media, which may have caused infections to which the proximal temporal lobe was most vulnerable.

There is also evidence that dendritic branching processes are more complex in neurons from the left hemisphere language cortex than in neurons from the homologous right hemisphere areas (Scheibel, 1983). If, as Scheibel hypothesized, this difference in dendritic branching between the hemispheres is related to language capability, then developmental processes that impede dendritic branching in the left cortex may have serious repercussions on language acquisition.

Another possible sex difference in the cortical representation of language is indicated by evidence from cortical stimulation experiments (Ojemann, 1983). It was observed that cortical stimulation interfered with naming responses over greater areas of the cortex in males than in females. It appears that, in males, a larger area of lateral frontal and parietal lobes is involved in language processes. This observation may relate to another tentative conclusion reached from the same kind of experiment conducted with bilingual subjects. Naming in the less competent language of these subjects was affected by stimulation over a substantially larger area than was naming of the same objects in the more competent language. One interpretation of this result suggested by Ojemann is that with increasing language competence, simple processes like naming require smaller primary cortical areas. Perhaps language processes are more diffusely represented in the male cortex because males tend to be less competent in language. As a consequence of this diffuse representation, males are more likely to suffer language disturbance following damage to various areas of the brain.

Does a genetic–hormonal conspiracy thus place boys at risk for impairments of communicative functions, which are preferentially based in the left hemisphere? Of course, it is too early to say with any degree of confidence. However, Geschwind and his colleagues have pointed to an intriguing result of autopsy on a male dyslectic patient who died in an accident. The normal disparity in size between the left and right planum temporale was much reduced, and a large island of cortex was abnormally situated below the left planum. The possibility that the left hemisphere is preferentially vested with communicative functions also is supported by studies showing that aphasia in deaf persons usually results from left hemisphere damage rather than right hemisphere damage (Chiarello, Knight, & Mandell, 1982; Leischner, 1943; Underwood & Paulson, 1981). Thus, auditory experience in language learning is not essential to a left hemisphere lateralization of language.

Although auditory processing difficulties are not established as causal factors in speech and language disorders, it is remarkable that depressed performance on tasks of dichotic listening or tasks of rapid auditory processing has been reported for stutterers (see citations in Andrews et al.), developmentally dysphasic children (Stark & Tallal, 1979, and articles cited in their paper), and children with learning disabilities (Tobey, Cullen, Ramp, & Fleischer-Gallagher, 1979).

FLUENCY-INDUCING CONDITIONS: COMMON ROOTS

Many writers have been interested in identifying the factor(s) common to fluency-inducing conditions. Andrews et al. concluded that the common factor was simplification, which can be expressed as reduced central demands (as in the situation of chorus reading, shadowing, singing, prolonged speech, and adaptation), restriction of information from external feedback (as in the conditions of lipped speech, whispering, and masking), or reduction of event or decision rate (as in the conditions of slowed speech, rhythmic speech, speaking with rhythmic movement, and "probably" speaking alone). The major exception to this conceptualization is response contingent stimulation, which Andrews et al. supposed forces the stutterer to use additional capacity at the expense of other functions. That is, response contingent stimulation requires more "work" from the stutterer whereas the other methods listed above reduce the "work" of speaking. However, simplification itself is a vague term, because simplification can be achieved in several different ways. We might say with some gain in precision that most of the fluency-inducing conditions reduce the uncertainty of verbal/motor formulation in the speaking task. Even more precisely, we might say that most of the fluency-inducing conditions lead to *a reduction of uncertainty in the temporal pattern of speech motor control.*

Recent experiments on repeated performances of hand tapping (Povel, 1981) or spoken utterances (Weismer & Cariski, in press) have shown that long sequences sometimes have a greater temporal stability than short sequences. The greater consistency of temporal patterning for selected longer sequences was explained by proposing that the central nervous system can code some temporal structures more reliably than others. The effects of temporal structure sometimes can override the effects of increased length. Perhaps a similar explanation applies to certain fluency-inducing conditions (especially those involving rhythmic patterns), for which variations in temporal structure seem to be the key element.

STUTTERING AS A DEFICIT IN TEMPORAL PROGRAMMING

In their theory of stuttering, Andrews et al. offer the crux statement that "due to inadequate central capacity, stutterers have a diminished ability to deal with the relationship between motor activity and the associated sensory or reafferent activity produced during speech. " This statement implies that the critical disorder is one of integrating motor and sensory activities. But if the central disturbance is one that affects integration, then why should stutterers tend to be poorer than non-stutterers in tasks of central auditory function for which integration of motor and sensory events is not particularly critical (except, of course, that some kind of motor response is required of the subject). In addition, it is not clear why this model accounts for some special conditions which immediately reduce stuttering, such as speaking alone, delayed auditory feedback, masking, change in pitch, or whispering. Although Andrews et al. suggest that two of these conditions (whispering and masking) are explained by simplifying the sensory feedback for the model update task, it is not clear why reducing the information to a defective integrator is an effective strategy, unless the reduction of information applies to sources of information that are redundant or particularly difficult to manage. Andrews et al. do not comment on why speaking alone should reduce the stutter except to speculate that speech rate may be reduced to give more time for model update or that linguistic complexity may be decreased. This possibility is easily tested by asking the stutterer to speak alone at different rates. I predict that rate will not be a potent factor. Andrews et al. make no comment on pitch change, and I see no reason why their model accommodates this effect on stuttering (unless the change in pitch is accompanied by a reduction in overall prosodic variation).

My own suspicion is that the central disturbance in stuttering involves a reduced ability to generate temporal patterns, whether for perceptual or productive purposes, but especially the latter. From the definition of stuttering as an impairment in the rhythm or fluency of speech, one immediately grasps the essence of stuttering as a disorder of the temporal regulation of speech. Normal speech is uttered, with occasional disruptions or sequencing errors, at rates that rival the rehearsed repetition of simple nonsense strings (Tiffany, 1980). Thus, speech is a brisk motor activity. In addition, speech is a perishable auditory signal that is complexly structured in time.

Van Riper (1971) expressed a similar idea when he wrote about stuttering:

> If we ignore for the moment the entire complex overlay of reactions to this experience, we find the essence of the disorder in this fracturing and disruption of the motor sequence of the word. The integrity of a spoken word demands great precision in the timing of its components. When for any reason, that timing is awry and askew, a temporally distorted word is produced, and when this happens, the speaker has evidenced a core stuttering behavior. (p. 404)

More recent studies reviewed by Andrews et al. show that minor timing abnormalities can be detected even in the fluent productions of stutterers. This observation leads to a tentative conclusion that stutterers almost continually contend with a faulty or unreliable mechanism for control of temporal structure.

It has long been assumed that the production and perception of speech share certain control mechanisms. Although this idea remains as much in the realm of assumption as fact, experimental work indicates that a good candidate for such a common mechanism is one handling temporal patterns, such as voice onset time (Gordon & Meyer, 1982). Additional evidence for common temporal processing in speech perception and production comes from experiments on rhythmicity of syllable sequences (Fowler, 1979). When subjects are asked to produce rhythmic sequences of syllables or to judge perceptually the rhythm of syllable sequences, the results deviate systematically from a strict temporal regularity (i.e., the syllabic patterns are not uniformly spaced in time). Moreover, the optimal or ideal rhythmic sequences deviate from strict temporal regularity in exactly the same way for production and perception. Stark and Tallal (1979) demonstrated that dysphasic children who had difficulty in perceiving initial stop consonants also had abnormal timing patterns in their productions of these consonants. They interpreted their results as indicating that these dysphasic children had "a lack of precise control over the timing of speech events" (p. 1703).

Temporal patterns come to our attention again with respect to an intriguing factor in the etiology of stuttering—sex differences. McGuinness (1981) suggested that a critical distinction between the sexes lies in the *capacity to generate temporal programs*. These temporal programs figure importantly in fine motor sequencing ability, verbal fluency, speed of verbal coding from visual display, singing in tune, and awareness of musical dynamics, all of which show a female superiority, at least at certain ages. Males, on the other hand, are better than females in tasks of visual problem solving in three dimensions, Piagetian conservation tasks, and various tasks involving visuo–gross motor systems. McGuinness concluded that females' superiority in auditory and fine motor tasks is the basis for their favored *communicative* mode of information acquisition. In contrast, males' superiority in visuo–gross motor systems tends to give them an advantage in an *action* mode of information acquisition. The female edge in sensorimotor substrates of language extends even to signing, for which girls are superior in complex linguistic aspects of syntax, word order, inflection, and interrogation (Gattney, 1977).

Fluency-inducing conditions generally reduce temporal uncertainty (hence, chorus reading, rhythmic speaking, singing, adaptation) or allow more time for the preparation of temporal programs (slowed speech, speaking with rhythmic movement, and to some extent speaking with DAF). Thus, conditions that involve "simplification" or slowing of rate become explainable by the same construct, one of reduced capacity to generate temporal programs. Generation of these programs is positively affected either by reducing the task complexity (that is, reducing temporal uncertainty in the speaking task) or giving more time for the processing of information needed to construct the programs.

The idea of temporal uncertainty is similar to the discoordination hypothesis which holds that stuttering will tend to decrease for any condition which facilitates the initiation of phonation in coordination with articulation and respiration (Perkins, Rudas, Johnson, & Bell, 1976). The discoordination hypothesis was broadened by Perkins, Bell, Johnson, and Stocks (1979) to an effective planning time hypothesis. This hypothesis asserts that "effective planning time for voice onset coordinations is the common element that explains the power of retarded phone rate, reduction of phonatory complexity, and rhythm virtually to eliminate stuttering" (p. 747). The temporal uncertainty hypothesis takes still one more step by proposing a general deficiency in temporal patterning for speech production and perception.

This is not to say that reduction of temporal uncertainty is the only way to reduce disfluencies, or that temporal uncertainty is the only factor to be considered in the precipitation of stuttering moments. Stuttering may increase as the combination of pressures or strains, including social or communicative anxiety, language formulation, and temporal uncertainty in utterance formulation. The locus of disfluency is to some degree syntactically constrained (Bernstein, 1981; Bloodstein, 1974). Bernstein's data for disfluencies in stuttering and normally fluent children showed that sentential constituent structure governs the location of many disfluencies for both stuttering and nonstuttering subjects. The major difference between the two groups was that the stutterers had an additional point of disfluency—the initiation of the verb phrase. The verb phrase appears to be a major point of linguistic uncertainty, as indicated by experiments reported by Lindsley (1975, 1976). These experiments showed that sentence production may begin before information about the verb is completely processed and that "subject phrases can always be counted on to provide at least a two-syllable delay by their overt utterance, a delay which may be generally sufficient to permit enough verb information processing to assure fluency" (Lindsley, 1976, p. 349; see Bernstein, 1981, and Kempen & Huijbers, 1983, for further discussion). It can be concluded that both linguistic uncertainty in sentence formulation and temporal uncertainty in speech production may interact to precipitate moments of disfluency.

Why does stuttering vary with propositionality of the speaking situation, with anxiety, or with response contingencies? First, it may be important to recognize that anxiety and reinforcement contingencies also can affect reading scores, at least in males (Cotler & Palmer, 1971). One possibility is that skills required for speaking and reading are susceptible to affective modulation, especially in males and in fewer females. (Generally, females develop language and reading skills that are relatively uninfluenced by socioeconomic status, emotional distress, or size or sex constitution of the family, whereas males tend to be strongly influenced by these factors; McGuinness, 1981.) Anything that reduces the affective modulation can yield increased fluency. Speaking alone obviously reduces propositionality or anxiety. Response contingent stimulation may serve to break temporarily the maladaptive modulation of perceptual and motor systems by affective neural circuits or, as Andrews et al. suggest, to force the stutterer to expend more capacity on speaking and thus alter the peculiar conditions that lead to stutter.

The means by which anxiety can influence cognitive and motor systems are speculative, but much has been learned about the neuropsychology of anxiety and other emotions. With respect to stuttering, it is particularly interesting to examine interactions between anxiety and language. Gray (1982) writes as follows on this interaction.

> In man a particularly important role in anxiety is apparently played by the prefrontal and cingulate regions of the neocortex... Within the present theory the role of these areas is twofold. First, they supply to the SHS [septo-hippocampal system] information about the subject's own ongoing motor programmes; this information is essential if the SHS (together with the Papez circuit) is to generate adequate predictions of the next expected event to match against actual events. Second, they afford a route by which language systems in the neocortex can control the activities of the limbic structures which are the chief neural substrate of anxiety. In turn, these structures, via subicular and hippocampal projections to the entorhinal cortex, are able to scan verbally coded stores of information... In this way, human anxiety can be triggered by stimuli that are largely verbal (relatively independently of ascending monoaminergic influences) and verbally coded search strategies can be used to cope with perceived threats. (Gray, 1982, p. 483)

Various proposals have been made to explain how anxiety can affect behavioral responses. Gray (1982) developed the concept of a "behavioral inhibition system" that reacts to novel stimuli or to stimuli enjoined to punishment or nonreward by inhibiting current behavior and by increasing arousal and attention to external stimuli. Obviously, such a system could interfere with motor planning and execution for an activity like speech. Other mechanisms have been proposed for interaction of anxiety with behavior, but suffice it to say that the neuropsychology of anxiety may hold some important answers. This literature may hold implications for the identification of neurotransmitter imbalances, if such are found to be factors in the etiology of stuttering. In addition, this literature may help to explain the actions of certain drugs in the improvement of fluency. For example, it is not clear whether improvement of stuttering through administration of haloperidol (Crookson & Wells, 1973; Murray, Kelly, Campbell, & Stefanik, 1977; Prins, Mandelkorn, & Cerf, 1980; Wells & Malcolm, 1971) is attributable to anxiolytic influences or to specific effects on motor function.

SUMMARY

I have tried to tie facts about stuttering to facts about sex differences, about laterality, and about other disorders. My impression is that facts about stuttering, considered in isolation from other facts, give us only a small part of a large picture of communicative competence and risk for communicative disorder.

Drawing largely on the arguments of Geschwind and McGuinness reviewed above, one might argue that males are at risk for developmental speech and language disorders because they (as a population) are less adept than females at tasks of auditory sequencing and fine motor control. These tasks underlie the acquisition and performance of speech as a precisely regulated motor skill. Boys may be at risk because testosterone slows the growth of the left hemisphere, which is more likely than the right hemisphere to process rapid auditory patterns and intricate motor sequences, perhaps because of a cytoarchitectonic biasing (Seldon, 1981a, 1981b).[5] A genetic factor emerges in the possibility of an inherited oversecretion of, or hypersensitivity to, testosterone in males. If genetic factors apply as strongly to females as males, then some other explanation may be required, unless a left hemisphere sensitivy to testosterone is just one feature of a genetic complex that predisposes to stuttering and other communicative disorders. The peculiar weakness that underlies stuttering (and perhaps other disorders such as developmental dysphasia or dyslexia) is a reduced capability to generate fine temporal programs that are necessary for motor regulation, for efficient auditory perception, and for language expression. Most fluency-inducing conditions reduce the temporal uncertainty of the speaking task (or slow its rate) and thereby contribute to increased success in the preparation of temporal structures for speaking and listening. The generation of temporal programs also is influenced by affective input. The stutterer is aided toward fluency by conditions that diminish or alter affective influences. The vulnerability of males and a smaller number of females to environmental circumstances during development explains why stuttering results from the combination of a genetic predisposition and a host of social and psychological forces.

Dr. William H. Perkins, Dr. Gary Weismer, and Dr. Richard F. Curlee offered helpful suggestions on drafts of this chapter.

NOTES

[1] Although the generalization that girls acquire language earlier than boys has been questioned (Maccoby & Jacklin, 1974), Schachter, Shore, Hodapp, Chalfin, & Bundy (1978) reported that young toddler girls (mean age of about 2 years) were significantly advanced over boys in mean length of utterance and upper bound, length of longest utterance. These results confirm the results of studies done in the 1930s and 1940s (McCarthy, 1954).

[2] For a recent review of apraxia of speech, see Rosenbek, Kent, and LaPointe (1984). Acoustic evidence of dyscoordination in apraxia of speech has been presented by Kent and Rosenbek (1983) who argued that motor control deficits are a primary feature of this disorder.

[3] Flor-Henry (1978) proposed that males have a relatively superior nondominant hemisphere but a more vulnerable dominant hemisphere. Females were thought to have a

relatively superior dominant hemisphere but a more vulnerable nondominant hemisphere. Superiority of the nondominant hemisphere in males is indicated by their high performance in visuospatial tasks, whereas superiority of females' dominant hemisphere is associated with their verbal and language accomplishments. Dominant hemisphere vulnerability in males is marked by relatively higher incidence of schizophrenia, psychopathy, conversion hysteria, conduct disturbances, reading retardation, developmental dyslexia, developmental aphasia, infantile autism, and childhood epilepsy (associated with left hemisphere lesions). Vulnerability of the nondominant hemisphere in females is linked with affective psychoses, hysteria, atypical depressions, paranoid melancholias, mixed "neurotic–psychotic" disorders, "anxiety–depression" states, and "neurotic" depression, all of which occur more frequently in females than in males. However, the preponderance of females in depression samples is called into question by a recent study of the Amish (Egeland & Hostetter, 1983). The Amish study showed equal proportions of females and males for both mania/hypomania and depression. The authors suggested that in the Amish sample, the incidence of male affective disorders may not be masked by alcoholism and sociopathy, as they presumably are in the general population. For further discussion of gender and psychopathology, see Al-Issa (1982).

[4] This is not to argue that auditory processing disorders are the only causative factors linked to dyslexia. Dyslexia is a complex disorder and several dyslexic syndromes have been described (Hier, LeMay, Rosenberger, & Perlo, 1978; Mattis, French, & Rapin, 1975; Mattis, 1981; Pirozzolo, 1979).

[5] Although the possibility of cortical abnormalities has been emphasized in this chapter, it is highly possible that subcortical structures also may be involved in neurologic explanations of stuttering. Lateralization is not unique to the cerebral cortex but applies as well to subcortical structures involved in the regulation of speech (see review in Kent, 1984).

REFERENCES

Al-Issa, I. *Gender and psychopathology. Personality and psychopathology.* New York: Academic Press, 1982.

Andrews, G., Craig, A., Feyer, A. M., Hoddinott, S., Howie, P., & Neilson, M. Stuttering: A review of research findings and theories circa 1982. *Journal of Speech and Hearing Disorders,* 1983, *48,* 226–246.

Bernstein, N. E. Are there constraints on childhood disfluency? *Journal of Fluency Disorders,* 1981, *6,* 341–350.

Blinkov, S. M., & Glezer, I. I. *The human brain in figures and tables.* New York: Plenum Press, 1968.

Blood, G. W., & Seider, R. The concomitant problems of young stutterers. *Journal of Speech and Hearing Disorders,* 1981, *46,* 31–33.

Bloodstein, O. The rules of early stuttering. *Journal of Speech and Hearing Disorders,* 1974, *39,* 379–394.

Caplan, L. An investigation of some aspects of stuttering-like speech in adult aphasic subjects. *Journal of the South African Speech and Hearing Association,* 1972, *19,* 52–66.

Chiarello, C., Knight, R., & Mandel, M. Aphasia in a prelingually deaf woman. *Brain,* 1982, *105,* 29–51.

Cotler, S., & Palmer, R. J. Social reinforcement, individual difference factors, and the reading performance of elementary school children. *Journal of Personality and Social Psychology,* 1971, *18,* 97–104.

Cooper, M. H., & Allen, G. D. Timing control accuracy in normal speakers and stutterers. *Journal of Speech and Hearing Research,* 1977, *20,* 55–71.

Crookson, L. B., & Wells, P. G. Haloperidol in the treatment of stutterers. *British Journal of Psychiatry,* 1973, *123,* 491.

Delis, D. C., Wapner, W., Gardner, H., & Moses, J. A., Jr. The contribution of the right hemisphere to the organization of paragraphs. *Cortex,* 1983, *19,* 43–50.

Dwyer, J. H., & Rinn, W. E. The role of the right hemisphere in contextual inference. *Neuropsychologia,* 1981, *19,* 479–482.

Egeland, J. A., & Hostetter, A. M. Amish study, I. Affective disorders among the Amish, 1976–1980. *American Journal of Psychiatry,* 1983, *140,* 56–61.

Flor-Henry, P. Gender, hemispheric specialization and psychopathology. *Social Science and Medicine,* 1978, *12*B, 155–162.

Fowler, C. A. "Perceptual centers" in speech production and perception. *Perception and Psychophysics,* 1979, *25,* 375–381.

Fromkin, V. A. The non-anomalous nature of anomalous utterances. *Language,* 1971, *47,* 27–52.

Galaburda, A. M., & Kemper, T. L. Cytoarchitectonic abnormalities in developmental dyslexia: A case study. *Annals of Neurology,* 1979, *6,* 94–100.

Gattney, D. W. Assessing receptive language skills of five to seven year old deaf children. *Dissertation Abstracts International,* 1977, *38,* 1665–1666.

Golden, G. S. Neurobiological correlates of learning disabilities. *Annals of Neurology,* 1982, *12,* 409–418.

Gordon, P. C., & Meyer, D. E. *Shared mechanisms for perceiving and producing speech.* Paper presented at the meeting of the Midwestern Psychological Association, Minneapolis, Minnesota, May 1982.

Gray, J. A. Precis of The neuropsychology of anxiety: An enquiry into the functions of the septo-hippocampal system. *The Brain and Behavioral Sciences,* 1982, *5,* 469–484.

Hammond, G. R. Hemispheric differences in temporal resolution. *Brain and Cognition,* 1982, *1,* 95–118.

Hier, D. B., LeMay, M., Rosenberger, P. B., & Perlo, V. P. Development dyslexia: Evidence for a subgroup with a reversal of cerebral asymmetry. *Archives of Neurology,* 1978, *35,* 90–92.

Ibbotson, N. R., & Morton, J. Rhythm and dominance. *Cognition,* 1981, *9,* 125–138.

Jackson, M. D., & McClelland, J. L. Processing determinants of reading speed. *Journal of Experimental Psychology (General),* 1979, *108,* 151–181.

Jarvis, E. O. Auditory abilities of primary school children. *Dissertation Abstracts International,* 1974, *35*A, 890–891.

Johns, D. F., & Darley, F. L. Phonemic variability in apraxia of speech. *Journal of Speech and Hearing Research,* 1970, *13,* 556–583.

Keele, S. W. Movement control in skilled motor performance. *Psychological Bulletin,* 1968, *70,* 387–403.

Kempen, G., & Huijbers, P. The lexicalization process in sentence production and naming: Indirect election of words. *Cognition,* 1983, *14,* 185–209.

Kent, R. D. Brain mechanisms of speech and language with special reference to emotional interactions. In R. Naremore (Ed.), *Language Science: Recent advances.* San Diego: College-Hill Press, 1984.

Kent, R. D. Facts about stuttering: neuropsychologic perspectives. *Journal of Speech and Hearing Disorders,* 1983, *48,* 249–255.

Kent, R. D., & Rosenbek, J. C. Acoustic patterns of apraxia of speech. *Journal of Speech and Hearing Disorders,* 1983, *26,* 231–248.

Leischner, A. Die 'aphasie' der Taubstummen. *Archiv fur Psychiatrie und Nervenkrankheiten,* 1943, *115,* 469–548.

Lexier, K. A. Auditory discriminability, blending and phoneme segmentation ability: Exploring basic skills in reading acquisition. *Dissertation Abstracts International,* 1979, 2469A–2470A.

Lindsley, J. R. Producing simple utterances: How far ahead do we plan? *Cognitive Psychology,* 1975, *7,* 1–19.

Lindsley, J. R. Producing simple utterances: Details of the planning process. *Journal of Psycholinguistic Research,* 1976, *5,* 331–353.

Maccoby, E. E., & Jacklin, C. N. *The psychology of sex differences.* Stanford, CA: Stanford University Press, 1974.

Marx, J. L. Autoimmunity in left-handers. *Science,* 1982, *217,* 141–144.

Mattis, S. Dyslexia syndromes in children: Toward the development of syndrome-specific treatment programs. In F. J. Pirozzolo & M. C. Wittrock (Eds.), *Neuropsychological and cognitive processes in reading.* New York: Academic Press, 1981.

Mattis, S., French, J., & Rapin, I. Dyslexia in children and young adults: Three independent neuropsychological syndromes. *Developmental Medicine and Child Neurology,* 1975, *17,* 150–163.

Mazzucchi, A., Moretti, G., Carpeggiani, P., & Parma, M. Clinical observations on acquired stuttering. *British Journal of Disorders of Communication,* 1981, *16,* 19–30.

McCarthy, D. Language development in children. In L. Carmichael (Ed.), *Manual of child psychology* (2nd. ed.). New York: Wiley, 1954.

McClelland, C. J., Craig, B. F., & Crockard, H. A. Brain abscesses in Northern Ireland: A 30 year community review. *Journal of Neurology, Neurosurgery and Psychiatry,* 1978, *41,* 1043–1048.

McGuinness, D. Auditory and motor aspects of language development in males and females. In A. Ansara, M. Albert, A. Galaburda, & N. Gartrell (Eds.), *The significance of sex differences in dyslexia.* Towson, MD: The Orton Society, 1981.

Mirabile, P. J., Porter, R. J., Hughes, L. F., & Berlin, C. I. Dichotic lag effect in children 7–15. *Developmental Psychology,* 1978, *14,* 227–285.

Moore, W. H., Jr., & Haynes, W. O. Alpha hemispheric asymmetry and stuttering: Some support for a segmentation dysfunction hypothesis. *Journal of Speech and Hearing Research,* 1980, *23,* 229–248.

Murray, T. J., Kelly, P., Campbell, L., & Stefanik, K. Haloperidol in the treatment of stuttering. *British Journal of Psychiatry,* 1977, *130,* 370–373.

Nasrallah, H. A., Keelor, K., Schroeder, C. Van, & Whitters, M. M. Motoric lateralization in schizophrenic males. *American Journal of Psychiatry,* 1981, *138,* 1114–1115.

Ojemann, G. Brain organization for language from the perspective of electrical stimulation mapping. *The Behavioral and Brain Sciences,* 1983, *6,* 189–206.

Paolozzi, C. Hemispheric dominance and asymmetry related to vulnerability of cerebral hemisphere. *Psychiatric Digest,* 1970, *31,* 61.

Perkins, W. H., Bell, J., Johnson, L., & Stocks, J. Phone rate and the effective planning time hypothesis of stuttering. *Journal of Speech and Hearing Research,* 1979, *22,* 747–755.

Perkins, W., Rudas, J., Johnson, L., & Bell, J. Stuttering: Discoordination of phonation with articulation and respiration. *Journal of Speech and Hearing Research,* 1976, *19,* 509–522.

Prins, D., Mandelkorn, T., & Cerf, F. A. Principal and differential effects of haloperidol and placebo treatments upon speech disfluencies in stutterers. *Journal of Speech and Hearing Research,* 1980, *23,* 614–629.

Pirozzolo, F. J. *The neuropsychology of developmental reading disability.* New York: Praeger, 1979.

Povel, D. J. Internal representation of simple temporal patterns. *Journal of Experimental Psychology: Human Perception and Performance,* 1981, *7,* 3–18.

Reed, E. S. An outline of a theory of action systems. *Journal of Motor Behavior,* 1982, *14,* 98–134.

Rosenbek, J. C. Apraxia of speech-relationship to stuttering. *Journal of Fluency Disorders,* 1980, *5,* 233–253.

Rosenbek, J. C., Kent, R. D., & LaPointe, L. L. Apraxia of speech: An overview and some perspectives. In. J. C. Rosenbek, M. R. McNeil, & A. Aronson (Eds.), *Apraxia of speech: Physiology, acoustics, linguistics, and management.* (pp 1-72). San Diego: College-Hill Press, 1984.

Rosenberger, P. B., & Hier, D. P. Cerebral asymmetry and verbal intellectual deficits. *Annals of Neurology,* 1980, *8,* 300–304.

Ross, E. D., Harney, J. H., deLacoste-Utamsing, C., & Purdy, P. D. How the brain integrates affective and propositional language into a unified behavioral function. *Archives of Neurology,* 1981, *38,* 745–748.

Schachter, F. F., Shore, E., Hodapp, R., Chalfin, S., & Bundy, C. Do girls talk earlier? Mean length of utterance in toddlers. *Developmental Psychology,* 1978, *14,* 388–392.

Scheibel, A. [Paper presented to the Biological Foundations of Cerebral Dominance Conference, Harvard Medical School and Institute for Child Development Research.] Boston, MA, April 4-6, 1983.

Seldon, H. L. Structure of human auditory cortex. I. Cytoarchitectonics and dendritic distributions. *Brain Research,* 1981, *229,* 277–294. (a)

Seldon, H. L. Structure of human auditory cortex. II. Axon distributions and morphological correlates of speech perception. *Brain Research,* 1981, *229,* 295–310.

Shtremel, A. K. Stuttering in left parietal lobe syndrome. *Zhurnal Nevropatologii i Psikhiatrii imeni S S. Korsakova,* 1963, *63,* 828–832.

Stark, R. E., & Tallal, P. Analysis of stop consonant production errors in developmentally dysphasic children. *Journal of the Acoustical Society of America,* 1979, *66,* 1703–1712.

Sternberg, S., Monsell, S., Knoll, R. L., & Wright, C. E. The latency and duration of rapid movement sequences: Comparisons of speech and typewriting. In G. E. Stelmach (Ed.), *Information processing in motor control and learning,* (pp. 117–152). New York: Academic Press, 1978

Sussman, H. M. Contrastive patterns of intrahemispheric interference to verbal and spatial concurrent tasks in right-handed, left-handed and stuttering populations. *Neuropsychologia,* 1982, *20,* 675–684.

Tiffany, W. R. The effect of syllable structure on diadochokinetic and reading rates. *Journal of Speech and Hearing Research,* 1980, *23,* 894–908.

Tobey, E. A., Cullen, J. K., Ramp, D. R., & Fleischer-Gallagher, A. M. Effects of stimulus-onset asynchrony on the dichotic performance of children with auditory-processing disorders. *Journal of Speech and Hearing Research,* 1979, *22,* 197–211.

Trost, J. E. *Apraxic dysfluency in patients with Broca's aphasia.* Paper presented to the Annual Convention of the American Speech and Hearing Association, Chicago, IL, 1971.

Underwood, J. K., & Paulson, C. J. Aphasia and congenital deafness: A case study. *Brain and Language,* 1981, *12,* 285–291.

Van Lancker, D., & Canter, G. J. Impairment of voice and face recognition in patients with hemispheric damage. *Brain and Cognition,* 1982, *1,* 185-195.

Van Riper, C. *The nature of stuttering.* Englewood Cliffs, NJ: Prentice-Hall, 1971.

Wapner, W., Hamby, S., & Gardner, H. The role of the right hemisphere in the apprehension of complex linguistic materials. *Brain and Language,* 1981, *14,* 15-33.

Weismer, G., & Cariski, D. On speakers' abilities to control speech mechanism output: Theoretical and clinical implications. In N. Lass (Ed.), *Speech and language: Advances in basic research and practice* (Vol. 9). New York: Academic Press, in press.

Wells, P. B., & Malcolm, M. T. Controlled trial of the treatment of 36 stutters. *British Journal of Psychiatry,* 1971, *119,* 603-604.

Whitaker, H. A., Bub, D., & Leventer, S. Neurolinguistic aspects of language acquisition and bilingualism. In H. Winitz (Ed.), *Native language and foreign language acquisition. Annals of the New York Academy of Sciences,* Vol. 379. New York: New York Academy of Sciences, 1981.

Wynne, M. K., & Boehmler, R. M. Central auditory function in fluent and disfluent normal speakers. *Journal of Speech and Hearing Research,* 1982, *25,* 54-57.

Clinical management of stutterers

Chapter 15

Assessment Strategies for Stuttering

Janis M. Costello and Roger J. Ingham*

The purpose of this chapter is to describe a behavioral methodology that has been found useful and comprehensive in the pretreatment (and continuing) assessment of persons who stutter. Although several such assessment protocols have been described in the literature (i. e., Brutten, 1975; Riley, 1972; Ryan, 1974; Wertheim, 1972; Williams, 1978), there is yet to emerge a "science of assessment," so there is little information available to verify the clinical worth of any currently used procedure. This chapter endeavors to describe, then, some new directions for an optimum, idealized set of measures—appropriate for a range of therapy methods and philosophies—that will be available for future systematic studies of its sensitivity and usefulness. It is a methodology that relates to the authors' previously described treatment outcome evaluation procedure (Ingham & Costello, 1984).

Pretreatment assessment of children and adults is, first, a diagnostic process. That is, the assessment procedure should make it possible to determine whether the person in question is, in fact, a stutterer. Although the behavioral manifestations of stuttering are quite obvious and easy to detect in the vast majority of adult stutterers, this is not necessarily the case for young children. Further, it is not unusual for stuttering to occur in the presence of other disorders, thus requiring stuttering to be distinguished from them. Beyond this, the pretreatment process is even more valuable when it aids in the selection of treatment strategies that are likely to be successful. And another characteristic of a comprehensive pretreatment assessment strategy is that it initiate a

*This chapter was prepared while Dr. Ingham was a visiting professor at the University of California, Santa Barbara.

continuous outcome evaluation process that will provide sensitive, reliable, and relevant measures of stuttering behavior. These measures should be regularly and consistently implemented, not only during a pretreatment interval, but also throughout the acquisition, transfer, generalization, maintenance, and follow-up phases of therapy.

This chapter, therefore, seeks to describe an assessment protocol that meets the above requirements. The procedure described is appropriate for both children and adults, and is designed to provide comprehensive and sensitive measures of all relevant dimensions of stuttering, irrespective of the treatment methods that might be put in place. For the purposes of this chapter, children are considered to be persons under the age of seven or eight, and everyone older is generally referred to as adults. Although it has been observed (e. g., Bloodstein, 1960; Luper & Mulder, 1964) that stuttering often begins to become more adult-like during the young elementary school ages, our dividing line is somewhat arbitrary and is based primarily upon reading skills and the various kinds of assessment tasks that are most appropriate to each age group. Users of this system may find it helpful to pick and choose activities from the child and adult versions of the assessment protocol for children in the seven-to-twelve-year-old range.

Obtaining talking samples

As the authors have described elsewhere (Costello, 1981; Ingham & Costello, 1984), the most important information to be gained from pretreatment assessment procedures comes from samples of the client's speech, and the more samples that are procured, the better. The purpose of obtaining talking samples is, obviously, to find out if the person's speech contains stuttering to any significant degree.

Most human behavior, and especially stuttering, is known to be variable; that is, it does not display itself in exactly the same form or frequency on every occasion (Bloodstein, 1981). Therefore, the assessment procedure should seek to capture the boundaries, the peaks and valleys, of that variability in order to adequately describe the form and frequency of stuttering or, conversely, to convincingly demonstrate that no stuttering is present. When stuttering is present, a representative picture cannot be drawn unless wide ranging sampling has been made; and later, when treatment has been instigated, its effect cannot be adequately judged unless one can demonstrate that stuttering has been reduced below the levels displayed during the valleys of the pretreatment samples.

The extent of the variability of an individual's stuttering can only be assessed through repeated, direct measures of that behavior across two dimensions: environments and time. First, clinicians select several environments within and beyond the confines of the clinic, from which talking samples can be regularly made. Second, measures are obtained from those several environments regularly across time. In practice, an individualized set of standard talking samples (STSs) is developed for each client, and these are then obtained routinely throughout the course of pretreatment assessment, establishment of nonstuttered speech in the clinic environment, transfer and generalization of stutter-free speech to the natural environment, and maintenance and follow-up periods. This set of measures, then, provides a consistent evaluation of the progress of therapy, tapping the variability of the client's performance throughout all stages of treatment. As described in more detail elsewhere (Ingham, 1984, chap. 12; Ingham & Costello, 1984), this procedure follows a time series quasi-experimental research model (Hersen & Barlow, 1976; McReynolds & Kearns, 1983) by requiring standard repeated measures prior to the initiation of treatment, during treatment, and following treatment. (See Ingham, 1984, chap. 12; and Ingham & Costello, 1984, for a more elaborate description and rationale for this repeated measures treatment outcome evaluation model.) Andrews and Harvey (1981) reported that stutterers' first assessments may produce data that indicate the client's problem is worse than it normally is because people are typically moved to seek treatment when their speech is at its worst. Although stuttering subsequently returns to its normal level, if this occurs during the early stages of treatment, measures of treatment effect could be confounded. This "regression to the mean" phenomenon makes even more obvious the need to establish stable baserates during the pretreatment assessment period, before treatment is initiated. That is, one set of baseline measures is not enough.

Standard talking samples for children: Within clinic. It is recommended that at least two within-clinic talking samples be obtained from children who are being evaluated as potential stutterers: a 10-min conversation between the child and parent and a 10-min conversation between the child and the clinician. Whenever possible, these conversations are videotaped for analysis, but they are always at least audiotaped. Parents are instructed beforehand that a conversation with their child will be a part of some sessions, and they are asked to bring some of the child's favorite toys along so that natural conversation can be easily evoked. The parent and child are instructed to carry on a normal, typical conversation, although the parent is reminded that the purpose of the conversation is to allow the clinician to hear as much of the child's talking as possible.

The same rules apply to the conversation that occurs between the child and the clinician except that the clinician makes sure to introduce into the interaction variables common to conversations so that their influence on stuttering may be observed, and so that the conversation is representative of natural conversations. Therefore, the clinician will occasionally interrupt the child, disagree with the child's statements, overlap the child's speech with her own talking, ask questions, and change the topic. Most of the time, however, the clinician attends to the child's talking in a positive and responsive manner and refrains from talking as much as possible so that an adequate sample of the child's speech is obtained.

Standard talking samples for children: Beyond clinic. Because the ultimate measure of the success of treatment is based upon the way the client talks outside of the clinic setting, the most crucial measures are those that are obtained from outside the treatment environment. For children, regular sampling of beyond-clinic speech in 10-min conversations in at least four STSs is suggested: (1) with the clinician outside of the clinic room; (2) at home with the other parent or with another caretaker who is familiar and routinely accessible to the child; (3) at home with a sibling or frequent playmate; (4) in a regularly occurring activity in the preschool, kindergarten, or regular school setting. (Items 2, 3, and 4 must be arranged for and carried out by the parents, and they are made aware of this responsibility when their child is scheduled for assessment. They are also required to provide cassette recorders and tapes and are trained by the clinician in their proper operation.)

It is unfortunate that research and experience so consistently tell us that speech behavior in the clinic is not necessarily representative of speech performance beyond the clinic; but nonetheless, this is oftentimes the case; and clinical researchers have not, as yet, found a way to measure what speech is like in the natural environment without measuring it directly in that environment. So, rather than lament the absence of information regarding the child's speech outside the clinic—or worse, assume that within-clinic samples accurately reflect beyond-clinic performance—clinicians must arrange to obtain regular, repeated beyond-clinic talking samples. Once this fact of clinical life is fully appreciated, clinicians find that they can become quite facile at designing convenient ways of obtaining and analyzing (or training others to analyze) such samples.

Standard talking samples for adults: Within clinic. Ryan's (1974) protocol for sampling stutterers' speech provides a useful method for obtaining within-clinic STSs. That is, recordings are made of 5-min each of oral reading, conversation with the clinician, and monologue, with the clinician absent from the room and the client talking aloud about any topic. (In all of these STSs the majority of the allotted time is filled with client speech, thereby approximating the amount of talking time children produce in a 10-min conversation.) Although oral reading is not a common daily talking activity for most persons, it is often a useful starting place for treatment. Further, reading tasks may serve to highlight occasions of word avoidance. For these reasons, reading appears to have value as an STS in pretreatment (and continuing) assessment procedures. The monologue task, similar to Johnson, Darley, and Spriestersbach's (1963) job task, has become almost a universal assessment task and has particular value because it requires self-formulated speech similar to that used in conversation, yet is less complex than conversational speech, which requires the client to formulate the semantic and syntactic components of a message while applying conversational rules appropriate to dyadic interaction.

Standard talking samples for adults: Beyond clinic. Beyond-clinic talking samples are required for adult clients for the same reasons noted above for children. In fact, clinicians will depend exclusively upon measures from these STSs as indicators of treatment effectiveness for all post acquisition phases of an adult client's total treatment time. The four beyond-clinic 5-min STS conversation tasks recommended for adult clients are as follows: (1) conversation with the clinician outside the clinic setting, (2) conversation with a spouse or close friend, (3) telephone conversation with a friend, and (4) conversation occurring with someone in the workplace. A different conversation partner is selected for each STS, and that person remains as the partner for these samples throughout the course of treatment. The adult client is made responsible for providing the recorder and tapes and for recording the last three listed beyond-clinic talking samples on the schedule determined by the clinician. This is part of the client's obligation to the treatment contract, and oftentimes turns out to be an excellent indicator of the client's commitment to treatment.

For both child and adult clients, talking tasks beyond or different from the ones described herein may be appropriate and necessary, either because the client reports certain situations to be especially difficult and/or because certain situations are frequently encountered by the client and are convenient to record. What is most important to the selection of within- and beyond-clinic STSs is that they are individually determined for each client to provide representative and broad samples of the client's speech.

Covert assessments. It is possible that some stutterers will be able to control their manner of talking under the demand characteristics of the overt kinds of assessment tasks described above, and this will be especially true the longer the client has been engaged in treatment. The presence of the clinician or a tape recorder can exercise powerful stimulus control and thus subvert the ability of the talking tasks to provide a representative sample of the client's natural, unmonitored speech. Therefore, it is important to obtain, at least occasionally, covert measures of the client's speech in natural settings. Although Andrews and Craig (1982) found no differences between overt and covert assessments for groups of stuttering subjects, they apparently agree with Ingham (1975; 1980), who has demonstrated that, in comparison to performance in overt talking samples, covert data may yield a different picture of speaking performance for some individual clients. This is especially pertinent during the transfer, maintenance, and follow-up stages of treatment. There appear to be no data regarding differences that may appear between overt and covert samples of speech during pretreatment assessments, but it is wise to obtain at least one covert sample during pretreatment in order to identify yet another potential source of variability in the client's speech patterns. (Ingham & Costello, 1984, and Ingham & Onslow, 1983, describe the way in which they obtain client permission for covert assessments to be made.)

A definition of stuttering

Although this is obviously a fundamental component of the measurement process, defining and counting stutterings turns out not to be a simple matter. First, stutterings must be differentiated from disfluencies, those interruptions to the flow of speech that typify normally fluent talkers. And since the purpose of treatment is to remove stuttering, it is only stuttering that should be counted and subsequently reduced in frequency. MacDonald and Martin (1973) demonstrated that even unsophisticated listeners could reliably and unambiguously identify some behaviors as either stutterings or disfluencies, thus offering validity to the notion of their distinction in listeners' perceptual codes. However, Bloodstein (1974) countered that MacDonald and Martin

> systematically defined away as neither stuttering nor normal disfluency a large number of behaviors, the very ones on which disagreement existed on that score, and have concluded that stuttering and normal disfluencies are reliable and unambiguous response classes. Unfortunately, it is not that easy. The ambiguous instances are still there. (p. 750)

Further, Curlee's (1981) systematic replication of MacDonald and Martin (1973) found that listeners were not able to make such clear differentiations between stutterings and disfluencies, thus leading to his conclusion that "the perceptual boundaries of stuttering are not clear" (p. 600).

Webster (1979) sidestepped this definitional problem by simply counting "*all* instances of disfluency and avoiding the selection of assumed 'stuttering disfluencies' and the rejection of assumed 'normal disfluencies' " (p. 231). This seems an extreme tactic just to preserve reliability and complicates unnecessarily the interpretation of such measures. For example, if a stutterer began treatment with 11% syllables disfluent and completed treatment with 3% syllables disfluent, is the client still a stutterer (albeit improved)? If the remaining disfluent syllables were all "normal" disfluencies, one would have to say "no" to that question. However, if some or all of those speech interruptions would be judged as stutterings, some, including the client, might suggest that the treatment had not been completely successful. The two outcomes are clearly clinically different.

It might be expected that listeners would be better able to reliably identify stuttering if they were provided with a definition of stuttering (Wingate, 1977). Many writers have developed and/or studied such definitions (e.g., Boemhler, 1958; Floyd & Perkins, 1974; Huffman & Perkins, 1974; Johnson, 1961; Schiavetti, 1975; Voelker, 1944; Williams & Kent, 1958; Young, 1961), but the most often cited definition is that offered by Wingate (1964). He described particular topographies of behaviors that are the kernel characteristics of stuttering—audible and silent repetitions of sounds or syllables and audible and silent prolongations—one or more of which are found in the speech of all persons who stutter. Wingate further suggested that a wide range of accessory features—speech-related movements, ancillary body movements, and verbal features—can also characterize the speech patterns of persons who stutter, but that their occurrence is not universal among stutterers and so not pertinent to the definition of stuttering for all stutterers. Both Curlee (1981) and Martin and Haroldson (1981) assessed the contribution of Wingate's (1964) standard definition of stuttering to listener agreement for identification of stuttering, and both studies found its contribution to be insignificant. That is, when listeners were provided with a written version of Wingate's kernel characteristics and instructed to rely on that definition to identify stutterings, they were not more likely to agree on the occurrence and location of specific moments of stuttering than were listeners for whom no definition was supplied. Both studies agreed, as well, that not only did listeners not agree among themselves regarding the location of moments of stuttering (interobserver reliability), but the listeners' agreement with themselves (intraobserver reliability) was also poor.

Wingate (1981) suggested that the provision of a definition of stuttering for one group of listeners did not enhance inter- or intraobserver agreement because the definition that was provided to the listeners was incomplete and misleading, and not an accurate representation of Wingate's own (1964) definition. Although the following was not a directly expressed concern of Wingate's, it can be noted that both studies (Curlee, 1981; Martin & Haroldson, 1981) provided listeners only with descriptions of Wingate's kernel characteristics. However, the stuttering samples to which the subjects listened were obtained from adult stuttering speakers and probably included accessory features as well. In fact, Martin and Haroldson (1981, p. 62) provide descriptions of some of the utterances reliably and unambiguously identified as stutterings by their listeners, and they were almost exclusively composed of accessory features. Therefore, it is possible that the definition did not aid listeners' identification of stutterings because it was an incomplete definition that did not include descriptions of the kinds of behaviors perceived as stuttering in the experimental samples.

Curlee (1984) has thoroughly reviewed the literature relevant to these issues and has pointed out that there appear to be two different kinds of definitions of stuttering: perceptual and behavioral. Although Martin and Haroldson (1981) concluded that stuttering is best identified as a "threshold phenomenon" (a perceptual definition), Curlee (1984) points out that behavioral and perceptual definitions appear to generate comparable levels of recognition of moments of stuttering, so that either may be used by clinicians.[1] It might make sense to utilize both of these kinds of definitions to aid clinicians (and others) to accurately recognize moments of stuttering. That is, a clinician might first listen to a variety of talking samples of a client and perceptually determine which interruptions to the flow of speech sound like stutterings. After stutterings have been pinpointed perceptually, the clinician could then formulate a topographical description of the responses identified. Such behavioral definitions of stuttering are, then, individualized for each client and might serve to aid the clinician to produce consistent measures of

---

[1] Another interpretation of the findings of these studies might lead one to believe that listeners operate at the perceptual level when required to identify stutterings and that the addition of a definition (at least when that definition lists only Wingate's (1964) kernel characteristics) either has no added effect (Curlee, 1981) or has a negative effect (Martin & Haroldson, 1981) on listener agreement. The research conducted thus far has not attempted to determine whether listeners who were given the definition actually attended to it or whether their "gut level" perceptions overrode the guidance provided by the definition.

stuttering. At the least they would provide a broad description of the client's stuttering for the clinical records.[2]

Reliability of the measurement of stuttering

The above-described studies illustrated that listeners agreed rather poorly among and with themselves when they were required to identify the exact loci of moments of stuttering. However, in clinical settings interobserver and intraobserver agreements are typically calculated on the basis of a comparison of total counts of stutterings. That is, percentage agreement between total counts is generally the more convenient and useful indicator of measurement reliability for talking samples such as the STSs described above.[3] Research has indicated that frequency counts of stuttering are able to be made with quite satisfactory levels of listener agreement (e.g., Curlee, 1981; Young, 1969; Young & Downs, 1968). Since the data abstracted from the standard talking samples are used to provide information regarding trends in the frequency counts of stuttering over time, the potential reliability of such a measure suggests that the data will be appropriately sensitive to clinically significant changes in stuttering frequency.

The dependent variables

In the section to follow, measures of stuttering, speed of speech, stutter-free utterances, and speech quality are described. All are considered necessary in the pretreatment assessment stage to piece together a composite picture of the stutterer's manner of talking. Therefore, each of these measures is calculated for the several STSs established for the

[2] Perkins (1983) argues that the *validity* of any *listener's* definition of stuttering moments may be questioned because a key factor in the definition of stuttering, at least from the stutterer's perspective and from that of some theorists as well, is the accompanying feeling of a momentary *involuntary* loss of speech motor control. If this is a critical component of stuttering, then such a "private behavior" might not be reliably observed unless the observation or recording procedure is in some way linked to the stutterer's judgment of his or her stuttering behavior. It is possible that the validity *and* reliability of assessments of stuttering may be enhanced by the development of such a procedure.

[3] Also to enhance reliability, stuttering is typically measured in global fashion, that is, a *moment of stuttering*. One moment of stuttering is counted for each of the speaker's attempts to produce a given syllable, irrespective of the duration of that attempt. For example, in an attempt to say "The weather is cold" one stutterer might produce the following response: "The wwwwwweather is cold" while another might say, "The THROAT CLEARING, the THROAT CLEARING, the wəwəwəweather is cold." Both stutterers would be counted as having produced one moment of stuttering, or one syllable stuttered. Further, most clinical researchers and clinicians have given up the practice of atempting to record stutterings according to different forms or topographies, since research has shown those divisions not to be clinically meaningful (e.g., Costello & Hurst, 1981).

client across the four or more pretreatment assessment sessions. (Appendix A provides specific instructions regarding how to calculate each.)

Percentage syllables stuttered. Probably the most popular and the most sensitive measure of stuttering is its frequency of occurrence. In the current treatment research literature, frequency of stuttering is most commonly reported as percentage syllables stuttered (%SS) or percentage words stuttered (%WS).[4] Whatever one selects as a measure of stuttering frequency, such a measure is clearly necessary (but not sufficient) for the quantification of a client's talking samples. The clinician, the client, and society expect that stuttering treatment will produce a clinically and socially significant reduction in stuttering frequency.

Duration of moments of stuttering. Data based on the talking samples of two different stutterers might reveal similar information regarding %SS, but listeners might still perceive differences in the severity of stuttering between the two speakers. This might be because they differed regarding the length of their moments of stuttering. Or, stuttering frequency could be quite low for a given stutterer, but his or her infrequent stutterings might be long and therefore as debilitating as the more frequent, shorter, stutterings of another speaker. Therefore, another useful measure of stuttering is its duration (see Appendix A). One method of measurement is to calculate the length in seconds of the client's typical moments of stuttering and report, as well, the actual length of the three longest moments of stuttering in the given talking sample. This measure captures a dimension of stuttering that is lost in %SS. Although decreases in stuttering frequency usually parallel decreases in the length of stutterings as treatment progresses, it is possible for these aspects of stuttering to be somewhat independent of one another (Martin & Haroldson, 1979); therefore, both measures are necessary.

Speed of speech. Moments of stuttering take up time in the flow of the speaker's speech and, therefore, often serve to slow speaking rate.

---

[4] The authors prefer %SS because, in terms of motor production, syllables are considered to be the basic physiologic units of utterances. Further, counting syllables allows one to assign more than one moment of stuttering to multisyllable words, and syllable counts are unaffected by variation in word length (all syllables are composed of about the same number of phonemes [Umeda & Quinn, 1980]) or by big differences in speakers' vocabulary levels. The early treatment literature frequently reported stuttering frequency in stutters per minute, a measure that is not independent of word output and can be improperly influenced by it. Reducing word output produces an apparent, but spurious, decrease in stutters per minute. This may be an inadvertent byproduct of slowed speech which is known to reduce stuttering frequency, or simply the numerical consequence of producing fewer stutters because fewer syllables are uttered. The calculation of %SS controls for fluctuating syllable output.

The more frequent and longer are stutterings, the slower is overall speaking rate. The *overall speaking rate* (see Appendix A), measured in syllables spoken per minute (SPM), could be considered an indication of the efficiency of the speaker's communication since, in some ways, it reflects the amount of information the stutterer conveys in a given interval. In general, one would expect abnormally low overall speaking rates prior to treatment (Bloodstein, 1944) and increases in speaking rate as successful treatment progresses. At the termination of treatment, of course, it is not enough to observe a low or absent frequency of stuttering. The client's speech rate should also be within the range of nonstuttering talkers. As a matter of fact, there is increasing evidence that the often reported perceived differences between the posttreatment speech of stutterers and normally fluent speakers (Ingham & Packman, 1978; Runyan & Adams, 1978) may be caused by differences in speech rate (Prosek & Runyan, 1982, 1983). For adults, normal rates are typically between 190 and 210 SPM (Ingham, 1984, chap. 2; Bernard, 1965). For children, less is known about normative overall speaking rates, although data collected by Kowal, O'Connell, and Sabin (1975) suggest that at kindergarten level the child's utterance rate should be about 50% of adult speaking rates, and adult rates are reached by the onset of adolescence.

Although the measurement of overall speaking rate may indicate that a given person's word output is low, this measure does not necessarily present an accurate picture of the actual speed at which a person is talking. Because the calculation of overall speaking rate includes time-consuming moments of stuttering, pauses used for sentence formulation time, and pauses used to emphasize or convey subtleties of meaning, this measure is not entirely satisfactory. An indication of how fast a person is talking is important before treatment is introduced, and subsequently, because the literature indicates that stuttering is reduced when speech rate is reduced (Adams, Lewis, & Besozzi, 1973; Ingham, Martin, & Kuhl, 1974; Johnson & Rosen, 1937; Perkins, Bell, Johnson, & Stocks, 1979), and some experimental research suggests that some stutterers' abilities to coordinate the speed with which they can use their articulators and/or respiratory and laryngeal mechanisms is slower than that of nonstutterers. Therefore, a second measure of the speed of speech has been advocated by Perkins (1975) and Adams (1976), referred to here as *articulatory rate*. Articulatory rate can also be measured in SPM (see Appendix A) but is calculated from speech samples that contain no stutterings or disfluencies and from which pauses greater than 2 sec have been eliminated. Although no articulatory rate normative data for either children or adults has yet been reported, it is clear that information in this realm is necessary for a composite picture of the client's talking performance. As research progresses, it may be found that stutterers as a group or individually may evidence an optimal or even maximum articulatory rate that facilitates the production and maintenance of stutter-free speech. This is unlikely to be discovered, however, if articulatory rate is not customarily measured. Such rates should be consistently calculated from the periodic STSs obtained throughout pretreatment, treatment, generalization, maintenance, and follow-up periods. Generally, overall speaking rate tends to increase as the stutterer's speech improves, but for many clients a concurrent decrease in articulatory rate is also an appropriate treatment goal.

Length of stutter-free utterances. The measures described thus far have concentrated on providing quantified information regarding the occurrence of stuttering in the client's speech and should be regularly calculated. Other measures are useful during pretreatment and intermittently thereafter. The reciprocal of stuttering, that is, the occurrence of periods of nonstuttered speech,[5] is such a measure. The length of typical stutter-free periods of speech can be measured in both seconds and syllables (see Appendix A), and the length of the three longest stutter-free utterances in the client's speech sample can also be reported. From pretreatment measures of such utterances it is possible to determine whether frequent enough and long enough nonstuttered utterances are available as treatment targets (see Costello, 1983; chap. 18, this volume). Further, comparison over time of these measures from the client's STSs provides yet another measure of speech improvement that may result from the imposition of a given treatment strategy. Of course, the length of stutter-free utterances should progressively increase under such conditions.

[5] The terms *fluency* and *fluent speech* are oftentimes used on occasions where the terms *stutter-free* or *nonstuttered speech* appear in this chapter. As Hegde (1978) and Starkweather (1980) among others have so eloquently stated, research has yet to supply us with an adequate description of exactly what is meant by the term. In fact, fluency is usually defined indirectly—as a period of talking time or a given number of syllables or words produced without any occurrences of stuttering (and, sometimes, without disfluencies as well). As we have stated previously (Costello, 1981), "The fact that we can't describe, behaviorally or physiologically, the components of a fluent utterance is a clear indication of the primitive level at which we are still operating regarding our understanding of fluent speech production. It seems likely that if we could precisely describe and measure the behaviors, and movements, and coordinations, and transitions which produce a fluent utterance, we might select these as treatment targets and thereby begin to teach our clients to speak fluently. (This is the approach advocated by Adams & Runyan, 1981, and Webster, 1974.) Instead, most of what we do is teach clients to talk without stuttering." At any rate, because the precise meaning and measure of fluency or fluent speech is as yet unspecified, we prefer to use the more descriptive terms *stutter-free* and *nonstuttered speech*.

Speech quality. Speech that ·is free of stutterings and that displays appropriate overall and articulatory rates may or may not be speech that sounds like "normal speech" to listeners. That is, there is yet another dimension of speech production that is only partially overlapped by these other measures: a measure of the quality of speech. The need for a measure of speech quality is obvious in the case of treatments that rely on speech patterns such as rhythmic speech or prolonged speech and its numerous variants (Ingham, 1984, chap. 5 & 10). Indeed, there is increasing evidence from various treatments that differences noted between the treated speech of stutterers and nonstutterers may be attributed to subtle differences in speech quality (Runyan & Adams, 1978). A number of relatively impractical procedures have been suggested as means of evaluating speech quality (Ingham & Packman, 1978; Jones & Azrin, 1969; Perkins, 1973). However, one of the most promising practical approaches to the task of measuring this dimension has emerged from a recent study by Martin, Haroldson, and Triden (1984). They found that listeners could produce remarkably reliable ratings (within one scale value) of "naturalness" of speech samples when asked to rate for this dimension on a 9-point scale (with 1 = highly natural and 9 = highly unnatural). This has provoked a series of investigations by Martin and Haroldson and the present authors to determine whether it might be possible to use this measure to evaluate speech quality. (We are also studying whether it is possible to use the feedback of such ratings to shape the naturalness quality in a client's speech during treatment.) The findings of Martin et al. (1984) suggest a host of possible avenues for research, including determination of the reliability and validity of a stutterer's own judgments of naturalness.

Appendix B illustrates a data sheet that is convenient for presenting a consolidated view of all the data collected from one set of STSs.

Talking logs

Thus far quantifiable measurements made from the STSs gathered periodically for each client have been described. Even though some of these measures are taken from beyond the clinic environment, it is still informative to know more about the stutterer's speech in the natural environment, for much of the client's talking is beyond our ability to measure conveniently and unobtrusively. One solution is to ask clients to maintain talking logs. Such logs are kept by the parents (often assisted by the child's teacher) or by the clients themselves when they are old enough to record the required information accurately. A talking log is simply a record of all of a person's talking episodes in a given 24-hr. period. The record shows the time of the talking episode, the person(s) with whom the client was talking, the setting in which the exchange occurred, the approximate length of time the exchange required, and a rating of the client's stuttering (0 = no stuttering; 1 = less stuttering than usual; 2 = stuttering about the same as usual; 3 = more stuttering than usual). Perusal of talking log data gives the clinician at least some approximate indication of the amount and nature of talking in which a client typically engages in a day, particular conversation partners and settings in which the client typically converses, and information about the variability of stuttering across these situations and over time. Further, rather than having clients complete paper and pencil questionnaires regarding their "avoidances" and "reactions" to various talking situations, talking log data can provide an informative and client-specific basis for constructing treatment task hierarchies and for measuring whether the client's number of interactions and talking situations expand over time.

Summary of the dependent variables

It should be evident that the above-mentioned measures are highly related and show consistent covariation. In a sense they overlap along the edges, yet each contributes a component not offered by the others. By viewing stuttering and "fluency" through this patchwork of inter-connected empirical measures, the slack in the reliability of these measures is offset, and the validity of the combined measures is fortified. Comparisons of all of these measures across each of the within- and beyond-clinic STSs provide the clinician and researcher with information regarding the complexity and severity of a person's stuttering, its uniqueness in comparison to other stutterers, and its variability across settings and conditions. Further, continued calculation of these measures provides a sensitive and generally objective evaluation of the effects of treatment at any given time.

Probes of the changeability of stuttering

The talking tasks and analyses described above provide information about the stutterer's speech in unmanipulated conditions. However, a variety of conditions that reliably produce changes, typically reductions, in the stuttering frequency of most stutterers have been described and tested. Testing a given client's performance under these conditions tells the clinician whether the person's stuttering behaves predictably under conditions known to alter stuttering. Further, each of these probes can be considered a preliminary test of a potential treatment technique. (Fields, 1980, has described an assessment rationale similar to this.)

In order to get information regarding the effects of each of the conditions described below, the effects of each on stuttering are probed in an "ABAB" fashion. That is, the client is first instructed to talk continuously in monologue[6] for a period of 1 min, the baseline or "A" period. After that time the probe condition is introduced and the client continues to talk for a 2nd min, the treatment or "B" period. Following this the clinician instructs the client to return to talking in the usual manner for another minute ("A" condition), and then the treatment probe is instituted again for a final 1-min period. As the client talks throughout each 1-min period, the clinician counts and records syllables and stutterings on-line so that %SS and SPM can be individually calculated for each segment at the conclusion of each 4-min probe. Conditions that produce reliable reductions in stuttering should be easily identified by comparisons between %SS in "B" periods and the preceding "A" periods. Of course, this cannot be considered a final test of a treatment's potential effects since some procedures may take much longer to produce effects with some clients.

Instructional control probe. Following the 1-min baseline period in this probe the clinician instructs the client (child or adult) to continue talking for another minute and to try as much as possible to talk without stuttering. No instructions regarding how to talk without stuttering are given, but the client is encouraged to use his or her very best speech and speak as well as possible. At the end of the minute the client is instructed to talk for another minute, returning to the regular way of talking. Then the instruction to talk without stuttering is re-presented prior to the last minute of the probe. Data on %SS and SPM indicate whether the client has the ability, under instructional control alone, to reduce stuttering frequency, and whether this is achieved independently of rate reduction strategies. The clinician will also want to note other changes that are perceived in the client's speech during this activity, especially ones related to the naturalness of any observed changes in speech pattern. Performance on this probe may be an indication of how easy it is for the client to improve speech simply by concentrating and trying to do so. Clients may also apply techniques learned in former treatment. At any rate, the effect of current treatment must be able to exceed the control exhibited by this task to ensure that the new treatment produces legitimate effects. The literature indicates that some stutterers

---

[6] It is often necessary to prepare the client to produce continuous monologue by providing topic cards (for adults) or picture stimuli (for children). These tasks can be conducted via reading, as well, but self-formulated continuous speech is preferred as a better approximation to natural speech.

reduce stuttering under instructions to do so, but that such reductions are of a temporary nature (Martin & Siegel, 1966; Martin & Harold-son, 1979).

Reduced speech rate probe. Before this probe is initiated the clinician models for the client (child or adult) a slowed rate of talking, one approximately one half to two thirds of the client's typical articulatory rate. The client then has the opportunity to practice this rate for an utterance or two until it is determined that the requirements of the task are understood and can be executed, at least briefly. Then the 4-min ABAB probe is conducted as above except that the "B" conditions are introduced by the clinician's instructions to the client to talk for the next minute at a slowed speech rate. When this probe is completed, the clinician will be able to note (1) whether the client is able to readily modify speed of speech and (2) whether reduced speech rate reduces stuttering frequency (%SS).

Prolonged speech probe. This probe is also initiated by the clinician modeling the kind of speech that will be required during the "B" conditions and by allowing the client (child or adult) a moment or two of practice. The speech modeled by the clinician and practiced by the client should be extremely prolonged, having each syllable stretched in duration and maintaining continuous voicing across phonetic transitions, with breaks in phonation occurring only for voiceless phonemes, for pauses between phrases, and for purposes of air intake (Howie, Tanner, & Andrews, 1981; Ingham & Andrews, 1973). An appropriate speed of speech for this probe is somewhere in the vicinity of 70 SPM. If the client has unusual difficulty executing this prolonged speech task, this kind of speech can be generated while the client is talking under 250 ms of continuous delayed auditory feedback (Goldiamond, 1965), where such equipment is available. Once again, the collected data will indicate whether the client was able to control this speech pattern adequately in order to produce sustained prolonged speech, and whether such speech was accompanied by reduced stuttering. If the client typifies most stut-terers (Is there such a client?), stuttering will be essentially eliminated while the client speaks in this fashion.

Rhythmic speech. Another condition known to reliably reduce stut-tering occurs when the stutterer speaks each syllable in time to a rhythmic stimulus (Brady, 1969, 1971; Johnson & Rosen, 1937). It is easiest to conduct this task with a metronome set at approximately 90 beats per minute, especially for children; but some clients are able to maintain a rhythmic speech pattern while talking in time with the clinician's auditory signal or with the assistance of an audiotape containing pre-recorded rhythmic signals. Rhythmic stimulation has been reported to produce quite dramatic reductions in stuttering for most stutterers (e.g., Martin & Haroldson, 1979).

Shadowing. Two additional probes are of interest for child clients. During shadowing (Cherry & Sayers, 1956; Kondas, 1967), the clinician first gives the child practice in concurrent talking. The child is instructed to repeat the words just spoken by the clinician, who speaks words and then sentences. The clinician can demonstrate the task by first shadowing some of the child's speech, and then by having the child repeat short utterances produced by the clinician in an imitative fashion and then, more quickly, overlapping the clinician's continuous talking. Very young children may find this task difficult, and it always requires some practice before the probe is initiated. Once again, %SS and SPM data are collected and calculated separately for each 1-min segment of the ABAB probe.

Verbal punishment probe. During this probe the child is instructed simply to talk in monologue on topics of his or her choice. After the first baseline minute the clinician introduces a response contingent (assumed) verbal punisher, such as "No!" or "Huh uh," immediately contingent upon every moment of stuttering (Quist & Martin, 1967). Several examples of the effectiveness of verbal punishers of this nature exist in the stuttering treatment literature (e.g., Martin, Kuhl, & Haroldson, 1972; Reed & Godden, 1977).

Self-recording probe. Three additional probes are of interest for adult clients. During self-recording (LaCroix, 1973) the task is first explained to the client and then a signal from the clinician is established that indicates when to begin self-recording. As in the previously described probes, a 1-min baseline is first established. Then, for the 2nd min, the client is required to continue talking but also concurrently to mark a sheet of paper each time a moment of stuttering occurs. During the 3rd min, the client returns to unmonitored talking, which is then followed by another minute of self-recording. During this task the clinician records total stutterings per minute and SPM. After the task is completed the clinician calculates percentage agreement by comparing her counts with the client's total stuttering counts for each "B" condition. These data will provide information regarding the client's awareness of stuttering as well as the effects of self-recording on stuttering frequency. It is of interest (but beyond current understanding) that the accuracy with which clients self-record stuttering does not correlate with the amount of reduced stuttering produced by self-recording (James, 1981).

Time-out probe. Response contingent interruptions in the flow of speech known as periods of time-out from positive reinforcement (assumedly, talking) have been repeatedly shown to produce significant decreases in frequency of stuttering (e.g., Costello, 1975; Haroldson, Martin, & Starr, 1968; Martin & Berndt, 1970). Before this probe is initiated the clinician tells the client to begin talking in monologue and to continue until the clinician says, "Stop." At that time the client is required to immediately refrain from continued talking, even in mid-word, until the clinician says, "Continue." During the "B" conditions of the ABAB probe, 5- to 10-s time-out periods are presented immediately contingent upon every moment of stuttering emitted during those periods. Data in the form of %SS and SPM are collected as above.

Chorus reading. Much like the shadowing task used with children, chorus reading has been shown to produce reductions in stuttering frequency for many stutterers (Barber, 1939; Johnson & Rosen, 1937). In this task, client and clinician simply orally read the same material simultaneously during the "B" conditions of the ABAB probe, while during the "A" conditions the client reads aloud alone. Data in the form of %SS and SPM continue to be calculated for each minute of the probe so that the effect of chorus reading on reading rate and stuttering frequency can be assessed. The literature has shown the effects of chorus reading to be independent of changes in reading rate (Ingham & Packman, 1979).

Summary of probes. When the six probes for children and the seven probes for adults have been completed, the data tell the clinician essentially three items of information. First, it gives the clinician (and the client) information about how readily changeable (or how intractable) the client's speech performance is. That is, if essentially all of the probe conditions produce ABAB stuttering reductions, one would note that the client's speech behavior appears malleable, and clients making this observation might be surprised and encouraged to note the ease with which their stuttering could be altered. If, however, the client had great difficulty in executing some or all of the probe tasks, and/or stuttering frequency was relatively unaffected by most of the probe conditions, one might anticipate that the client's speech may require longer and more extraordinary treatment procedures than those appropriate for clients whose speech changes more easily. (Of course, this question can be resolved best by research.)

Second, from the data gained from these probes, clinicians can gauge how similar a given client is to the imaginary "typical" stutterer whose stuttering would generally be reduced at least to some degree by many of these procedures. The more a client's performance differs from these "normative" data, the more unpredictable might be the effects of a given treatment—again, a question in dire need of research. Data such as these will promote better understanding, as well, of atypical stuttering in persons such as those with sudden and late onset, post cardiovascular accident onset, mental retardation, and even those whose stuttering continues following laryngectomy. At this point, no comprehensive descriptive or treatment data exist for such persons, so it is not possible to appreciate the consequences, if any, of their unusual stuttering histories.

Another obvious benefit of the data provided by these tasks is that they serve as tests of prospective treatments for each client, and their relative effects can be judged. Essentially all of these probe techniques have been developed into viable treatment procedures and reported in the treatment literature.

Other measures of interest

The reader is referred to other references such as Johnson et al. (1963) or Darley and Spriestersbach (1978) to be reminded of other components of pretreatment assessment that are no less important for stutterers than they are for persons with other potential disorders. For example, hearing screenings are appropriate for child and adult clients alike, even though one would probably not suggest a causal relationship between hearing acuity or discrimination and stuttering. Nonetheless, clinicians are responsible for determining the adequacy of all communication channels in any pretreatment assessment regimen, and the literature has suggested that children who stutter are more likely to display other concomitant speech and language disorders (e.g., Blood & Seider, 1981). Therefore, clinicians also gather genetic, birth, and developmental history information from the parents of child clients, and administer articulation, language, and cognitive screening measures as well. Although deficits in any of these areas may not be directly connected to the child's stuttering, such deficits would nonetheless influence the selection of treatment methods and even treatment targets (i.e., deficient language performance may be a more serious problem than a preschool child's incipient stuttering, or improvements in language may be seen as prerequisite to certain methods of treatment for stuttering). Of course, some writers have suggested that a language deficit may be at the heart of stuttering for some children (e.g., Wall & Myers, 1982; Westby, 1979), although firm evidence in this regard is still lacking.

It is interesting that birth and developmental histories are not typically regarded as important information to obtain from adult stuttering clients (with the exception of information regarding sudden onset), even though such information is typically discussed at length in regard to children.

This may be because such reports from adults have the reliability of hearsay evidence at best; or it may be because such information actually has little usefulness in providing information relevant to a description of the status of the client's speech, and does not lead the clinician to particular treatment procedures. Of more interest may be the knowledge of the adult client's previous treatment history, which may allow one to glean something about previous treatments that have and have not been beneficial, why the client did not continue in those reported to be beneficial, and whether treatment methods such as those about to be selected by the current clinician are known to the client.

Differential diagnosis

Distinguishing between stuttering and normally disfluent children. Many authors have written about the difficulties of correctly diagnosing stuttering in very young children—difficulties that largely stem from the apparent overlap in the disfluencies of normally talking children and the stutterings of young stutterers. The issues are well known and do not need reiterating here, although the interested reader is directed to a recent cogent review of that literature by Curlee (1984). Adams (1976, 1980) has offered rather specific guidelines to help clinicians recognize those children whose speech interruptions appear to be pathologic and, in a recent summary of his own writing and that of others (e.g., Curlee, 1980; Gregory & Hill, 1980; Johnson, 1980), Adams (1984) suggests the following profile as characteristic of a child who is becoming or is already a beginning stutterer.

> (1) Part-word repetitions and prolongations make up in excess of 7% of all words spoken; (2) the part-word repetitions are marked by at least 3 unit repetitions (e.g., "bee-bee-bee-beet" vs. "bee-bee-beet"); (3) the part-word repetitions are also perceived as containing the schwa in place of the vowel normally found in the syllable that is being repeated (e.g., "buh-buh-buh-beet" vs. "bee-bee-beet"); (4) the prolongations last longer than 1 second; and (5) difficulty in starting and/or sustaining voicing or air flow is heard in association with the part-word repetitions and prolongations. As more and more of these 5 signs are noted in a child's speech, a clinician can be increasingly confident that he or she is dealing with an incipient stutterer. Contrariwise, the fewer of these symptoms that are noted, the more likely that the youngster is normally disfluent. Whichever choice is made, it ought to be based on the foregoing and other behavioral data, be compatible with case history information that bears on the incidence of stuttering in the child's family, [and] take into account any current trends in the frequency of occurrence of the young-ster's disfluency (i.e., has it been steadily increasing or decreasing?). (p. 263)

Although Adams (1984) suggests that the validity of these charac-teristics as hallmarks of beginning stuttering is enhanced by the fact

that a group of authors working independently came to similar conclusions, no research has yet shown whether children displaying this
profile actually turn out to be stutterers, while those whose behavior
is different along some dimensions do not. As was pointed out earlier
when the problem of defining stuttering was addressed, rather than
attending to specific speech interruptions, the clinician (or parent) may
simply make perceptual judgments regarding whether the child's speech
interruptions sound like stuttering or not. These perceptual first impressions might then be confirmed by obtaining repeated measures across
a variety of conditions, as described above, and by observing whether
the perceived stutterings are altered by conditions that usually reduce
stuttering (although most of them have been reported to reduce disfluencies as well). A pattern of behavior usually emerges from this
abundance of observations so that a diagnostic decision often becomes
obvious.

On the other hand, it is well known that some unknown proportion
of young stutterers may be expected to recover without formal treatment
(see Ingham [1983] for a review and critique of this literature). Therefore, the view could be taken that, where there remains doubt regarding
the diagnosis of stuttering, the conservative route would be simply to
continue periodic observations based on STSs within and beyond the
clinic until the child's speech pattern changed to unequivocal stuttering
or unquestionably normal speech. It is also interesting to note that,
despite the warning of clinicians such as Johnson and Bloodstein, no
evidence exists to show that enrolling a normally disfluent child in
stuttering treatment has negative consequences for that child, although
such an extravagant use of precious treatment time is certainly not
recommended.

Classifying stutterers into subgroups. It has often been suggested that
stuttering may be an inordinately difficult disorder to understand
because it may, in fact, be several disorders. That is, some authors (most
notably Van Riper, 1971) have hypothesized that stutterers may stutter
for different reasons; that is, different etiologies might underlie the
stuttering observed among a group of stutterers. Following the logic of
this argument, one could subsequently hypothesize that different kinds
of stuttering would be amenable to different kinds of treatments.

Probably the most elaborate delineation of this concept of subcate-
gories is found in the work of Riley and Riley (1979, 1980, 1983). On
the basis of a combination of test scores and behavioral observations
of highly inferential nature, the Rileys described nine components of
stuttering (neurologic components including attending problems,

auditory processing problems, sentence formulation problems, and oral–motor problems; intrapersonal components including high self-expectations and manipulative stuttering; and interpersonal components including a disruptive communicative environment, high expectations by the parents, and abnormal parental need for the child to stutter). They subsequently developed somewhat differing treatment strategies that depended upon the "loading" of one or more of these factors. Although they report success from these treatments, the rigor with which the treatment data were gathered and reported leaves something to be desired. Further, in order to evaluate whether different treatments were really necessary, it would seem mandatory to administer, for example, oral–motor treatment to children exhibiting problems of high self-expectations. One would expect that treatment to be ineffective for those children whereas the same treatment should be shown to produce improvement for children classified as primarily oral–motor disabled. Conversely, one could delineate several groups of stutterers by the Rileys' diagnostic categories and administer the same treatment regimen to all of them. If the different groups responded in the same fashion to one treatment approach, then the concept of separate subgroups of stutterers would be suspect, at least for treatment purposes. These crucial experiments have not been conducted.

The clinical writings of Adams (1980, 1984; Adams & Runyan, 1981) have also been directed to the issue of differential assessment of stutterers. For example, Adams (1980) suggested the implementation of particular treatment strategies based on certain observations made during the pretreatment assessment (for example, the use of a treatment program that concentrates on breath stream management for children who exhibit "problems in commencing and sustaining voicing or air flow" [1980, p. 219]), or teaching prevoicing during the implosion phase of stop consonants when voiceless phonemes are substituted for voiced ones, illustrating problems of slowed voice onset time (Adams & Runyan, 1981).

Others have suggested that indications of maladjusted communicative attitudes should lead one to treatment directed toward those attitudes (Guitar & Bass, 1978; Guitar & Peters, 1980), even though convincing evidence to support this supposition is completely lacking. Ingham (1982) raised the same issues regarding Adams and Runyan's (1981) method of making a priori selection of specialized treatment components, and the undocumented report of the effects of such treatments.

In contrast to this symptom-specific treatment view, Costello (1983; chap 18, this volume) has recommended that treatment begin first with "the basics", and that additions to this treatment regimen be based first on empirical treatment data that show that the basics are not sufficient. That is, treatment designed to establish nonstuttered utterances through precise manipulations of consequences for stutterings and stutter-free responses (such as time-out or verbal reinforcers and punishers), perhaps with the addition of control over progressively longer utterances (such as Ryan's 1974 GILCU program or Costello's 1980, 1983 ELU treatment), may be all that is necessary to significantly alter stuttering patterns. However, if the *data collected during treatment* indicate small or innocuous treatment effects from these most simple, basic procedures, then, based on data gathered during pretreatment and subsequently, the clinician can append to the basic treatment procedures "additives" directed to the particular deficiency noted (such as decreased speed of speech for clients with high articulatory rates). The philosophy underlying this view is to keep treatment regimens as simple as possible and to *test* one's assumptions about the relevance of potential independent variables by empirical means.

Summary

The pretreatment assessment procedures described herein present an ambitious, yet clinically realistic, set of procedures designed to provide a quantitative analysis of stuttering and related phenomena. Further, the protocol is designed not only to provide relevant pretreatment data, but also to generate a consistent set of data to be systematically gathered throughout the subsequent course of treatment and followup. In addition, many of the measures described are also ones collected on-line during treatment (e.g., %SS and SPM), so there exists a congruence between assessment and treatment measures.

At this point in its development, the pretreatment assessment system described herein is logically, but arbitrarily, constructed. Extensive research is needed regarding how instrumental each of the tasks and measures is to the assessment process, the effectiveness of the treatments derived from the process, the gaps that may exist in terms of crucial variables left unmeasured, the reliability of clinicians' and others' use of the system, and the social validity of this set of measures as a comprehensive and sensitive indicator of the changing status of stuttering across time and conditions.

REFERENCES

Adams, M. R. Some common problems in the design and conduct of experiments in stuttering. *Journal of Speech and Hearing Disorders*, 1976, *41*, 3–9.

Adams, M. R. The young stutterer: Diagnosis, treatment and assessment of progress. *Seminars in Speech, Language and Hearing*, 1980, 1, 289–299.

Adams, M. R. The differential assessment and direct treatment of stuttering. In J. M. Costello (Ed.), *Speech disorders in children: Recent advances.* San Diego: College-Hill Press, 1984.

Adams, M. R., Lewis, J. I., & Besozzi, T. E. The effect of reduced reading rate on stuttering frequency. *Journal of Speech and Hearing Research,* 1973, *16,* 671–675.

Adams, M. R., & Runyan, C. M. Stuttering and fluency: Exclusive events or points on a continuum? *Journal of Fluency Disorders,* 1981, *6,* 197–218.

Andrews, G., & Craig, A. Stuttering: Overt and covert measurement of the speech of treated subjects. *Journal of Speech and Hearing Disorders,* 1982, *47,* 96–99.

Andrews, G., & Harvey, R. Regression to the mean in pretreatment measures of stuttering. *Journal of Speech and Hearing Disorders,* 1981, *46,* 204–207.

Barber, V. Studies in the psychology of stuttering: XV. Chorus reading as a distraction in stuttering. *Journal of Speech Disorders,* 1939, *4,* 371–383.

Bernard, J. R. L. Rates of utterance in Australian dialectic groups. Occasional Paper No. 7, The University of Sydney, Australian Language Research Center, August, 1965.

Blood, G. W., & Seider, R. The concomitant problems of young stutterers. *Journal of Speech and Hearing Disorders,* 1981, *46,* 31–33.

Bloodstein, O. Studies in the psychology of stuttering: XIX. The relationship between oral reading rate and severity of stuttering. *Journal of Speech Disorders,* 1944, *9,* 161–173.

Bloodstein, O. The development of stuttering: II. *Journal of Speech and Hearing Disorders,* 1960, *25,* 366–376.

Boodstein, O. Continuity, overlap, and ambiguity in stuttering: A reaction to MacDonald and Martin (1973). *Journal of Speech and Hearing Research,* 1974, *17,* 748–750.

Bloodstein, O. *A handbook on stuttering* (3rd ed.). Chicago: National Easter Seal Society, 1981.

Boehmler, R. M. Listener responses to non-fluencies. *Journal of Speech and Hearing Research,* 1958, *1,* 132–141.

Brady, J. P. Studies on the metronome effect on stuttering. *Behaviour Research and Therapy,* 1969, *7,* 197–205.

Brady, J. P. Metronome-conditioned speech retraining for stuttering. *Behavior Therapy,* 1971, *2,* 129–150.

Brutten, G. J. Stuttering: Topography, assessment, and behavior-change strategies. In J. Eisenson (Ed.), *Stuttering: A second symposium.* New York: Harper & Row, 1975.

Cherry, C., & Sayers, B. McA. Experiments upon the total inhibition of stammering by external control, and some clinical results. *Journal of Psychosomatic Research,* 1956, *1,* 233–246.

Costello, J. M. The establishment of fluency with time-out procedures: Three case studies. *Journal of Speech and Hearing Disorders,* 1975, *40,* 216–231.

Costello, J. M. Operant conditioning and the treatment of stuttering. *Seminars in Speech, Language and Hearing,* 1980, *1,* 311–325.

Costello, J.M. Pretreatment assessment of stuttering in young children. *Communicative disorders: An audio journal for continuing education.* New York: Grune & Stratton, 1981.

Costello, J. M. Current behavioral treatments for children. In D. Prins & R. J. Ingham (Eds.), *Stuttering in early childhood. Treatment methods and issues.* San Diego: College-Hill Press, 1983.

Costello, J.M., & Hurst, M. R. An analysis of the relationship among stuttering behaviors. *Journal of Speech and Hearing Research,* 1981, *24,* 247–256.

Curlee, R. A case selection strategy for young disfluent children. *Seminars in Speech, Language and Hearing*, 1980, *1*, 277–287.

Curlee, R. Observer agreement on disfluency and stuttering. *Journal of Speech and Hearing Research*, 1981, *24*, 595–600.

Curlee, R. Stuttering disorders: An overview. In J. M. Costello (Ed.), *Speech disorders in children: Recent advances*. San Diego: College-Hill Press, 1984.

Darley, F. L., & Spriestersbach, D. C. *Diagnostic methods in speech pathology.* New York: Harper & Row, 1978.

Fields, T. A. An individualistic approach to the evaluation and remediation of stuttering. *Journal of Fluency Disorders*, 1980, *5*, 115–136.

Floyd, S., & Perkins, W. H. Early syllable dysfluency in stutterers and nonstutterers: A preliminary report. *Journal of Communication Disorders*, 1974, *7*, 279–282.

Gregory, H., & Hill, D. Stuttering therapy for children. *Seminars in Speech, Language and Hearing*, 1980, *1*, 351–364.

Guitar, B., & Bass, C. Stuttering therapy: The relation between attitude change and long-term outcome. *Journal of Speech and Hearing Disorders*, 1978, *43*, 392–400.

Guitar, B., & Peters, T. J. *Stuttering: An integration of contemporary therapies.* Memphis: Speech Foundation of America, 1980.

Haroldson, S. K., Martin, R. R., & Starr, C. D. Time-out as a punishment for stuttering. *Journal of Speech and Hearing Research*, 1968, *11*, 560–566.

Hersen, M., & Barlow, D. H. *Single-case experimental designs.* New York: Pergamon, 1976.

Hegde, M. N. Fluency and fluency disorders: Their definition, measurement, and modification. *Journal of Fluency Disorders*, 1978, *3*, 51–71.

Howie, P. M., Tanner, S., & Andrews, G. Short- and long-term outcome in an intensive treatment program for adult stutterers. *Journal of Speech and Hearing Disorders*, 1981, *46*, 104–109.

Huffman, E. S., & Perkins, W. H. Dysfluency characteristics identified by listeners as "stuttering" and "stutterer." *Journal of Speech and Hearing Disorders*, 1974, *7*, 89–96.

Ingham, R. J. A comparison of covert and overt assessment procedures in stuttering therapy outcome evaluation. *Journal of Speech and Hearing Research*, 1975, *18*, 346–354.

Ingham, R. J. Modification of maintenance and generalization during stuttering treatment. *Journal of Speech and Hearing Research*, 1980, *23*, 732–745.

Ingham, R. J. Some comments on "Stuttering and fluency: Exclusive events or points on a continuum?" *Journal of Fluency Disorders*, 1982, *7*, 303–307.

Ingham, R. J. Spontaneous remission of stuttering: When will the emperor realize he has no clothes on? In D. Prins & R. Ingham (Eds.), *Treatment of stuttering in early childhood: Methods and issues.* San Diego: College-Hill Press, 1983.

Ingham, R. J. *Stuttering and behavior therapy: Current status and experimental foundations.* San Diego: College-Hill Press, 1984.

Ingham, R. J., & Andrews, G. Details of a token economy stuttering therapy programme for adults. *Australian Journal of Human Communication Disorders*, 1973, *1*, 13–20.

Ingham, R. J., & Costello, J. M. Stuttering treatment outcome evaluation. In J. M. Costello (Ed.), *Speech disorders in children: Recent advances.* San Diego: College-Hill Press, 1984.

Ingham, R. J., Martin, R. R., & Kuhl, P. Modification and control of rate of speaking by stutterers. *Journal of Speech and Hearing Research*, 1974, *17*, 489–496.

Ingham, R. J., & Onslow, M. *Stuttering treatment evaluation manual.* Sydney: Cumberland College of Health Sciences, 1983.

Ingham, R. J., & Packman, A. C. Perceptual assessment of normalcy of speech following stuttering therapy. *Journal of Speech and Hearing Research,* 1978, *21,* 63–73.

Ingham, R. J., & Packman, A. C. A further evaluation of the speech of stutterers during chorus- and nonchorus-reading conditions. *Journal of Speech and Hearing Research,* 1979, *22,* 784–793.

James, J. E. Self-monitoring of stuttering: Reactivity and accuracy. *Behaviour Research and Therapy,* 1981, *19,* 291–296.

Johnson, L. Facilitating parental involvement in therapy for the disfluent child. *Seminars in Speech, Language and Hearing,* 1980, *1,* 301–310.

Johnson, W. Measurements of oral reading and speaking rate and disfluency of adult male and female stutterers and nonstutterers. *Journal of Speech and Hearing Disorders* (Monograph Suppl. No. 7), 1961, 1–20.

Johnson, W., Darley, F. L., & Spriestersbach, D. C. *Diagnostic methods in speech pathology.* New York: Harper & Row, 1963.

Johnson, W., & Rosen, L. Studies in the psychology of stuttering: VII. Effect of certain changes in speech pattern upon frequency of stuttering. *Journal of Speech and Hearing Disorders,* 1937, *2,* 105–109.

Jones, R. J., & Azrin, N. H. Behavioral engineering: Stuttering as a function of stimulus duration during speech synchronization. *Journal of Applied Behavior Analysis,* 1969, *2,* 223–229.

Kondas, O. The treatment of stammering in children by the shadowing method. *Behaviour Research and Therapy,* 1967, *5,* 325–329.

Kowal, S., O'Connell, D. C., & Sabin, E. F. Development of temporal patterning and vocal hesitations in spontaneous narratives. *Journal of Psycholinguistic Research,* 1975, *4,* 195–207.

LaCroix, Z. Management of disfluent speech through self-recording procedures. *Journal of Speech and Hearing Disorders,* 1973, *39,* 272–274.

Luper, H. L., & Mulder, R. *Stuttering therapy for children.* Englewood Cliffs, NJ: Prentice-Hall, 1964.

MacDonald, J. D., & Martin, R. R. Stuttering and disfluency as two reliable and unambiguous response classes. *Journal of Speech and Hearing Research,* 1973, *17,* 691–699.

Martin, R. R., & Berndt, L. A. The effects of time-out on stuttering in a 12 year old boy. *Exceptional Children,* 1970, *36,* 303–304.

Martin, R. R., & Haroldson, S. K. Effects of five experimental treatments on stuttering. *Journal of Speech and Hearing Research,* 1979, *22,* 132–146.

Martin, R. R., & Heraldson, S. K. Stuttering identification: Standard definitions and moment of stuttering. *Journal of Speech and Hearing Research,* 1981, *24,* 59–63.

Martin, R. R., Haroldson, S. K., & Triden, K. A. Stuttering and speech naturalness. *Journal of Speech and Hearing Disorders,* 1984, *49,* 53–58.

Martin, R. R., Kuhl, P., & Haroldson, S. K. An experimental treatment with two preschool stuttering children. *Journal of Speech and Hearing Research,* 1972, *15,* 743–752.

Martin, R. R., & Siegel, G. M. The effects of simultaneously punishing stuttering and rewarding fluency. *Journal of Speech and Hearing Research,* 1966, *9,* 466–475.

McReynolds, L. V., & Kearns, K. *Single-subject experimental designs.* Baltimore: University Park Press, 1983.

Perkins, W. H. Behavioral management of stuttering. Final report. Social and Rehabilitation Services Research Grant 14-P-55281, 1973.

Perkins, W. H. Articulatory rate in the evaluation of stuttering treatments. *Journal of Speech and Hearing Disorders,* 1975, *40,* 277–278.

Perkins, W. H. The problem of definition: Commentary on "stuttering." *Journal of Speech and Hearing Disorders,* 1983, *48,* 246–249.

Perkins, W. H., Bell, J., Johnson, L., & Stocks, J. Phone rate and the effective planning time hypothesis of stuttering. *Journal of Speech and Hearing Research,* 1979, *22,* 747–755.

Prosek, R. A., & Runyan, C. M. Temporal characteristics related to the discrimination of stutterers' and nonstutterers' speech samples. *Journal of Speech and Hearing Research,* 1982, *25,* 29–33.

Prosek, R. A., & Runyan, C. M. Effects of segment and pause manipulations on the identification of treated stutterers. *Journal of Speech and Hearing Research,* 1983, *26,* 510–516.

Quist, R. W., & Martin, R. R. The effect of response contingent verbal punishment. *Journal of Speech and Hearing Research,* 1967, *10,* 795–800.

Reed, C. G., & Godden, A. L. An experimental treatment using verbal punishment with two preschool stutterers. *Journal of Fluency Disorders,* 1977, *2,* 225–233.

Riley, G. D. A stuttering severity instrument for children and adults. *Journal of Speech and Hearing Disorders,* 1972, *37,* 314–322.

Riley, G. D., & Riley, J. A component model for diagnosing and treating children who stutter. *Journal of Fluency Disorders,* 1979, *4,* 279–294.

Riley, G. D., & Riley, J. Motoric and linguistic variables among children who stutter: A factor analysis. *Journal of Speech and Hearing Disorders,* 1980, *45,* 504–514.

Riley, G. D., & Riley, J. Evaluation as a basis for intervention. In D. Prins & R. J. Ingham (Eds.), *Treatment of stuttering in early childhood: Treatment methods and issues.* San Diego: College-Hill Press, 1983.

Runyan, C. M., & Adams, M. R. Perceptual study of the speech of "successfully therapeutized" stutterers. *Journal of Fluency Disorders,* 1978, *3,* 25–39.

Ryan, B. P. *Programmed therapy for stuttering in children and adults.* Springfield, IL: Thomas, 1974.

Schiavetti, N. Judgments of stuttering severity as a function of type and locus of disfluency. *Folia Phoniatrica,* 1975, *27,* 26–37.

Starkweather, C. W. Speech fluency and its development in normal children. In N. J. Lass (Ed.), *Speech and language: Advances in basic reasearch and practice* (Vol. 4). New York: Academic Press, 1980.

Umeda, N., & Quinn, A. M. S. Some notes on reading: Talkers, materials and reading rate. *Journal of Speech and Hearing Research,* 1980, *23,* 56–72.

Van Riper, C. *The nature of stuttering.* Englewood Cliffs, NJ: Prentice-Hall, 1971.

Voelker, C. H. A preliminary investigation for a normative study of fluency: A clinical index to the severity of stuttering. *American Journal of Orthopsychiatry,* 1944, *14,* 285–294.

Wall, M. J., & Myers, F. L. A review of linguistic factors associated with early childhood stuttering. *Journal of Communication Disorders,* 1982, *15,* 441–449.

Webster, R. L. A behavioral analysis of stuttering: Treatment and theory. In K. S. Calhoun, H. E. Adams, & K. M. M. Mitchell (Eds.), *Innovative treatment methods in psychopathology.* New York: Wiley, 1974.

Webster, R. L. Empirical considerations regarding stuttering therapy. In H. H. Gregory (Ed.), *Controversies about stuttering therapy.* Baltimore: University Park Press, 1979.

Wertheim, E. S. A new approach to the classification and measurement of stuttering. *Journal of Speech and Hearing Disorders,* 1972, *37,* 242–251.

Westby, C. E. Lauguage performance of stuttering and nonstuttering children. *Journal of Communication Disorders,* 1974, *12,* 133–145.

Williams, D. E. The problem of stuttering. In F. L. Darley & D. C. Spriestersbach (Eds.), *Diagnostic methods in speech pathology.* New York: Harper & Row, 1978.

Williams, D. E., & Kent, L. R. Listener evaluations of speech interruptions. *Journal of Speech and Hearing Research,* 1958, *1,* 124–131.

Wingate, M. E. A standard definition of stuttering. *Journal of Speech and Hearing Disorders,* 1964, *29,* 484–489.

Wingate, M. E. Criteria for stuttering. *Journal of Speech and Hearing Research,* 1977, *20,* 596–606.

Wingate, M. E. Knowing what to look for: Comments on "Stuttering identification— Standard definition and moment of stuttering." *Journal of Speech and Hearing Research,* 1981, *24,* 622–623.

Young, M. A. Predicting ratings of severity of stuttering. *Journal of Speech and Hearing Disorders* (Monograph Suppl. No. 7), 1961, 31–54.

Young, M. A. Observer agreement: Cumulative effects of repeated ratings of the same samples and of knowledge of group results. *Journal of Speech and Hearing Research,* 1969, *12,* 144–155.

Young, M. A., & Downs, T. D. Testing the significance of the agreement among observers. *Journal of Speech and Hearing Research,* 1968, *11,* 5–17.

APPENDIX A: CALCULATIONS FOR THE MEASUREMENT OF STUTTERING

For some years now, clinical researchers in this country, and in Australia and Canada, have used a relatively simple dual button press electronic counter-timer that can be used to record the raw data required for calculations of %SS and SPM. Pressing one button registers nonstuttered syllables and the other registers stuttered syllables. Articulatory rate is measured by arranging for the unit to cease recording time if a syllable count is not registered within a specified time period. During overall speaking rate measures, the counter-timer is set to record uninterrupted time periods. When such equipment is available, these measures (%SS stuttered and SPM) can be made quite conveniently from the entire talking sample so that the approximate measures described below can be avoided. Details on this equipment may be obtained by writing the authors. If one does not have such equipment, however, the sampling and calculation techniques described below can be used to produce reliable and relatively accurate data from the talking samples within reasonable time constraints, once the data collector has become proficient. Each of the dependent variables described below is to be calculated separately for each STS.

1. Percent syllables stuttered (%SS)

$$\%SS = \frac{\text{total number of stutterings}}{\text{total number of syllables spoken}} \times 100$$

The *total number of stutterings* is obtained by counting the entire number of moments of stuttering (see Footnote 2) in the talking sample. Stutterings can occur between words and within words. Further, more than one stuttering can occur in a word; when this occurs, each moment of stuttering should be counted separately. When all moments of stuttering have been tallied from listening to the entire sample, a total count equals the total number of stutterings in the sample.

In order to calculate an approximation of *total number of syllables spoken,* one must first calculate the *total amount of client talking time (CTT)* in the sample and the *average number of syllables spoken per minute.* To measure the total amount of CTT in the sample, listen to the entire sample and activate a stopwatch any time the client is talking. If the client pauses for more than 2 s (for example, between sentences or thoughts, while turning the pages of a book or manipulating a toy, or when another person is talking), turn off the stopwatch until the client once again begins talking. Use the stopwatch so that it cumulates the CTT so that the total amount of CTT shows on the stopwatch at the end of the sample. Record this number in minutes and seconds in the appropriate place on the Stuttering Data Sheet (see Appendix B).

Calculation of the *average number of syllables spoken per minute* requires first a count of the total number of syllables spoken during the entire sample. Because this is a tedious and time-consuming measurement task when many analyses are to be made (unless one has the electronic counter described above), a somewhat less precise, but adequate and reliable, shortcut has been developed. Listen to the entire talking sample again and this time listen carefully to randomly selected intervals of the client's uninterrupted talking. Using the stopwatch, time each talking interval and count the number of syllables spoken in each interval until a minimum of 2 min of CTT is accumulated. It is important that the intervals represent the entire sample, so they should be selected from sections throughout the length of the sample. Moments of stuttering that are interjections of words or syllables or repetitions of words or phrases are counted only once. When the total number of syllables spoken during the 2 min of accumulated talking time is recorded, divide that number by 2 (or by the amount of talking time that has been accumulated if it is different from 2 min). Now the *approximate number of syllables spoken per minute* has been determined. To calculate the *total number of syllables spoken* in the entire sample for the above formula, multiply the number of syllables spoken per minute by the CTT as determined above.

Now both total number of stutterings and the (approximate) total number of syllables spoken are known. Use these numbers to calculate %SS in the above formula.

2. Average duration of stutterings

Listen to the speech sample throughout once again and time the length of 10 different stutterings, randomly selected but with an ear to their representativeness regarding length. Sum the total times and divide by 10 to estimate the length of the average or typical moment of stuttering.

3. Duration of the three longest stutterings

Pick out what you judge to be the three longest stutterings occurring in the talking sample. Time each with a stopwatch and note their length on the Stuttering Data Sheet.

4. Overall speaking rate (approximate) calculated in syllables per minute (SPM)

$$\frac{\text{overall speaking rate}}{\text{(SPM)}} = \frac{\text{number of syllables spoken in 2 min}}{2}$$

This measure has already been calculated in 1 above.

5. Articulatory rate

$$\frac{\text{articulatory rate}}{\text{(SPM)}} = \frac{\text{total number of nonstuttered syllables}}{\text{total amount of talking time}}$$

Articulatory rate (or phone rate) is the measure of the client's speaking rate unimpeded by disfluencies or stutterings. It is also measured in SPM. To calculate articulatory rate, count the number of syllables spoken from 10 randomly selected intervals of the client's talking sample (or as many as you can reliably identify and count). These must be intervals that do not contain stuttering or disfluencies and from which pauses greater than 2 s are eliminated. Record the time and the number of syllables uttered separately for each utterance. Next, measure the total amount of talking time produced during these intervals. Put these numbers into the above formula. (Severe stutterers may not exhibit nonstuttered intervals of sufficient number or length to allow calculation of this measure prior to the initiation of treatment.)

6. Average duration of nonstuttered intervals

$$\frac{\text{duration of}}{\text{average nonstuttered utterance}} = \frac{\text{total amount of nonstuttered talking time}}{10}$$

From the measures of 10 nonstuttered intervals collected in 5 above, the total amount of talking time required to produce those 10 nonstuttered intervals has already been calculated. When this number is divided by 10 (or by the number of nonstuttered utterances actually measured if it is different from 10), average duration of the "typical" nonstuttered interval is determined.

7. Duration of the three longest nonstuttered intervals

Separately time the duration of what you judge to be the three longest periods of speaking without stuttering that occur in the sample and indicate those times in minutes and seconds on the Stuttering Data Sheet.

8. Average length of nonstuttered intervals

$$\frac{\text{length of}}{\text{average nonstuttered utterance}} = \frac{\text{total number of nonstuttered syllables}}{10}$$

From the measures of 10 nonstuttered intervals collected in 5 above, the total number of nonstuttered syllables emitted in those utterances is already calculated. When this number is divided by 10 (or by the actual number of utterances measured if different from 10), the length of the "typical" nonstuttered interval is determined.

9. Length of the three longest nonstuttered intervals

This measure is based on the same three nonstuttered utterances used in 7 above. For each of these utterances, the longest observed in the sample, count the number of syllables emitted and record these three numbers in the appropriate place on the Stuttering Data Sheet.

10. Naturalness rating

On the Stuttering Data Sheet record your own overall impression of the naturalness of the client's speech throughout the talking sample using a 9-point scale (1 = highly natural; 9 = highly unnatural). It is also useful to obtain naturalness ratings from lay persons as well, and especially from the client, given that these evaluations are found to be valid and reliable.

APPENDIX B
STUTTERING DATA SHEET
(ADULT)

Client name_____

Birthdate_____

Kernel characteristics:

Accessory features:

	Stuttering	Speaking Rate		Nonstuttered Utterances	Naturalness Ratings
% SS	Length in seconds avg. stutter/ 3 longest	Overall spkg. rate (SPM)	Artic. rate (SPM)	Length in seconds Length in syllables 1 = highly natural avg. flu. utt./ avg. flu. utt./ 9 = highly unnatural 3 longest 3 longest	

IN-CLINIC STUTTERING DATA

5 minute Reading

Passage

Client talking time (CTT)

date_____

5 minute Monologue

CTT_____

date_____

5 minute conver. with Clinician

location_____

CTT_____

date_____

EXTRACLINIC STUTTERING DATA

5 min. conver. with Clinician

location_____

CTT_____

date_____

5 min conver. with Friend/Spouse

other person_____

location_____

CTT_____

date_____

5 min conver.: Telephone

other person_____

CTT_____

date_____

5 min conver.: Workplace

other person_____

CTT_____

date_____

Covert assessment description

_____

_____

_____

CTT_____

date_____

Chapter 16

Prevention of Stuttering: Management of Early Stages

Hugo H. Gregory

As professionals interested in stuttering, some of our most fruitful and rewarding activity focuses on prevention. Advances during recent years in our understanding of the nature of children's disfluency and the factors that contribute to increased disfluency and stuttering have enabled us to intervene more appropriately (Cooper, 1979; Gregory, 1979a, 1979b; Gregory & Hill, 1980; Prins & Ingham, 1983; Van Riper, 1973). Also, the general public may be acquiring more of the kind of information that leads to normal development of speech, including fluency, in children. I tell my students that work on prevention is our "highest calling."

When parents express concern that their child is "stuttering" or "beginning to stutter," a speech–language pathologist does an evaluation to determine (1) whether there should, or should not, be concern about the child's speech, and (2) if there is concern, what developmental or environmental factors should be focused upon to prevent the development of stuttering, or in some cases, to "stem the tide" of a developing problem. The process involved has been called differential evaluation (Gregory, 1973; Gregory & Hill, 1980). This chapter shows how treatment strategies are determined from the evaluation process, taking into account each child's specific needs. Information about the development of speech fluency in children, and factors related to increased disfluency and the development of stuttering also are reviewed. The discussion of treatment strategies focuses upon our experience and reports from other clinics.

OVERVIEW OF DIFFERENTIAL EVALUATION

Several contributors, among them Van Riper (1973), Gregory (1973), Riley and Riley (1979), Gregory and Hill (1980), and Daly (1981), have advocated systems for differential evaluations based on the belief that it is important to recognize individual differences from child to child. The diagram in Figure 16-1 illustrates the differential evaluation procedure utilized at Northwestern University and shows, in general, how a clinician chooses appropriate treatment procedures. In this system, the level of initial evaluation is determined by information received from the parent, often by telephone. Gregory and Hill state:

> During initial contacts, approximately 50 percent of parents we have seen expressed concern about a perceived disfluency difference that had existed for less than a year, and reported no other concern about speech and language development or behavioral characteristics (for example, auditory, attentional, motor, and social). In these cases, the children were referred for the screening examination. In the other 50 percent, parents described disfluency patterns of concern that had persisted beyond a year, or reported other concerns about speech, language, or behavior. Children in this group were referred directly for a more comprehensive evaluation. (pp. 381–382)

The screening evaluation consists of four main parts: (1) a brief case history of speech, language, and fluency development and other factors, such as illness, that may be important; (2) an analysis of fluency as noted in monologue, play, play with pressure, and parent–child interaction; (3) an analysis of parent–child interactive behaviors, such as parental interrupting or asking one question and then another before the child has answered the first; and (4) an assessment of speech, language, and hearing. Decisions following this evaluation may result in utilizing Treatment Strategy 1 (Preventive Parent Counseling) or 2 (Prescriptive Parent Counseling and Limited Involvement of the Child), or in scheduling an in-depth speech and language evaluation (see Figure 16-1). The in-depth speech and language evaluation includes more extensive assessment in each of the four areas already mentioned with attention given to a comprehensive evaluation of speech, language, oral motor, auditory, and visual motor skills and observation of the child's response to the clinician's model of a more easy, relaxed speech pattern. Ordinarily, an in-depth evaluation leads to the child and parents' involvement in Treatment Strategy 3 (Comprehensive Therapy Program; Involvement of Both Parents and Child) (see Figure 16-1).

Since our evaluation procedures are similar to diagnostic procedures widely used, they are not reviewed in detail. Only those features that are of particular value to a valid differential evaluation and their rationales will be discussed.

FIGURE 16-1. Overview of Differential Evaluation and Therapy

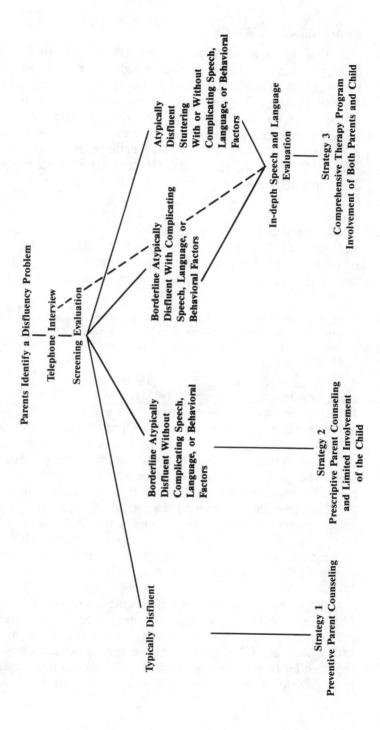

Parents Identify a Disfluency Problem

Telephone Interview

Screening Evaluation

Typically Disfluent

Borderline Atypically
Disfluent Without
Complicating Speech,
Language, or Behavioral
Factors

Borderline Atypically
Disfluent With Complicating
Speech, Language, or
Behavioral Factors

Atypically
Disfluent
Stuttering
With or Without
Complicating Speech,
Language, or Behavioral
Factors

In-depth Speech and Language
Evaluation

Strategy 1
Preventive Parent Counseling

Strategy 2
Prescriptive Parent Counseling
and Limited Involvement
of the Child

Strategy 3
Comprehensive Therapy Program
Involvement of Both Parents and Child

(From Gregory and Hill, 1980)

ANALYSIS OF FLUENCY

As language is acquired and as articulatory proficiency develops during the years of childhood, there are also changes in the flow of speech, noted mainly by the quality and quantity of speech disfluency. Before suggesting an approach to evaluating a child's fluency, the following summary statements about our knowledge of nonstuttering and stuttering children's disfluency are provided as a frame of reference.

1. There is great intersubject variability in the occurrence of disfluency (DeJoy, 1975; Haynes & Hood, 1977; Wexler & Mysak, 1982; Yairi, 1981, 1982). In other words, we can expect considerable variability from child to child. Gottfred (1979) and Yairi (1982) reporting on longitudinal studies of 2-year-olds, have shown that the amount of total disfluency and the prevalence of types of disfluency varies considerably from one evaluation of a child to the next, separated by 3 or 4 months. Yairi (1982) concluded that alternations of a large magnitude in the number of disfluencies (both increases and decreases) occur in the speech of many young children at this age. He stated:

> Unlike several other aspects of speech and language such as sound acquisition, articulatory precision, and syntactic skills that usually assume a one-way developmental course, disfluency stands out as a phenomenon which is prone to alternating reversals. (p. 159)

2. Pauses, revisions, and interjections (nonrepetitious disfluencies) occur most frequently (Brownell, 1973; DeJoy, 1975; Wexler & Mysak, 1982). In general, part-word sound and syllable repetitions and prolongations of sounds are the least frequent (Brownell, 1973; DeJoy, 1975; Haynes & Hood, 1977; Wexler & Mysak, 1982). However, data from Johnson (1955) and Yairi (1981) indicate that 2-year-olds may show considerable part-word repetition. Yet, most studies show that part-word repetitions begin to decrease during the 3rd year (Johnson, 1955; Yairi, 1982). Single-syllable word repetitions are fairly frequent in a child's speech, especially during years 2 and 3 when relational language is developing rapidly (Yairi, 1981). Based on data presently available, there is reasonably good evidence that disfluency, especially repetitious types, decreases generally following the 3rd year (DeJoy, 1975; Wexler & Mysak, 1982).

3. Situational differences affect the frequency and type of disfluency. Although clinical evidence supports the existence of such differences in children's responses, research results have been equivocal (Johnson, 1942; Silverman, 1972). In a study that may illustrate an important approach for future research, Gottfred (1979) showed that children 24 to 30 months of age responded to standardized speech pressure by

producing more prolongations. In addition to situational differences, syntactic context appears to influence the occurrence of disfluency. Most studies of either nonstuttering or stuttering preschool children have revealed a greater than expected number of disfluencies on function words and pronouns at the beginning of syntactic units (Bloodstein & Gantwerk, 1967; Silverman, 1973; Helmreich & Bloodstein, 1973). Bloodstein (1981) notes that children probably respond to these syntactic units as the basic units of speech formulation and motor speech production.

4. Regarding sex differences, studies have shown there is a higher frequency of syllable repetitions in boys (Davis, 1939; Oxtoby, 1943; Yairi, 1981), but no differences have been statistically significant. Yairi (1981) reported a trend for boys to show more repetitions per instance of syllable repetition.

5. Listener reaction studies (Boehmler, 1958; Giolas & Williams, 1958; Williams & Kent, 1958), in which observers listened to disfluencies drawn from the speech samples of both nonstutterers and stutterers, have shown that there is greater agreement in classifying sound and syllable repetitions and disfluencies rated as more severe as stuttering. Revisions and interjections are judged infrequently as stuttering.

6. Several studies have shown that speakers who are considered to be stutterers demonstrate substantially greater amounts of sound and syllable repetitions and prolongations (Davis, 1939; Voelker, 1944). Johnson et al. (1959) summarized data showing that male stuttering children showed significantly more sound and syllable repetitions, word repetitions, phrase repetitions, and prolongations than male nonstuttering children. In the last of three studies of the onset and development of stuttering, Johnson et al. (1959) acknowledged that the parents of stuttering children reported the presence of sound and syllable repetition at the onset of stuttering significantly more often than was reported by parents of a matched group of nonstuttering children.

Such information about disfluency in children reveals that we are acquiring increased knowledge that helps us to be more precise in our evaluations of a child's speech. Nevertheless, defining the existence of a stuttering problem with reference to observations of a child's speech is far from being an "either-or" matter. Certain disfluencies, word and phrase repetitions, and most of the nonrepetitious disfluencies occur rather frequently in the speech of most children. Breaks in fluency at the word level (sound and syllable repetitions and prolongations of sounds) occur less frequently. Therefore, in general, we are more concerned about increases of the latter disfluency types in a child's speech. Furthermore, we are more concerned about one-syllable word repetitions or part-word syllable repetitions if there is a high frequency of repetition per instance and even more so if the tempo among repetitions is irregular. We are also more concerned if there is disruption of air flow or phonation between repetitions or if a schwa-sounding vowel is substituted for the one ordinarily used in the repetition of a syllable (Adams, 1977; Cooper, 1973; Curlee, 1980; Gregory & Hill, 1980; Van Riper, 1982). Of course other signs of increased tension in the lips, jaw, larynx, or chest are more obvious characteristics that create additional concern and point more definitely to a problem.

Having said this, the information on children 24–42 months of age indicate that we should be mindful that fluency is ordinarily quite unstable within a child (greater intrasubject variability) during this period of rapid speech development. Increases in disfluency may be cyclic, and the clinician should note if there is a change toward longer or shorter periods of increased disfluency, obviously the latter being a positive development. Preventive strategies that are described later are aimed toward creating conditions that are conducive to a normal developmental reduction of disfluency and cyclic variations.

For use in clinical evaluations and parental guidance lectures, we have generated a continuum of disfluent speech behaviors from *More Usual* at one end to *More Unusual* at the other (see Figure 16-2). More typical disfluencies are followed on the continuum by borderline atypical disfluencies, then more atypical disfluencies. Quantitative and qualitative guidelines based on our experience and on reports in the literature have been used (Cooper, 1973; Van Riper, 1982). We like the continuum idea because it reflects our present knowledge about children's disfluency, and we are comfortable with the use of "concern" in describing our evaluation, because it lends itself to the consideration of degree.

EVALUATING ENVIRONMENTAL FACTORS

Most contributors, regardless of their point of view, have considered environmental influences to be important in the development of stuttering. Likewise, modifications of the environment have been considered important in the prevention of stuttering and in early intervention. Those who have examined the role of genetic factors also assume that environmental conditions interact with genetic predispositions (Kidd, 1977). Thus, our evaluations of children include procedures for obtaining information about communicative stress (the way the parents and others talk to the child) and interpersonal stress (general interaction among family members). In my opinion, a particularly important and useful approach during the last 15 years has been the investigation of parent–child interactive behaviors in a more objective manner. Kasprisin (1970) and

FIGURE 16-2. Continuum of Disfluent Speech Behaviors

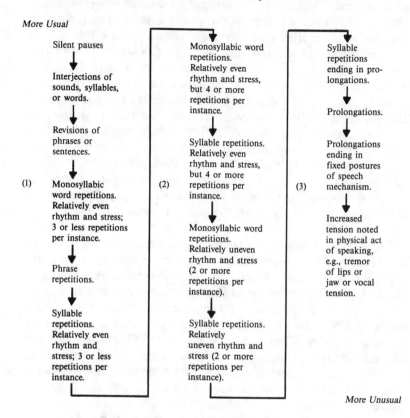

More Usual

(1)
- Silent pauses
- Interjections of sounds, syllables, or words.
- Revisions of phrases or sentences.
- Monosyllabic word repetitions. Relatively even rhythm and stress; 3 or less repetitions per instance.
- Phrase repetitions.
- Syllable repetitions. Relatively even rhythm and stress; 3 or less repetitions per instance.

(2)
- Monosyllabic word repetitions. Relatively even rhythm and stress, but 4 or more repetitions per instance.
- Syllable repetitions. Relatively even rhythm and stress, but 4 or more repetitions per instance.
- Monosyllabic word repetitions. Relatively uneven rhythm and stress (2 or more repetitions per instance).
- Syllable repetitions. Relatively uneven rhythm and stress (2 or more repetitions per instance).

(3)
- Syllable repetitions ending in prolongations.
- Prolongations.
- Prolongations ending in fixed postures of speech mechanism.
- Increased tension noted in physical act of speaking, e.g., tremor of lips or jaw or vocal tension.

More Unusual

(1) Typical disfluencies that occur in preschool children's speech. Listed on the continuum in general order of expected frequency (silent pauses the most frequent).

(2) Borderline atypical disfluencies that occur less frequently in the speech of children. For frame of reference, in a speech sample of 500 words or more, if there are 2 or more of any one of these behaviors per 100 words, this should be considered a basis for concern and especially so if air flow or phonation is disrupted between the repetitions or if a schwa sounding vowel is substituted for the one ordinarily used in the repetition of a syllable (for example, "Mə Mə Mə Ma Ma"). May be referred to as "cross-over behaviors" on the continuum between *More Usual* and *More Unusual* speech disfluencies.

(3) Atypical disfluencies that are very infrequent in the speech of children. More characteristic of what listeners perceive as stuttering. If 1 or more prolongations occur per 100 words in a speech sample of 500 or more, this should be considered a basis for considerable concern. Of course, fixed postures or other signs of increased tension and fragmentation of the flow of speech should be a basis for immediate attention.

(From Gregory and Hill, 1980)

Kasprisin–Burrelli, Egolf, and Shames (1972) trained observers to reliably identify parents' positive and negative child-directed verbal behaviors. Observations indicated that parents of stuttering children exhibited more negative verbal profiles than parents of nonstuttering children. They also reported that the verbal profiles of parents talking to stuttering children became less negative following treatment in which the parents participated. Mordecai (1979) conducted a study in which parent–child triads (mother, father, child) were videotaped during a prescribed period that was designed to provide opportunities for parents to instruct, compete, converse, and play with their preschool children. Parents of children evaluated as beginning to stutter were found to allow inadequate opportunities for their child to respond to questions before asking another question or making another statement. Parents of nonstuttering children were found to comment more frequently upon the content of their child's preceding utterance, which was generally regarded as a positive behavior.

We have found interactive analyses of audiotaped samples of parent–child interactions helpful in determining appropriate topics for counseling and intervention. The following interactive behaviors are examples of those that may be significant in the development and maintenance of stuttering (Gregory & Hill, 1980): interruption, filling in words, finishing the child's statement, guessing what the child is about to say, asking multiple questions at once, constant correction of a child's verbal and nonverbal behavior, and speech models of rapidly paced conversation including quickly changing topics. Although an interaction analysis is more objective, environmental factors associated with increased disfluency may be recognized through case history discussions of communication and interpersonal variables. A parent may have excessively high expectations related to speech development or to behavior in general such as table manners and neatness. Sheehan (1970, 1975) recommends considering how much support a child is receiving relative to how much is demanded, in what he terms the demand/support ratio. Other factors, such as hectic or inconsistent family routine and crisis within the family (Wyatt, 1969) can also be discovered through an interview.

EVALUATING SPEECH, LANGUAGE, AND OTHER BEHAVIOR

During recent years, speech–language pathologists have examined receptive–expressive language and articulation in beginning stutterers with increasing care. This is attributable to two circumstances: (1) increased interest in the effects of specific characteristics of the communicative message (ideas, word selection, syntax) on fluency (Bloodstein & Gantwerk, 1967; Helmreich & Bloodstein, 1973; DeJoy, 1975;

Colborn & Mysak, 1982) and (2) continuing reports that a notable number of stuttering children are delayed in language development, have specific language problems, or have articulation problems (Berry, 1938; Bloodstein, 1958; Andrews & Harris, 1964). Information about general development and health is considered by many speech–language pathologists to be important because delayed physical development and motor coordination or illness may be associated with delayed speech and language development or impaired control of the speech mechanism, which may contribute to disrupted fluency. The finding of an auditory processing disorder or a problem of oral motor coordination means that these factors should be considered in planning intervention.

Children who have attentional problems or who are passive and withdrawn may need therapy for these problems before beginning more specific work on speech development and fluency. Children who are fearful or perfectionistic may require therapy directed to these characteristics as we give attention to speech. If such characteristics are not modified within a reasonable length of time in the course of speech therapy, referral to a clinical psychologist should be considered. If patterns of different subject variables and environmental variables contribute to the onset and development of stuttering, a child's evaluation and subsequent treatment may involve a close working relationship between the speech–language pathologist and other child specialists.

DIFFERENTIAL TREATMENT STRATEGIES

At a conference on the prevention of stuttering, sponsored by the Speech Foundation of America at Northwestern University in 1982, there was general agreement that clinicians are working with the following factors during intervention aimed toward prevention of stuttering or stemming the tide of beginning stuttering: (1) Communicative stress in the environment, the way the parents and other adults talk to the child and the rate of the parents' speech; (2) interpersonal stress, that is, general interaction among family members; (3) linguistic and motor developmental differences; and (4) speech fluency. It is assumed that the first three factors influence the fourth, speech fluency, but consideration is also given to procedures that help the young child modify speech flow. Differential therapy is based on differential evaluation (Gregory, 1973; Gregory & Hill, 1980; Riley & Riley, 1979). Commonalities exist in intervention, but procedures are modified, to some extent, for each child. In general, most clinicians intervene to modify communicative stress first. More in-depth evaluation and intervention may or may not be necessary.

In the following sections, treatment strategies are discussed based on Gregory and Hill's system (Gregory & Hill, 1980). Reference is made to the ways in which other contributors' approaches are similar or different. Finally, data on treatment outcome is provided.

Treatment Strategy 1. Preventive parent counseling

Even when in the examiner's judgment, parents are concerned about disfluency that seems to be within normal limits, there appears to be general agreement among clinicians that some short-term parent counseling should be done. Such counseling proceeds along the following lines:

1. Take time to listen to the parents' concerns with a genuine desire to understand their thoughts and feelings. Reward them for sharing observations of their behavior and feelings, as well as observations of the child. Say such things as, "You have made some very important observations, and telling me about them helps me understand."

2. Describe how speech develops and include information about the occurrence of disfluency, perhaps by using the continuum. Help the parents to understand the basis for your present judgment that their child's disfluency is typical for his age.

3. Describe some communicative and interpersonal situations that have been related to increased disfluency in children. (See previous section, Evaluating Environmental Factors). Being careful to keep counseling oriented to a conversational interaction, not "talking at" but "talking with" the parents, relate the discussion to situations the parents have mentioned or observations from the parent–child analysis. Reinforce some appropriate and positive behaviors on the parents' part before turning attention to some behaviors that could interrupt fluency development.

4. Discuss the concept of time pressure in communication. Present time pressure as a natural part of communication. Show how children, during their preschool years when speech and language are developing and important emotional and social development is taking place, may respond by showing increased disfluency as they attempt to compete. Give a concrete example such as an adult asking a second question before a child has finished answering the first.

5. Explain the demand/support ratio (Sheehan, 1970, 1975, 1979). Encourage the parents to give attention and time to their children, to express appreciation for what they do in the way of childhood tasks, and to be reasonable in their demands based on the child's age and readiness.

6. Have parents read sections on speech interaction and nonverbal communication in *If Your Child Stutters: A Guide for Parents* (Ainsworth & Gruss, 1981) and *Between Parent and Child* (Ginott, 1969).

On the average, four counseling sessions are usually sufficient. Afterward, maintain a schedule of telephone contacts to confirm that the child's speech is developing normally and that the parents are comfortable. The parents are asked to call at any time they observe disfluent behaviors of concern or have questions about how to respond to the child.

Treatment Strategy 2. Prescriptive parent counseling, brief therapy with the child

If a child is judged to be demonstrating what we classify as borderline atypical disfluencies, the parents have been aware of the differences for less than a year, and the screening evaluation did not indicate the need for attention to any other speech, language, or behavioral characteristics, then our decision is to counsel the parents and work briefly with the child. In counseling parents, the general procedure of being a careful, interested listener, of giving information about speech and language development, and of describing our knowledge about the characteristics of children's disfluency are, in general, the same as discussed under Strategy 1. The following procedures are specific of Strategy 2.

1. Based on observations made and information gained in the Screening Evaluation, provide feedback about our judgment of the child's disfluency and other speech and language skills. Train the parents to identify the different types of repetitious and nonrepetitious disfluencies through use of videotaped examples.

2. Discuss environmental factors that experience indicates may contribute to increased disfluency and the beginning of stuttering. Include in this discussion, the concepts of time pressure in communication and the demand/support ratio as mentioned under Strategy 1. Give instruction in the charting of episodes of unusual disfluency using a recording form. Table 16-1 from Gregory and Hill (1980) illustrates this charting. Have parents bring their charts to counseling sessions and use them in either individual counseling with a mother and father or in a group of parents. In the example, Table 16-1, the mother can be complimented for the way she handled this situation. Of course, the mother should be certain to carry through on her commitment to talk when she gets off the phone. A parent may report increased word and syllable repetition when the child is reprimanded for not picking up his toys. This can lead

TABLE 16-1. Chart of Disfluent Episodes

Person	Message	Type of Disfluency	Child Awareness	Listener Reaction	Fluency Disrupters
Mother was talking on the phone	B interrupted his mother and wanted her attention	Irregular rhythm on syllable repetitions in the first word of the sentence	Overall tense, but not aware of disfluencies	Mother said she would talk as soon as she finished	Getting listener attention, not tolerant of delay

(From Gregory and Hill, 1980)

to a discussion of how to get children to understand what you want them to do by explaining to them, working along with them, and rewarding them for taking responsibility—"Johnnie, you are much better about cleaning up after you play."

3. The child is seen by a clinician for 30- to 50-minute sessions twice a week. The clinician models an easy, relaxed, somewhat slower speaking rate with an emphasis on pausing between phrases, being a responsive listener as the child talks, showing the child how we take turns—you don't interrupt and neither does the child. The clinician reads stories in the same relaxed manner, stopping to talk about the story whenever the child wishes.

4. A key in our successful work during the last 10 years has been that parents have practiced and learned improved interactive behaviors. Gradually, in successive sessions with the parents and child, they take over more of the clinician's role and become the primary model. Modeling (Bandura, 1969; Gregory, 1973b) is a powerful approach and one easily understood by clinicians and by parents. Most parents want to learn to respond appropriately, and once they get into the process of change, it is usually rewarding. Also, it is good for the children to know that their parents are learning too.

5. Ordinarily, four to eight weekly sessions are sufficient to accomplish the preventive measures necessary. Plans are made for monthly follow-up phone contacts and post-treatment observations as indicated. If, at any time, parents have concerns about increased disfluency, we advise by telephone or see the family as soon as possible.

Treatment Strategy 3. Comprehensive therapy program

As shown in Figure 16-1, we are describing therapy for the borderline atypically disfluent child with complicating speech, language, or behavioral problems, and also the atypically disfluent child (demonstrating more unusual disfluencies, more definite stuttering behaviors) in whom we may or may not have found contributing speech, language, or behavioral factors. Oftentimes, parents report concern about speech disfluencies that have persisted for a year or longer with decreasing cyclic variation. Of course, greater cyclic variation indicates a better prognosis. The child should be seen two to four times a week for 30- to 50-minute sessions, and the parents should have two counseling sessions a week, with perhaps one of these being a group session with other parents. The child should be included in a children's group as change occurs and as the children can model for each other.

Most of what has been said in discussing Strategies 1 and 2 about parent counseling, aimed toward reducing communicative and more general interpersonal stress, is true for Strategy 3. In brief, the clinician should be an understanding, interested listener who describes how such speech develops in a child and how disfluency occurs, discusses time pressure in communication and demands from the child compared to support and other factors that contribute to increased disfluency and stuttering, and teaches the parents to recognize differing types of disfluencies and to chart environmental situations that are associated with increases and decreases in disfluency (see the discussion Strategies 1 and 2). The following principles and procedures are more specific to Strategy 3.

Differential treatment. Based on results of a differential evaluation, plan a general approach for working with the child and parents that is based on factors believed to contribute to the problem. For illustrative purposes, consider two children:

A.   Brad, Age 3 years, 7 months.
      Onset—Parents first noted "sound repetition" at 2 years, 6 months.
      Speech analysis—Evaluation revealed moderately severe stuttering—a high frequency of sound and syllable repetitions, sound prolongations, and laryngeal tension (loud, hard glottal attacks). Avoidance of speaking observed. Considerable situational variation in frequency of disfluency.
      Developmental factors—Language, articulation, hearing, and motor skills within normal limits.
      Environmental factors—Parent-child interaction revealed that mother spoke with a rapid rate and used demanding questions frequently. At times, two or three consecutive questions were asked without allowing time for Brad to respond. Mother interrupted Brad's comments. Parent and child appeared to have a positive emotional relationship, and there were no signs of significant parent-child conflict.

B.   John, Age 3 years, 6 months.
      Onset—Stuttering noticed when sentences began to develop at Age 2 years, 6 months.
      Speech analysis—Moderately severe stuttering problem that included sound prolongations, and repetitions of sounds, syllables, and words. Syllable and word repetition were generally easy and regular and prolongations were brief. Very little situational differences.
      Developmental factors—Receptive language was at age level, but expressive language below age level and characterized by the use of presentence constructions, the omission of verbs and so on. Intelligibility of connected speech reduced due to frequent omissions and substitutions of sounds. Some difficulty in sequencing consonant-vowel combinations involving more than one place of production.
      Environmental factors—Child has few peers with whom to play. Very dependent on playing with 6-year-old sister and her friends. Mother admits difficulty disciplining her son. He shows rapid swings in behavior from "calm and loving" to "mean and destructive." Parents concerned about this.

In Child A, Brad, the emphasis was on counseling the parents about communicative stress, modeling improved interactive behaviors, and rewarding the parents for modifying their behavior. In working with Brad the clinician modeled a more easy, relaxed speech pattern going from shorter to longer utterances, and from less to more meaningful (naming, description, interpretation). The parents were taught to modify their speech rate and to pause more frequently. Therapy began in March 1980 and ended in December 1980.

In Child B, John, there were both developmental and environmental contributing factors to be considered. Speech therapy focused on modeling procedures in which more easy, relaxed responses were developed gradually from one word to longer utterances and from less meaningful to more meaningful. As John began to respond positively to modeling, work on specific language structures began. The clinic psychologist evaluated John and interviewed the parents. Suggestions were made for counseling the parents about John's behavior, but a recommendation for psychotherapy was not made. Parents participated in therapy and learned to change their speech pattern and interactive behavior. Therapy began in June 1977 and ended in March 1979.

These two brief examples illustrate how differential evaluation leads to different treatment approaches. The remainder of this chapter describes in greater detail some of the procedures mentioned in these examples.

Facilitating the child's fluency. An analysis of the literature on early intervention and attendance at recent short-course presentations indicates a trend toward the use of more specific fluency-enhancing procedures ranging, in terms of direct speech modification, from Ryan's gradual increase in length and complexity of normally fluent utterances (Ryan, 1974, 1979) to Cooper's use of fluency-enhancing gestures (Cooper, 1976, 1979). Gregory (1973), Van Riper (1973), Perkins (1979), Gregory and Hill (1980), and Shine (1980) describe the use of modeling by clinicians to modify the child's speech so that normal fluency results. Such models typically focus on only a minimal number of parameters. For example, a slower rate with easy initiations and smooth movements may be all that is needed. However, a particular child may, for example, require special help to reduce vocal tension which could begin with practice saying isolated vowels using a breathy approach. Clinicians should read Cooper (1979), Adams (1980), Gregory and Hill (1980), Johnson (1980), and Costello (1983) for more detailed descriptions of fluency-enhancing procedures to be used with young children beginning to stutter. Just to keep a balance in point of view, it should be noted that Williams (1983) has recently said that direct fluency shaping is contraindicated until it has been found that modifying psychosocial factors does not produce desired speech improvement.

In using modeling procedures, it is important that clinicians practice what they want to model until they are proficient. If the target behavior is "more easy relaxed speech," then clinicians should use this pattern throughout a therapy session. To the degree necessary, the clinician may direct a child's attention to cues by saying, "Watch me and listen as I ——."

In most cases, we have found it best to make the cues clearly discernible and to reinforce a child for listening to and looking at the clinician. Hill (Gregory & Hill, 1980) gives the following example: "I want you to do just what I do. I'll name the picture, then you say just what I do," and "Good, you told me the name of the picture. I like the way you told me."

As a child's fluency stabilizes, specialized desensitization procedures, as first described by Van Riper (1954), are applied as it seems appropriate. Based on analyses of parent–child interactions and observations of the child during therapy, the clinician constructs a hierarchy of factors that disrupt the child's fluency. At first, disruptors of lower strength are applied, and gradually as the child's fluency remains stable when these stimuli are introduced, disruptors higher on the hierarchy are introduced in a systematic manner. These procedures increase the child's tolerance of factors that once disrupted fluency and should be done only by the clinician, not the parents.

The development of language and articulation. We have implied that procedures to facilitate fluency are carried out in the context of a language activity program. Thus, various syntactic structures, depending on the developmental status of the child's language, can be practiced as we work on fluency. In addition, once a child is responding positively in therapy, ordinarily with improved fluency, articulation problems can be managed with a relaxed, developmental approach. Hill (Gregory & Hill, 1980) gives the following examples of target responses of the same length that can be used in stabilizing syntactic structures and articulation as work is done on fluency. (1) Early developing syntactic structures are stabilized in the utterances; "The dog *is running*." "*She* is very big." "He *took* the box." (2) The carry-over of prevocalic /k/ is facilitated by varying four-word utterances: "I found a *key*." "*K*eep the yellow *c*up." "The *k*ite was *c*aught." Development of vocabulary is integrated into activities by associating the names of objects and pictures in terms of semantic attributes such as function, size, shape, color, and taste, and by creating situations in which these words are used by the child. These are examples of the many ways in which a clinician who knows language and articulation therapy can weave all of this activity together.

Generalization and transfer. Most discussions of stuttering therapy for children and adults now emphasize that provisions should be made for modified responses to be generalized and transferred to real life speaking situations (Adams, 1980; Boberg, 1981; Gregory, 1979; Van Riper, 1973). With references to the treatment strategies for early developmental stages and our philosophy of developmental intervention, generalization should occur more readily than in an adult.

A useful frame of reference for generalization and transfer has been described by Griffiths and Craighead (1972). In what they term intratherapy generalization, the child learns to modify speech first in isolated words, then two-word combinations, then phrases and sentences. At first, in terms of communicative responsibility, the response may be an imitated naming response, then naming without a model, then naming one object or picture when the model is given on another one, and so on. This kind of successive approximation activity has been referred to throughout this chapter. Extratherapy generalization refers to the child generalizing change from individual therapy to a group session with other children or to a different listener (e.g., the mother) in the therapy setting. As noted earlier, we have observed success in generalization and transfer when parents and sometimes other children (depending on our judgment of the probable success of doing so) are brought into the therapy situation. At first, they observe the clinician and the child and follow the clinician's model. In the usual progression, the parents are given assignments to do at home what they have done at the clinic. Thus, both parents and child are experiencing generalization and transfer.

Maintenance of change must be followed by telephone checks with the parents, and rechecks of the child at the clinic or in the home. In the case of a child with complicating speech, language, or behavior problems, a more formal reevaluation session should be scheduled about a year following dismissal.

PROGRESS REPORT

Recent reports on the results of intervention with preschool children have been optimistic, and clinicians seem encouraged that this is a fruitful therapeutic endeavor (Gregory & Hill, 1980; Johnson, 1980; Prins, 1983; Shine, 1980). Johnson (1980) reported on seven children seen in a home prevention program, stating that it ordinarily required about four months for the parents to express confidence in their ability to manage the program resulting in decreased frequency of disfluency and changes in quality toward more normal disfluency. Shine (1980) provided results for 16 children, concluding that one may anticipate that, on the average, a child will need to be seen twice a week for 9 months to reach what he terms "fluent." Treatment up to approximately 2 years may be required for some children. Gregory and Hill (1980) state:

> An assessment of results indicates that 70 per cent of the children we see develop normal fluency that is maintained following 9 to 18 months in the comprehensive therapy program. In the other cases, factors interfering with the maintenance of normal fluency are identified, and recommendations such as referral for psycho-educational evaluation or family counseling are made.

As noted earlier in this chapter, Preventive Parent Counseling and Prescriptive Parent Counseling with Limited Involvement of the Child is often successful after four to eight sessions on a weekly basis.

REFERENCES

Adams, M. A clinical strategy for differentiating the normally nonfluent child and the incipient stutterer. *Journal of Fluency Disorders,* 1977, *2,* 141-149.

Adams, M. The young stutterer: Diagnosis, treatment and assessment of progress. In W. Perkins (Ed.), *Strategies in stuttering therapy.* New York: Thieme-Stratton, 1980.

Ainsworth, S., & Gruss, J. *If your child stutters: A guide for parents.* Memphis: Speech Foundation of America, 1981.

Andrews, G., & Harris, M. *The syndrome of stuttering.* London: Spastic Society, Levenham Press, 1964.

Bandura, A. *Principles of behavior modification.* New York: Holt, Rinehart & Winston, 1969.

Berry, M. F. Developmental history of stuttering children. *Journal of Pediatrics,* 1938, *12,* 209-217.

Bloodstein, O. Stuttering as an anticipatory struggle reaction. In J. Eisenson (Ed.), *Stuttering: A symposium.* New York: Harper & Row, 1958.

Bloodstein, O., & Gantwerk, B. Grammatical function in relation to stuttering in young children. *Journal of Speech and Hearing Research,* 1967, *10,* 786-789.

Bloodstein, O. *A handbook on stuttering.* Chicago: National Easter Seal Society, 1981.

Boberg, E. (Ed.) *Maintenance of fluency.* New York: Elsevier, 1981.

Boehmler, R. M. Listener responses to nonfluencies. *Journal of Speech and Hearing Research,* 1958, *1,* 132-141.

Brownell, W. *The relationship of sex, social class, and verbal planning to the disfluencies produced by nonstuttering preschool children.* Unpublished doctoral dissertation; Buffalo, State University of New York, 1973.

Colburn, N., & Mysak, E. Developmental disfluency and emerging grammar. II. Co-occurrence of disfluency with specified semantic syntactic structures. *Journal of Speech and Hearing Research,* 1982, 421-427.

Cooper, E. B. The development of a stuttering chronicity prediction checklist for school aged stutterers: A research inventory for clinicians. *Journal of Speech and Hearing Research,* 1973, *38,* 215-223.

Cooper, E. B. *Personalized fluency control therapy: An integrated behavior and relationship therapy for stutterers.* Austin, TX: Learning Concepts, 1976.

Cooper, E. Intervention procedures for the young stutterer. In H. Gregory (Ed.), *Controversies about stuttering therapy.* Baltimore: University Park Press, 1979.

Costello, J. Current behavioral treatments for children. In D. Prins & R. Ingham (Eds.), *Treatment of stuttering in early childhood: Methods and issues.* San Diego: College-Hill Press, 1983.

Curlee, R. A case selection strategy for young disfluent children. In W. Perkins (Ed.), *Strategies in stuttering therapy.* New York: Thieme-Stratton, 1980.

Daly, D. Differentiation of stuttering subgroups with Van Riper's developmental tracks. *Journal of National Student Speech Language Hearing Association,* 1981, 89–101.

Davis, D. The relation of repetitions in the speech of young children to certain measures of language maturity and situational factors. Part I. *Journal of Speech Disorders,* 1939, *4,* 303–318.

DeJoy, D. *An investigation of the frequency of nine individual types of disfluency and total disfluency in relation to age and syntactic maturity in nonstuttering males, three and one half years of age and five years of age.* Unpublished doctoral dissertation, pp. 155–158. Evanston, IL: Northwestern University, 1975.

Ginott, H. G. *Between parent and child.* New York: McMillan, 1965.

Giolas, T., & Williams, D. Children's reactions to nonfluencies in adult speech. *Journal of Speech and Hearing Research,* 1958, *1,* 86–93.

Gottfred, K. *A longitudinal analysis of type and frequency of disfluency, related to communicative pressure and length of utterance, in children 24 to 36 months of age.* Unpublished doctoral dissertation, Evanston, IL: Northwestern University, 1979.

Gregory, H. Applications of learning theory concepts in the management of stuttering. In H. Gregory (Ed.), *Learning theory and stuttering therapy.* Evanston: Northwestern University Press, 1968.

Gregory, H. *Stuttering: Differential evaluation and therapy.* Indianapolis: Bobbs-Merrill, 1973.

Gregory, H. Controversial issues: Statement and review of the literature. In H. Gregory (Ed.), *Controversies about stuttering therapy.* Baltimore: University Park Press, 1979. (a)

Gregory, H. Controversial issues: Analysis and current status. In H. Gregory (Ed.), *Controversies about stuttering therapy.* Baltimore: University Park Press, 1979. (b)

Gregory, H., & Hill, D. Stuttering therapy for children. In W. Perkins (Ed.), *Strategies in stuttering therapy.* New York: Thieme-Stratton, 1980.

Griffiths, H., & Craighead, W. E. Generalization in operant speech therapy for misarticulation. *Journal of Speech and Hearing Disorders,* 1972, *37,* 485–495.

Haynes, W., & Hood, S. Disfluency changes in children as a function of the systematic modification of linguistic complexity. *Journal of Communicative Disorders,* 1977, *11,* 79–93.

Helmreich, H., & Bloodstein, O. The grammatical factor in childhood disfluency in relation to the continuity hypothesis. *Journal of Speech and Hearing Research,* 1973, *16,* 731–738.

Johnson, L. Facilitating parental involvement in therapy of the disfluent child. In W. Perkins (Ed.), *Strategies in stuttering therapy.* New York: Thieme-Stratton, 1980.

Johnson, W. A study of the onset and development of stuttering. *Journal of Speech Disorders,* 1942, *7,* 251–257.

Johnson, W. *Stuttering in children and adults.* Minneapolis: University of Minnesota Press, 1955.

Johnson, W. *The onset of stuttering.* Minneapolis: University of Minnesota Press, 1959.

Kasprisin, A. *Implications of parental verbal behavior for stuttering therapy with children.* Unpublished paper, American Speech and Hearing Association Convention, New York, 1970.

Kasprisin-Burrelli, A., Egolf, D., & Shames, G. A comparison of parental verbal behavior with stuttering and nonstuttering children. *Journal of Communication Disorders,* 1972, *5,* 335–346.

Kidd, K. K. A genetic perspective on stuttering. *Journal of Fluency Disorders,* 1977, *2,* 259–269.

Mordecai, D. *An investigation of the communicative styles of mothers and fathers of stuttering versus nonstuttering preschool children during a triadic interaction.* Unpublished doctoral dissertation, pp. 48–64. Evanston: Northwestern University, 1979.

Oxtoby, E. A quantitative study of the repetitions in the speech of three-year-old children. M.A. thesis, University of Iowa, 1943.

Perkins, W. From psychoanalysis to discoordination. In H. Gregory (Ed.), *Controversies about stuttering therapy.* Baltimore: University Park Press, 1979.

Prins, D. Continuity, fragmentation, and tension: Hypotheses applied to evaluation and intervention with preschool disfluent children. In D. Prins & R. Ingham (Eds.), *Treatment of stuttering in early childhood: Methods and issues.* San Diego: College–Hill Press, 1983.

Prins, D., & Ingham, R. *Treatment of stuttering in early childhood: Methods and issues.* San Diego: College–Hill Press, 1983.

Riley, G., & Riley, J. A component model for diagnosing and treating children who stutter. *Journal of Fluency Disorders,* 1979, *4,* 279–294.

Riley, G., & Riley, J. Evaluation as a basis for intervention. In D. Prins & R. Ingham (Eds.), *Treatment of stuttering in early childhood: Methods and issues.* San Diego: College–Hill Press, 1983.

Ryan, B. *Programmed therapy for stuttering in children and adults.* Springfield, IL: Thomas, 1974.

Ryan, B. Stuttering therapy in a framework of operant conditioning and programmed learning. In H. Gregory (Ed.), *Controversies about stuttering therapy.* Baltimore: University Park Press, 1979.

Sheehan, J. (Ed.) *Stuttering: Research and therapy.* New York: Harper & Row, 1970.

Sheehan, J. Conflict theory and avoidance-reduction therapy. In J. Eisenson (Ed.), *Stuttering: A second symposium.* New York: Harper & Row, 1975.

Sheehan, J. Current issues on stuttering and recovery. In H. Gregory (Ed.), *Controversies about stuttering therapy.* Baltimore: University Park Press, 1979.

Shine, R. Direct management of the beginning stutterer. In W. Perkins (Ed.), *Strategies in stuttering therapy.* New York: Thieme-Stratton, 1980.

Silverman, E. Generality of disfluency data collected from preschoolers. *Journal of Speech and Hearing Research,* 1972, *15,* 84–92.

Silverman, E. The influence of preschoolers' speech usage on their disfluency frequency. *Journal of Speech and Hearing Research,* 1973, *16,* 474–481.

Van Riper, C. *Speech correction: Principles and methods.* Englewood Cliffs, NJ: Prentice-Hall, 1954.

Van Riper, C. *The treatment of stuttering.* Englewood Cliffs, NJ: Prentice-Hall, 1973.

Van Riper, C. *The nature of stuttering.* Englewood Cliffs, NJ: Prentice-Hall, 1982.

Voelker, C. A preliminary investigation for a normative study of disfluency: A critical index to the severity of stuttering. *American Journal of Orthopsychiatry,* 1944, *14,* 285–294.

Wexler, K., & Mysak, E.   Disfluency characteristics of 2-, 4-, and 6-year-old males. *Journal of Fluency Disorders,* 1982, *7,* 37–46.

Williams, D., & Kent, L.   Listener evaluations of speech interruptions. *Journal of Speech and Hearing Research,* 1958, *1,* 124–131.

Williams, D.   Working with children in the school environment. In J. Gruss (Ed.), *Transfer and maintenance in stuttering therapy.* Memphis: Speech Foundation of America, 1983.

Wyatt, G.   *Language learning and communication disorders in children.* New York: Free Press, 1969.

Yairi, E.   Disfluencies of normally speaking two-year-old children. *Journal of Speech and Hearing Research,* 1981, *24,* 490–495.

Yairi, E.   Longitudinal studies of disfluencies in two-year-old children. *Journal of Speech and Hearing Research,* 1982, *25,* 155–160.

Chapter 17

Treatment of the Young Chronic Stutterer: Managing Stuttering

David A. Daly

Van Riper (1970, 1971), Bloodstein (1975), and Wingate (1976) have thoroughly reviewed and described early treatment procedures that were advocated for stutterers. This chapter focuses on procedures conceived since the 1930s that have been employed successfully with young, chronic stutterers and that are still in use today.

EARLY PROPONENTS OF VOLUNTARY STUTTERING PROCEDURES

Advancement of a specific-symptom modification approach to treating stuttering gained acceptance between the 1930s and 1950s and was characterized by Bloodstein (1975) as "the Iowa Development." The majority of these procedures involved the idea of "voluntary stuttering." Bryngelson is credited with conceptualizing this revolutionary notion in the 1930s. During stuttering, stutterers reported that their speech was "out of control" and claimed that a sound or word "got stuck" and "would not come out." These abnormal speech patterns "just happened" and were not the stutterer's fault. Stutterers frequently told their clinicians that "it" was involuntary and beyond control. Williams' (1957) point of view on the "it" of stuttering cogently describes this phenomenon and its role in the stutterer's problem.

Bryngelson

Patterning his intervention strategy after Dunlap's (1932) work on negative practice, Bryngelson (1944) maintained that stutterers should confront their speech disruptions by consciously and willingly practicing voluntary stuttering. In fact, Bryngelson insisted that stutterers simulate *their own* disfluent speech patterns as nearly as possible to their real ways of stuttering. By imitating and practicing their own behaviors openly, Bryngelson believed that stutterers would reduce their fears of the unknown and be better able to control stuttering when it did occur. This new thrust, coupled with Bryngelson's insistence on an objective attitude, forced stuttering individuals to accept some of the responsibility for changing and controlling their own speech. Because voluntary stuttering was something which stutterers could control, Bryngelson believed it was "healthier" than their old ways of stuttering.

Johnson

Wendell Johnson is credited with streamlining Bryngelson's voluntary stuttering strategy into a more normalized disfluency pattern called "the bounce." Rather than imitating exactly one's own stuttering block (as Bryngelson had advocated), Johnson (1955, 1956) trained stutterers to use an easy bouncing repetition of the feared sound or word as a therapeutic technique for confronting avoidance behavior and moving forward in speech. Many clinical training programs across the country embraced Johnson's bounce technique and incorporated it into their stuttering therapy programs. In later years, Johnson deemphasized bouncing and recommended that stutterers use any form of normal disfluency, rather than avoid or stutter in the old way. Nevertheless, Johnson's students, and others in the profession, have adhered to "the bounce" long after he moved on to other therapeutic strategies.

For example, I directed a summer speech camp between 1973 and 1979 which provided treatment for chronic, young stutterers from throughout the United States. Without question, one of the most frequently practiced speech therapy techniques clients reported having used before coming to camp was "the bounce."

One problem with the bounce technique is that stutterers, particularly adolescents, experience embarrassment when voluntarily repeating in public. Many of my adolescent stuttering clients have confessed that they had completed almost every outside speaking assignment, all but one. They had not, and would not, use a multisyllabic bounce speech pattern in public. Several youngsters who had used the bounce in my presence when accompanied on speaking assignments admitted never having used it when they were alone. Discussions with other experienced clinicians suggest that such reactions are typical. For example, Sheehan (1970) has reported that many stutterers admit completing assignments involving voluntary stuttering without any real self-involvement. That is, although stutterers performed their assignments, they only "went through the motions" in the most superficial way possible.

Research by Berlin and Berlin (1964) did not find widespread acceptance of a bounce pattern. They showed a film depicting a person using three types of control patterns: pullouts, prolongations, and bounce. The film was shown to 200 lay listeners, 95 speech clinicians, and 146 high school age stutterers. All groups clearly preferred the pullout pattern over the other two control patterns.

Considerable common sense should be employed when utilizing the bounce pattern to reduce tension, avoidance, and fear. I have observed stuttering youngsters "bouncing" effortlessly on the same syllable for three or four breath groups. Such clients obviously did not understand the rationale for using the bounce technique. Voluntary stuttering had taken neither the embarrassment nor the abnormality from their stuttering; they were merely substituting one unacceptably disfluent pattern for another.

Van Riper

Charles Van Riper's (1954) well-known therapeutic procedures of cancellation, pullout, and preparatory set were products of his systematic studies of stuttering therapy. His emphasis on therapy rather than theory (Van Riper, 1958) was unlike that of his teachers and colleagues from Iowa. But, like them, he was convinced that deliberate modification of overt stuttering was absolutely essential to reduce its abnormality and to attenuate the fears and anxieties which exacerbate it. Thus, Bloodstein (1981) included Van Riper with Bryngelson and Johnson as a leader of "the Iowa Development" that challenged the older, more indirect methods of treating this disorder.

Van Riper (1954) reported that considerable improvement occurred when clients could be taught to change or modify their stuttering pattern in a deliberate volitional way. That is, rather than struggling to speak fluently, clients were instructed to stutter in an easier, less effortful way. Rather than experiencing panic from their temporary loss of speech control, stuttering clients frequently were successful in their efforts to stutter with only a minimum of abnormality. Van Riper's approach to "stutter fluently" revolutionized the treatment of stuttering.

Among the changes that Van Riper advanced was his insistence that clients alter their speech patterns by repeating or prolonging the first sounds or syllables of nonfeared words. This differed markedly from Bryngelson's and Johnson's technique of voluntary stuttering on feared words. Van Riper's intent was to establish ongoing, forward-moving speech; his immediate goal was not normally fluent speech, but fluent stuttering. In addition to giving stutterers a more normal appearing disfluent speech pattern, pseudostuttering on nonfeared words often yielded a secondary benefit. The more proficient that stutterers became in pseudostuttering, the less frequent and less severe were their real moments of stuttering.

Confirmed stutterers, however, still frequently experienced their old, voluntary stuttering behaviors. Van Riper's cancellation technique was specifically designed to assist such clients. After stuttering, the client was to pause, analyze what he had done, and determine how he could stutter differently on the same word. Then he was to say the same word again, stuttering differently. The task was not to say the word fluently on the second trial, but to stutter volitionally with less abnormality.

Van Riper believed that the period immediately following stuttering was an important point of therapeutic attack. The cancellation technique, he argued, weakened involuntary symptom patterns and allowed learning of substitute forms of more fluent stuttering. Eleven specific examples of the cancellation technique were outlined by Van Riper in his 1954 text (pp. 422–423), with more detailed illustrations presented in his more recent treatment text (1973, pp. 442–443).

As stutterers became adept at analyzing and cancelling their old, involuntary stuttering acts, Van Riper introduced a pullout technique. This procedure allowed stutterers to modify stuttering acts in process by completing the word with a smooth, slow prolongation. In teaching this technique, Van Riper imitated the stutterer's disfluent speech before modeling a volitionally controlled prolongation pattern and practicing pullouts in unison with the client. In contrast to the easy onset or gentle onset procedure which many fluency shaping programs now teach, the pullout technique can be viewed as a slow, smooth, gentle exit from the stuttering act. Again, forward-moving speech is emphasized with voluntary speech behaviors being substituted for involuntary speech disruptions.

A third technique, preparatory set, was introduced for older stutterers who respond to expectation or fear of stuttering on specific words by tensing their muscles as they prepare to speak. Van Riper observed that many stutterers seemed to "preform" articulatory postures for an initial phoneme of a feared word or to produce an initial sound with such tension that a normal sequence of speech movements was not possible. Van Riper once again substituted one form of behavior for another. New preparatory sets, which carefully integrated airflow and phonation with slowed motoric sequences, were substituted for the preformations and hard contacts characteristic of the old involuntary stuttering pattern. New rehearsal behaviors were practiced during a client's period of anticipation; that is, during the period just before he expected to stutter. While he strongly advocated teaching cancellations and pullouts when treating a young, chronic stutterer, Van Riper maintained that preparatory sets should not be taught to young stutterers. In fact, he believed that the vigilance necessary to scan ahead and prepare preparatory sets might only serve to increase a child's sound and word fears (Van Riper, 1973, p. 445).

Voluntary stuttering in the form of faking, bouncing, cancelling, or pulling out are frequently used in stuttering therapy today. These techniques are especially worthwhile for stuttering children and adolescents who have begun to show obvious forms of avoidance behavior and concealment. Modifications and variations of these "traditional" procedures for managing stuttering in young stutterers are presented next.

ADDITIONAL PROCEDURES FOR MANAGING STUTTERING IN YOUNG CHRONIC STUTTERERS

The therapeutic techniques that follow have been advocated by a number of individuals. In some cases the contributions can be attributed to specific authors; in other cases this is not possible. Many clinicians use a combination of techniques when working with young, chronic stutterers.

The slide technique

Sheehan (1958, 1970) has advocated the use of the slide technique for many years. Basically, the slide is a form of voluntary stuttering which is employed prior to getting stuck on a feared word. Because most stutterers can scan ahead and identify words on which they expect to stutter, Sheehan uses the slide to intentionally prolong the initial sound of a feared word. By approaching a feared word with the notion that it can be controlled, stuttering either does not occur or its severity is markedly attenuated.

A study by Sheehan and Voas (1957) strongly supported use of the slide procedure. They compared the effects on stuttering adaptation of three different types of voluntary stuttering used in therapy. Stutterers were instructed to either imitate their own stuttering pattern, bounce (voluntary syllable repetition), or slide (voluntary prolongation) when they came to underlined words during oral readings of several passages. The experimenters had previously underlined all words each subject had stuttered during an initial oral reading. They found that the imitation task was significantly worse than the bounce or slide tasks in reducing the frequency of subsequent stuttering. The slide technique produced the greatest percentage of improvement, particularly when it was used on words just prior to a feared word. Thus, the slide response may be used effectively on either feared or nonfeared words.

Sheehan's slide technique is a form of voluntary stuttering employed before stuttering occurs; that is, just prior to getting stuck on a feared word. In contrast, Van Riper's pullout is utilized for smoothly and easily getting out of a stuttering block that has already occurred. Sheehan's stuttering modification program is similar to that of Van Riper's, in that it tries to reduce a client's avoidance of holding back tendencies by teaching him to stutter openly and easily in response to fear cues. Detailed rationales for his conflict therapy and avoidance reduction therapy have been presented elsewhere (Sheehan 1958, 1968) and will not be discussed here.

Loose contacts

A technique for teaching the chronic young stutterer to use his speech articulators more effectively is that of "loose contacts." Originally proposed by Van Riper (1954), this method consists of approaching feared words with reduced tension in the lips, tongue, and vocal cords. Luper and Mulder (1964) report that some young stutterers improve dramatically without further therapy once this technique is mastered. Their suggestions (p. 130) for teaching young children to stutter deliberately as they concentrate on keeping their articulators relaxed are especially useful. Other authors have used the term "light contact" to differentiate reduced tension from excessive tension. These terms are synonymous. Luper and Mulder's illustrations of cancellation and pullout techniques with older children and adolescents who stutter are also worthy of review. Their suggestions for helping a stuttering child cope with and replace his nonproductive anticipatory behaviors with more adequate phonetic attack skills are especially useful.

Easy talking versus hard talking

The concepts of easy talking and hard talking have been employed to heighten a stutterer's awareness of different ways of speaking. Williams (1971, 1979) has taken a leading role in applying these concepts to young stutterers. Initially, Williams focuses on awareness training; that is, he directs a young stutterer's attention to the specific things he does that interfere with talking and to those things he does that facilitate it. As therapy progresses, he teaches stutterers about the total process of talking. He shows clients that stuttering is not something that mysteriously happens to them but something they do. Voluntary stuttering, volitional tensing and not tensing, and instructions on doing more things that normal speakers do are stressed. Williams focuses on increased awareness of ways of talking, because he believes that most stutterers are only vaguely aware of what they do when they talk. Because stutterers direct much of their attention to what they are feeling, Williams contends that they suffer from a form of learned helplessness.

When older children and adolescents do show obvious avoidance behaviors, Williams (1958) deals directly with feelings and fears. He argues that "until these attitudes and emotional reactions are met constructively as part of the therapy program, the probability is reduced that the stutterer will maintain increased fluency after therapy is terminated" (pp. 298–299). Because such youngsters are helped to examine and confront their fears, as well as to learn new ways to speak, they are encouraged to develop an attitude of "what can I do to talk," rather than "what can I do to not stutter." Essentially, clients are taught through monitored practice of different speech parameters that their speech is governed by what they do and not by what they feel.

Modeling

Gregory (1968, 1973) uses modeling for contrasting different ways of talking and for teaching such techniques as light contacts or smooth transitions, to school-aged youngsters with chronic stuttering. Gregory advocates modeling because it allows a child to examine stuttering first in the clinician's speech. Not only is modeling used to countercondition fear and avoidance behavior related to sounds, words, or situations, but also to shape new psychomotor speech patterns.

The child copies the clinician's models precisely; first using word lists, then sentences and paragraphs. During therapy, Gregory often uses choral reading and a tape recorder to help teach voluntary stuttering patterns. Modeling also is used to contrast ways of tensing and fragmenting speech with ways of speaking at a slower phonetic rate using smooth transitions between sounds. The goal is to help the child evolve a pattern of speaking that is a "more easy relaxed approach with smooth movements" (Gregory & Hill, 1980, p. 361).

Gregory believes that modeling is similarly effective in helping parents of stuttering youngsters to understand the ways in which we are teaching their children to modify their speech. Through counseling and exposure to modeled relaxation and tenseness, parents are shown what is being taught to their children. Through modeling and role playing they learn how to reinforce such changes at home.

Forward speech flow

Numerous techniques have been suggested for teaching stuttering children the importance of keeping speech moving forward. Awareness training is used to assist young stutterers in recognizing what they are doing to interfere with talking. Concrete examples, especially with younger stutterers, may be needed. Conture's (1982) garden hose and nozzle analogies are particularly helpful for describing how it is possible to close off the flow of air and interfere with speech. Likening the faucet on the house to the larynx, the hose to the vocal tract, and the nozzle to the lips seems to help children grasp such concepts easily. This illustration can also be helpful when describing what happens during stuttering to adolescent stutterers and to parents.

Another analogy Conture uses in teaching a continuous flow of speech is cursive writing. Contrasting cursive writing to printing illustrates smooth transitions between sounds versus choppy speech. Conture also utilizes the VU meter on a tape recorder to help stutterers visualize what they are doing when they speak and to teach appropriate vocal initiations and transitions. His common-sense approach to stuttering describes novel variations for practicing clinicians and students who are training children to modify their stuttering.

Of course, there are many other writers and clinicians who have described direct treatment procedures for managing stuttering in children and adolescents. I have not tried to catalog every variation or technique but to highlight those strategies that are particularly useful in treatment. These procedures seem to have several common features—they all deal directly with the child and his stuttering; they try to heighten the child's awareness of what he is doing to interfere with smooth speech; and they teach the substitution and monitoring of new adaptive speech skills for old nonproductive, disruptive behaviors.

OTHER ASPECTS OF STUTTERING MANAGEMENT PROCEDURES

Programs designed to modify stuttering through identification, examination, discussion, and behavior change deal openly with a child's speech problem. Modeling, instruction, and practice of volitional bouncing, slides, or pullouts frequently lead to easier and easier disfluencies. These procedures encourage a stuttering youngster to acknowledge his speech problem and to deal directly with it. Knepflar (1978) and Riley and Riley (1979), among others, report frequent success with youngsters who are trained to bounce or slide. Starkweather (1980) maintains that voluntary stuttering is particularly valuable for those clients who show strong avoidance behaviors. In discussing desensitization experiences for clients with obvious fears he wrote: "pseudostuttering (faking) has been most effective in my practice, although it is met with resistance unless first approached gradually through identification and exploration of stuttering" (1980, p. 333).

By dealing directly with a child's stuttering, both his overt behaviors and his feelings about them are "put out on the table," so to speak, where they can be discussed. Young, chronic stutterers are frequently amazed that not only does a clinician respond unemotionally to his disrupted speech, but can somehow replicate it. By demonstrating that stuttering can be shared, the clinician seems to reduce the mystery of stuttering for a child, thereby creating an environment of camaraderie and trust. By sharing stuttering experiences and talking openly and honestly about such behaviors and feelings, the clinician sets the underpinnings for what many believe to be the single most important variable in stuttering therapy—the client–clinician relationship.

Clinicians advocating stuttering modification strategies explore, describe, and discuss the child's disfluencies. The process of identification begins with the first session. For children and adolescents who stutter, "the stuttering apple" (Cooper, 1965) has been used for identifying and cataloging various overt and covert features of a child's stuttering. The clinician suggests that the "core" of the problem is the child's getting stuck on words. As the child describes what he does when he stutters or because he stutters, the clinician writes (in the child's own words) around the core of the apple. With encouragement, youngsters may be able to list (perhaps for the first time) many behaviors and feelings specific to their stuttering. For example, "My throat tightens when I try to say words beginning with vowels" or "I don't answer in class even when I know the answer." The clinician acknowledges that other pieces of the apple may be identified later, but that part of what is done in therapy will involve specific activities directed toward getting to the "core" of the apple.

Other identification procedures can be used, of course, but it is important that the problem be concretely stated for the child and that a plan for doing something about it be described. Such descriptions may help reduce a child's fear regarding previously undefined communication problems. Advocates of such procedures also maintain that attention to feelings and attitudes should begin with the first session. Hood (1974), Emerick (1974), Cooper (1976), and Van Riper (1973), for example, focus on interpersonal sensitivity and the therapeutic relationship early in therapy. The clinician's willingness to identify and discuss the overt behavioral components of stuttering and to understand the child's feelings and concerns about his stuttering are believed to be very powerful in building a trusting relationship. Emerick (1974) contends that it is only after such trust is established that some clients are willing to "take a chance" and actually try the program. Other clinicians (e.g., Strupp, 1972) even maintain that, in the final analysis, clients change out of love for the clinician. Open, honest discussions about stuttering and feelings related to it are likely to foster such confidence and trust.

In managing young, chronic child stutterers, clinicians try to demonstrate an unreserved willingness to share a child's stuttering blocks and to show how feared sounds or words can be spoken in an easier, more acceptable way. They also try not to show disapproval, annoyance, or panic when a child regresses in therapy or has a particularly bad day. Procedures employed to manage stuttering concentrate on reducing fears, anxieties, and avoidances that often seem to be an integral part of the child's problem.

Clinicians using stuttering modification programs for children also provide instructions, modeling, and counseling for parents. They encourage parents and teachers not to be reticent in using the term "stuttering." As Emerick (1970) contended over a decade ago, pretending that stuttering does not exist, when indeed it does, may contribute immeasurably to a child's feelings of confusion, guilt, and frustration. As he put it, "Parents should not ignore the baby rhinoceros in the living room" (p. 14). Counseling parents by providing information about stuttering and the overall therapeutic plan, as well as by instructing and *showing* them ways in which they can help at home is an important ingredient of an effective treatment program. Specifically, parents may need to be shown how to reduce their own speech rates at home and how to focus on and reinforce the content of their child's message as well as his easily produced speech (Perkins, 1979). Parent counseling and training frequently may provide the extra support necessary for successful therapy. Booklets by Ainsworth (1977) and Cooper (1979b) offer many thoughtful suggestions for parents.

Most proponents of stuttering modification programs encourage group therapy for youngsters with chronic stuttering, in addition to individual therapy. Conture (1982) suggests that, "One should not only consider the age of the child with the problem, but the age of the problem with the child" (p. 71). A youngster who has been stuttering for 4 or more years, even though he is only 11 or 12 years of age, may benefit from the support of an empathetic peer group. Children and adolescents who stutter may have had little or no contact with other stutterers. The group therapy format offers such youngsters an opportunity to share experiences and feelings with others who often have similar fears. Clients see that they are not "freaks of nature" but that other people stutter, too; some similar to their way of stuttering and some differently. Different stuttering patterns observed in group sessions may be used to vary a client's stuttering during individual sessions.

Although quantitative data that document the benefits of group treatment for stutterers are not readily available, client reports and clinical experience indicate that structured group therapy for older children and adolescents who stutter can be a powerful component of effective treatment programs. Indeed, clients in our intensive summer program have always resisted attempts to reduce the number of their group sessions. Stutterers are not disfluent in vacuums. Whether at school or at play, youngsters who stutter learn, socialize, and communicate, in large measure, in groups. Treating stutterers in groups often helps motivate clients to change their ways of talking and their attitudes and feelings about themselves and their problems.

STUTTERERS WITH CONCOMITANT ARTICULATION AND LANGUAGE PROBLEMS

Conture (1982) highlighted speech articulation as a significant factor to consider and evaluate when treating older children and teenagers who stutter. He reported that two-thirds of 15 randomly selected youngsters he treated for stuttering also had shown, or still demonstrated, three or more articulation errors. Daly (1982) found that 52% of 138 youngsters seen for stuttering therapy in a remedial summer program also showed or had previously shown articulation disorders. Morley (1957), somewhat earlier, had reported a significant correlation between stuttering and articulation defects, with 50% of her group showing both problems. Recently, Thompson (1983) reported that articulation errors co-occurred among 45 and 35% of her two samples of stutterers. Riley and Riley (1979) and Andrews and Harris (1964) reported 33 and 30% figures, respectively. Darley (1955), Williams and Silverman (1968) and Van Riper (1971) reported that approximately 25% of their clients also misarticulated. Blood and Seider (1981) reported only a 16% prevalence of co-occurring articulation problems, but their data were gathered via questionnaires from clinicians who may or may not have tested their clients for such problems. I have personally experienced difficulty in convincing speech clinicians of the possible importance of testing for articulation and language problems in stutterers, particularly when they are not responding to treatment. Some clinicians seem to prefer to blame the ineffectiveness of a therapy program or to cite client disinterest, rather than to look for other variables that could interfere with therapeutic progress.

The repeated finding that stutterers often have concomitant articulation (and language) deficits may have important implications for treatment. As Bloodstein (1975) put it:

> There is hardly a finding more thoroughly confirmed in the whole range of comparative studies of stutterers and nonstutterers than the tendency of stutterers to have functional difficulties of articulation, 'immature' speech and the like. (p. 178)

Research (Daly, 1981; DeHirsh & Langford, 1950; Van Riper, 1971) has shown that stutterers fitting Van Riper's Track II category (i.e., late talkers, never very fluent, poor articulation, motor problems, cluttering, etc.) have a poorer prognosis for treatment than other stutterers. Recently, Daly (1982) reported that stutterers with concomitant articulation problems performed significantly poorer during 6 weeks of intensive therapy than stutterers without such problems.

Riley (1976) believes that clients' motor abilities should be considered in designing therapy for children who stutter. Riley and Riley (1979) designed differential therapy programs for children based on nine components that index neurologic and traditional factors believed to disrupt fluency. In a later study, Riley and Riley (1980) recommended testing, and possible treatment of oral motor problems, attending difficulties, auditory processing disorders, and central language processing disturbances along with treatment of stuttering. The Rileys' data support the hypothesis that differential treatment is needed for different stutterers' problems.

Gregory and Hill (1980) also utilize a differential evaluation and therapy model for stuttering children. In some cases, in-depth speech and language evaluations with particular attention to language, auditory, oral motor, visual motor, and gross motor skills may be necessary. For example, Gregory and Hill found that 55% of the 52 stuttering children they treated in a comprehensive therapy program demonstrated word retrieval difficulties. They advocate a problem-solving approach to treatment that may include language training, desensitization procedures, counseling, role playing, voluntary disfluencies, as well as the modeling of easy, relaxed, smooth speech movements.

Much remains to be learned about the significance of the association between stuttering and articulation defects. Perhaps, as Bloodstein (1975) suggests, they are caused to some extent by the same thing. Similar arguments can be made for the association among stuttering and language or motor problems. While the effects of remediation training for memory, motor, articulation, or language problems on stuttering are not yet known, investigations of the nature and treatment of such concomitant problems and their influence on stuttering remediation certainly appears warranted. Such efforts may be promising lines of scientific inquiry that will assist us in more fully appreciating and understanding the nature of stuttering.

FACTORS INFLUENCING TREATMENT DECISIONS

From information on managing stuttering presented thus far and information on managing fluency presented by Costello in the next chapter, the reader may conclude that either orientation can be effective for dealing with young confirmed stutterers. The question confronting a clinician, of course, is which procedures should be used with which clients. A definitive answer to this question does not exist; however, some investigators have begun to examine the issue.

Guitar and Peters (1980) contend that fluency management procedures are indicated when a stuttering youngster exhibits primarily short blocks and shows little awareness of his stuttering. They advocate a fluency management approach if the child responds well to a period of trial therapy using slow, prolonged speech and if the parents are willing to actively carry out a home management program.

Conversely, Guitar and Peters advocate a stuttering modification approach whenever a child shows considerable evidence of avoiding or disguising his stuttering, or if difficulty is encountered in producing prolonged, fluent speech during a trial therapy period. Their approach requires that the following questions be answered: (1) How does one determine how much avoidance and anxiety exists? and (2) How much trial therapy is appropriate to make a decision on treatment?

We have found the Perceptions of Stuttering Inventory (Woolf, 1967) particularly helpful for identifying avoidances of older children and adolescents. Clinicians should take care, however, not to interpret "normal" responses as abnormal. Nonstuttering children have fears and anxieties about speaking, too. Recent findings (Daly, Oakes, Breen, & Mishler, 1981) with 90 nonstuttering adolescent youngsters indicate than an average of 9.2 (SD = 6.0) items of the 60 possible responses on the Perception of Stuttering Inventory were checked as characteristic of their speech. These findings support Webster's (1975) contention that scores of 10 or less on the inventory indicate little concern with stuttering. In contrast, 55 adolescent stutterers (ages 13 to 18 years) checked an average of 27.4 items.

An assessment of perceptions, feelings, and attitudes about stuttering is desirable for clinicians using traditional approaches to managing stuttering. For youngsters 11 years of age and younger, the Perception of Stuttering Inventory is probably too difficult. Fortunately, other scales for young stutterers have recently been developed (e.g., Guitar & Peters, 1980; Thompson, 1983), and pertinent information may also be gathered during interviews and from therapy sessions. But clinicians are cautioned to explore responses carefully, for not all avoidances and fears should be attributed to stuttering.

In addition to inventories and scales, clinical experience suggests that poor eye contact, extraneous motor movements, and verbal distractions are readily observed signs of avoidance and fear in young children. Moreover, Emerick and Hatten (1974) contend that young stutterers with tonic type speech disruptions evidence more avoidance and escape than do clonic type stutterers; and that tonic stutterers have a poorer prognosis for therapeutic success. A recently developed disfluency description digest (Cooper, 1982) may have clinical application in this regard. Obviously, parent and teacher reports and comments from youngsters themselves can provide important information about their fears and feelings about stuttering.

TRIAL THERAPY

The issue of trial therapy raises more questions than answers. Intensity of treatment, structure of the program, clinician competencies, and number of trial sessions are only a few of the variables pertinent to such an evaluation. At a recent conference, Ingham (1982) proposed that a decision regarding the effectiveness of treatment might reasonably be made after 12 sessions. He suggested a trial period of about 4 weeks. While many clinical practitioners might be more comfortable if the number of sessions was increased to 16 and the time period extended to 6 weeks, most would likely agree with Ingham that guidelines for determining the length of trial therapy are needed. Some stuttering youngsters may be continued in one treatment program or another for months, even though improvement is not observed. Or, the same structured activities may be repeated week after week without success, because some improvement was noted during the first few sessions. Both situations can result in frustration and discouragement for client and clinician. Unfortunately, as Emerick and Hatten (1974) note, the longer a stutterer's history of therapeutic failure, the poorer the prognosis for future improvement.

Despite claims by some writers, no one therapy system or program works successfully for all stutterers. Most clinicians who treat chronic young stutterers agree with Perkins' (1973) contention that different facets of the problem may be treated effectively through different conceptual frameworks. At this juncture no single framework appears to cope adequately with all aspects of the problem.

MORE THOROUGH RECORD KEEPING

As more innovative evaluation and treatment programs for different types of stutterers are developed (e.g., Riley & Riley, 1979; Gregory & Hill, 1980), more accurate data will become available to make informed treatment decisions. To compare and contrast various treatment procedures effectively, however, it will become increasingly important for clinicians to document and catalog relevant information. Several formats are available that condense the array of information found in a stutterer's medical and school files into one manageable form. Williams' (1978) detailed case history outline is one format that clinical researchers and practitioners could employ to begin gathering such data; Webster's (1975) client information record is another. Daly (1981) and Thompson (1983) have described yet other inventories for coding information gleaned from parents and teachers as well as from school records, medical reports, and clinical folders. The results of previous therapies attempted, number of sessions, client attendance, extenuating circumstances, and so forth, should be recorded as accurately as possible. Such information, together with carefully documented longitudinal studies, may help us learn why some clients respond readily to treatment while others do not. Such data may also help identify critical common variables among stuttering children that can be used to guide clinicians in future treatment decisions.

FINAL COMMENTS

Despite some success in treating chronic young stutterers over the past 20 years, our clinical failures seem to be remembered more vividly than our successes. For some youngsters, fluency could not be maintained between sessions or, occasionally, even within sessions. Therapy for these children seemed to be continually "starting over" with each session. Although our clinical relationships and reinforcers seemed appropriate and parent training efforts in home programs had been emphasized, some children's struggle behaviors persisted or intensified. Their fears, avoidances, and frustrations were clearly evident; the treatment plan we were using with them was not working.

At times, we have blamed resistant clients, uncooperative parents, or even the unsatisfactory state of our clinical art for such failures. Only within the last few years have we systematically altered treatment plans when a persistent reduction in verbal output or increases in frustration and avoidance were observed. In such cases, we have focused on helping these children to cope with their highly feared moments of stuttering. Starkweather and Lucker's (1978) strategy of tangibly reinforcing bouncing and prolongation patterns has been used with dramatic results. Although stuttering continued, its severity and frequency attenuated. Sentence length and talking time increased. Previously stuttered words and sounds were approached with an attitude that "something could be done." In Van Riper's language, these stuttering management procedures took away the "pain of stuttering."

Changing our orientation did not force us to alter our goal of helping such children achieve normally fluent speech. Perhaps these youngsters needed time—time for maturation, time for learning. Perhaps, sometime in the future, a combination of stuttering and fluency management procedures, as Guitar and Peters (1980) propose, will provide a more effective framework for guiding young stutterers to fluent speech. After all, both approaches do have a number of mutually complementary objectives. Combining treatment approaches may well offer clinicians the flexibility to adopt critical elements of both orientations, and ultimately best serve their clients.

This chapter has provided an overview of procedures and strategies espoused by different clinical researchers who adhere to a stuttering management framework. Specific techniques believed to be valuable for treating stuttering youngsters, and the advantages of these tactics have been highlighted. Indications which suggest that a change of therapeutic approach may be warranted were presented, along with the possibility of integrating the various strengths of different remedial approaches. The view taken was that stuttering management and fluency management approaches can yield complementary treatment practices for young stutterers.

REFERENCES

Andrews, G., & Harris, M. *The syndrome of stuttering.* London: Heinemann Medical Books, 1964.

Ainsworth, S. *If your child stutters: A guide for parents.* Memphis: Speech Foundation of America, 1977.

Berlin, S., & Berlin, C. Acceptability of stuttering control patterns. *Journal of Speech and Hearing Disorders,* 1964, *29,* 436–441.

Blood, G. W., & Seider, R. The concomitant problems of young stutterers. *Journal of Speech and Hearing Research,* 1981, *46,* 31–33.

Bloodstein, O. *A handbook on stuttering.* Chicago: National Easter Seal Society for Crippled Children and Adults, 1975.

Bloodstein, O. *A handbook on stuttering.* Chicago: National Easter Seal Society for Crippled Children and Adults, 1981.

Bryngelson, B., Chapman, M. E., & Hansen, O. K. *Know yourself: A workbook for those who stutter.* Minneapolis: Burgess, 1944.

Conture, E. G. *Stuttering.* Englewood Cliffs, NJ: Prentice-Hall, 1982.

Cooper, E. B. A disfluency descriptor digest for clinical use. *Journal of Fluency Disorder,* 1982, *7,* 355–358.

Cooper, E. B. Intervention procedures for the young stutterer. In H. H. Gregory (Ed.), *Controversies about stuttering therapy.* Baltimore: University Park Press, 1979. (a)

Cooper, E. B. *Understanding stuttering: Information for parents.* Chicago: National Easter Seal Society for Crippled Children and Adults, 1979. (b)

Cooper, E. B. *Personalized fluency control therapy.* Hingham, MA: Teaching Resources Corp., 1976. (b)

Cooper, E. B. Structuring therapy for therapist and stuttering child. *Journal of Speech and Hearing Disorders,* 1965, *30,* 75–78.

Daly, D. A. *Considerations for treating stutterers with and without concomitant articulation disorders.* Paper presented at The American Speech-Language-Hearing Association annual convention, Toronto, 1982.

Daly, D. A. Differentiation of stuttering subgroups with Van Riper's developmental tracks: A preliminary study. *Journal of the National Student Speech Language and Hearing Association,* 1981, *9,* 89–101.

Daly, D. A., Oakes, D., Breen, K., & Mishler, C. *Perception of Stuttering Inventory: Norms for adolescent stutterers and nonstutterers.* Paper presented at the American Speech-Language-Hearing Association annual convention, Los Angeles, 1981.

Darley, F. L. The relationship of parental attitudes and adjustments to the development of stuttering. In W. Johnson & R. Leutenegger (Eds.), *Stuttering in children and adults.* Minneapolis: University of Minnesota Press, 1955.

De Hirsh, K., & Langford, W. S. Clinical note on stuttering and cluttering in young children. *Pediatrics,* 1950, *5,* 934–940.

Dunlap, K. *Habits: Their making and unmaking.* New York: Liveright, 1932.

Emerick, L. L. *Therapy for young stutterers.* Danville, IL: Interstate Printers & Publishers, 1970.

Emerick, L. L., & Hatten, J. T. *Diagnosis and evaluation in speech pathology.* Englewood Cliffs, NJ: Prentice-Hall, 1974.

Gregory, H. H. Applications of learning theory concepts in the management of stuttering. In H. Gregory (Ed.), *Learning theory and stuttering therapy.* Evanston, IL: Northwestern University Press, 1968.

Gregory, H. H. Modeling procedures in the treatment of elementary school children who stutter. *Journal of Fluency Disorders.* 1973, *1,* 58–63.

Gregory, H. H., & Hill, D. Stuttering therapy for children. In W. Perkins (Ed.), *Seminars in speech, language and hearing* (Vol. 1, pp. 351–364). New York: Thieme-Stratton, 1980.

Guitar, B., & Peters, T. J. *Stuttering: An integration of contemporary therapies.* Memphis: Speech Foundation of America, 1980.

Hood, S. B. Clients, clinicians and therapy. In L. L. Emerick & S. B. Hood (Ed.), *The client-clinician relationship.* Springfield, IL: Thomas, 1974.

Ingham, R. J. *Evaluation of assessment procedures.* Paper presented at Speech Foundation of America conference, Northwestern University, 1982.

Johnson, W. Stuttering. In W. Johnson, S. F. Brown, J. F. Curtis, C. W. Edney, & J. Keaster (Eds.), *Speech handicapped school children.* New York: Harper & Row, 1956.

Johnson, W. (Ed.) *Stuttering in children and adults: Thirty years of research at the University of Iowa.* Minneapolis: University of Minnesota Press, 1955.

Knepflar, K. L. *Stuttering: Intervention with children.* Paper presented at the American Speech and Hearing Association national convention, San Francisco, 1978.

Luper, H. L., & Mulder, R. L. *Stuttering: Therapy for children.* New York: Prentice-Hall, 1964.

Morley, M. E. *The development and disorders of speech in childhood.* Edinburgh: Livingstone, 1957.

Perkins, W. H. From psychoanalysis to discoordination. In H. H. Gregory (Ed.), *Controversies about stuttering therapy*. Baltimore: University Park Press, 1979.

Perkins, W. H. Replacement of stuttering with normal speech: I. Rationale. *Journal of Speech and Hearing Disorders*, 1973, *38*, 283–294.

Riley, G. D. *Riley Motor Problems Inventory*. Los Angeles: Western Psychological Services, 1976.

Riley, G. D., & Riley, J. A component model for diagnosing and treating children who stutter. *Journal of Fluency Disorders*, 1979, *4*, 279–293.

Riley, G. D., & Riley, J. Motoric and linguistic variables among children who stutter: A factor analysis. *Journal of Speech and Hearing Disorders*, 1980, *45*, 504–514.

Sheehan, J. G. Conflict theory of stuttering. In J. Eisenson (Ed.), *Stuttering: A symposium*. New York: Harper & Row, 1958.

Sheehan, J. G. Stuttering as self-role conflict. In H. Gregory (Ed.), *Learning theory and stuttering therapy*. Evanston, IL: Northwestern University Press, 1968.

Sheehan, J. G. *Stuttering: Research and therapy*. New York: Harper & Row, 1970.

Sheehan, J. G., & Voas, R. B. Stuttering as conflict. I. Comparison of therapy techniques involving approach and avoidance. *Journal of Speech and Hearing Disorders*, 1957, *22*, 714–723.

Starkweather, C. W. A multiprocess behavioral approach to stuttering therapy. In W. Perkins (Ed.), *Seminars in speech, language and hearing*, 1980, *1*, 327–338.

Starkweather, C. W., & Lucker, J. Tokens for stuttering. *Journal of Fluency Disorders*, 1978, *3*, 167–180.

Strupp, H. On the technology of psychotherapy. *Archives of General Psychiatry*, 1972, *26*, 270–278.

Thompson, J. *Assessment of fluency in school-age children*. Danville, IL: Interstate Printers & Publishers, 1983.

Van Riper, C. Experiments in stuttering therapy. In J. Eisenson (Ed.), *Stuttering: A symposium*. New York: Harper & Row, 1958.

Van Riper, C. Historical approaches. In J. G. Sheehan (Ed.), *Stuttering: Research and therapy*. New York: Harper & Row, 1970.

Van Riper, C. *Speech correction: Principles and methods*. Englewood Cliffs, NJ: Prentice-Hall, 1954.

Van Riper, C. *The nature of stuttering*. Englewood Cliffs, NJ: Prentice-Hall, 1971.

Van Riper, C. *The treatment of stuttering*. Englewood Cliffs, NJ: Prentice-Hall, 1973.

Webster, R. L. *Clinician's program guide: The precision fluency shaping program*. Roanoke, VA: Communications Development Corp., 1975.

Williams, D. E. A perspective on approaches to stuttering therapy. In H. H. Gregory (Ed.), *Controversies about stuttering therapy*. Baltimore: University Park Press, 1979.

Williams, D. E. A point of view about stuttering. *Journal of Speech and Hearing Disorders*, 1957, *22*, 390–397.

Williams, D. E. Stuttering therapy for children. In L. E. Travis (Ed.), *Handbook of speech pathology*. New York: Appleton–Century–Crofts, 1971.

Williams, D. E. The problem of stuttering. In F. L. Darley & D. C. Spriesterbach (Eds.), *Diagnostic methods in speech pathology*. New York: Harper & Row, 1978.

Williams, D. E., & Silverman, F. H. Note concerning articulation of school-age stutterers. *Perceptual and Motor Skills*, 1968, *27*, 713–714.

Wingate, M. *Stuttering: Theory and treatment*. New York: Wiley, 1976.

Woolf, G. The assessment of stuttering as struggle, avoidance, and expectancy. *British Journal of Disorders of Communication*, 1967, *2*, 158–171.

Chapter 18

Treatment of the Young Chronic Stutterer: Managing Fluency

Janis M. Costello*

The basic premise of this chapter is that stuttering in young children (even in very young children) *can* be treated and *should* be treated. Young children who stutter are not to be frightened of, or to be wary of. They can be, in fact, some of our most delightful clients; and for the most part, their stuttering is not particularly difficult to treat. If a child is old enough to use connected speech and to be noted as a stutterer (the youngest we have seen was just over Age 2), then that child is eligible for stuttering treatment targeted *directly* at stuttering and fluent utterances.

The problem is, however, that many clinicians today feel (probably accurately) that their education in the area of stuttering treatment is minimal, at best. They may know a great deal about theories of stuttering, but they feel they know very little about its treatment. And, of course, most clinicians do not have many stuttering children in their caseloads and may not, therefore, take the time to read the literature on stuttering or to become familiar with the ins and outs of stuttering and stutterers. These two factors together—lack of an academic background in which one feels confident where stuttering is concerned and lack of practice in dealing with clients who stutter, especially the little ones—leave speech–language pathologists feeling a bit nervous about working with young children who stutter. Further, the (nonexperimental) literature is replete with theories of stuttering and anecdotal stories that make one exceedingly cautious with such children for fear of heightening their awareness of stuttering or doing any of a myriad of other things that might make their stuttering worse instead of better. And since what makes them stutter in the first place still is not clearly understood, it

*Parts of this chapter were published in Prins and Ingham (1983) and are reprinted with permission.

seems difficult to guard against doing something that might precipitate a turn for the worse. Wingate (1971) wrote about such apprehensions saying, "I believe that one could develop impressive substantiation for the complaint that most speech clinicians are, in their own way, more afraid of stuttering than many of the stutterers they are called upon to treat" (p. 3). Wingate's statement is still true today.

Some substantiation for his comment was provided by St. Louis and Lass (1981). They administered the Clinicians' Attitudes Toward Stutterers Survey (CATS; Cooper, 1975) to undergraduate and graduate communicative disorders students throughout the country. They found that students generally believe that stutterers have serious psychosocial problems, that they do not have physiologic components to their stuttering, that counseling for stutterers and their families is a crucial component to treatment, that there is truth to Johnson's (1967) semantogenesis theory warning us not to label or draw attention to a child's disfluencies lest we cause stuttering, and they believe that clinicians lack competence where the treatment of stuttering is concerned. The data also indicated that these attitudes of speech-language pathology students become more ingrained as their level of education increases. Predictably, these findings parallel those of Cooper (1975), who studied practicing speech–language clinicians and summarized his results by pointing out that speech clinicians continue to be influenced by old attitudes that are unsubstantiated by research. Somehow these rumors about stuttering—what causes it, and how it should be treated—continue to be promulgated. Therefore, a goal of this chapter is to counter such beliefs with the view that conducting direct stuttering treatment with young children is not only possible, it is necessary and highly likely to be successful; and there is no reason in the world why we should not be doing it.

EARLY VIEWS OF STUTTERING TREATMENT FOR YOUNG CHILDREN

This chapter discusses the appropriateness of conducting treatment aimed *directly* at the way young stuttering children are speaking—at increasing their fluency and decreasing (eliminating) their stuttering. A more popular approach to treating the young stutterer (when one is advocated at all) is an indirect approach aimed at the alteration of environmental variables hypothesized to influence the occurrence of stuttering. Much of the literature, including pamphlets written for parents (Ainsworth, 1975; Ainsworth & Fraser-Gruss, 1981; Cooper, 1979; Johnson, 1967), contains authors' attempts at describing environmental factors that should be modified by the families of young stutterers. In general, these authors ascribe to the rule that one should be a good parent. There are obviously many ways to do this, but these writers typically suggest being a good listener, making sure the child knows he or she is loved, providing good speech models. They further suggest that parents should reduce the amount of punishment in the child's environment, increase the amount of reinforcement, and help the child develop an expanded vocabulary. Further, parents should not let the child get excited, let the siblings interrupt when the child is talking, call attention to the child's disfluencies, or demand perfect speech. All of the "do's" and "don'ts" of good parenting are invoked, which implicitly places responsibility for the child's stuttering squarely on the shoulders of the parents. Hence, responsibility for alleviating the child's problems then rests with them as well.

To my knowledge, there are no credible data to support any of the above-described contentions. That is, our literature is full of theoretical and philosophical pleas to common sense about environmental variables that could induce stuttering, but none of these variables has ever been clearly shown to be functionally related to stuttering. No rigorous experimental evidence exists to demonstrate that the presence or absence of any family-environment variable or composite of variables is a functional antecedent to stuttering. For example, if we were to believe that aversive or punishing interactions between a child and his or her parents produced stuttering, then we would need to see an experiment that demonstrated a high rate of stuttering during interactions that could be described as negative and a low rate of stuttering (preferably in the same child) when the environment was arranged so that no negative parent–child interactions occurred. (Actually, research on this variable was conducted by Egolf, Shames, Johnson, & Kaspirisin-Burrelli (1972) and by Kaspirisin-Burrelli, Egolf, & Shames (1972), although the design and clarity of the findings in these studies were less than adequate for demonstration of a causal relationship.)

To me, the issue is whether we have the right to ask families to rearrange their lives and alter their interactions with one another and to imply to them that their child's stuttering is a byproduct of their interactions with the child, when we do not *know*, with any level of empirical confidence, which, if *any*, of a large number of factors have, in fact, contributed to the child's stuttering. I believe that we do not have this right without convincing and replicated empirical evidence to guide us. Such evidence may eventually be gathered. When it is, the nature of our treatment for stuttering children would change in the direction dictated by the research findings.

A second issue of concern is the likelihood of such indirect treatment being effective. That is, how well are we able to affect family members' behaviors? When one is trying to produce change in a family's environment through treatment/counseling in the clinical environment, one is basically operating through advice and conversation. We try to get reports from family members about their behavior and the child's; but the accuracy of such reports is always open to question, no matter how well meaning family members may be. For any clinician, it is difficult to produce behavior change when one does not have control over many of the relevant variables that could influence family members, and when one cannot reliably observe (let alone measure) the behaviors of interest. This kind of long-distance, second-order treatment, aimed at changing family members' behaviors beyond the confines of the clinician's office, seems to me to be an inadequate method of effecting change. Further, if we add the uncertainties associated with the first problem—that of the clinician not clearly knowing what aspects of the stuttering child's family environment to change—the shaky ground on which this kind of treatment is built becomes even more obvious. A more suitable strategy for treating stuttering in young children, to me at least, is to teach them directly to produce fluent, nonstuttered speech, no matter what is going on in their natural environment.

DIRECT TREATMENT OF STUTTERING IN YOUNG CHILDREN

The relevant research can be divided into two categories: studies that concentrate on positive reinforcement of fluency and studies that include punishment of moments of stuttering. Since stuttering and fluency can be viewed as reciprocals of one another—a given syllable produced by a talker is either stuttered or produced fluently (without stuttering)—the problem has been addressed from both directions. That is, if treatment produces an increase in the proportion of nonstuttered syllables spoken, there will necessarily be less stuttering. And the reverse is also true; if treatment is directed at reducing the frequency of stuttering, the talker will necessarily be more fluent (as long as we describe a fluent utterance as one that contains no stuttering—an issue that turns out not to be as simple as it sounds [Adams, 1981; Few & Lingwall, 1972; Hegde, 1978; Ingham & Carroll, 1977; Ingham & Packman, 1978; Metz, Conture, & Caruso, 1979; Starkweather & Myers, 1979; Stephen & Haggard, 1980; Wendahl & Cole, 1961; Zimmerman, 1980]).

The positive reinforcement of fluent utterances

One of the early experimental studies of the reinforcement of fluency in children was accomplished by Shaw and Shrum (1972), although the philosophy was suggested earlier by Bar (1971) and described in an early clinical report by Rickard and Mundy (1965). In four 20-minute sessions, Shaw and Shrum treated three male stuttering children who were 9 and 10 years of age. In the first session, baseline data were collected while the child conversed freely with the clinician. During this time each child's speech was observed so that a fluency target for treatment could be pinpointed. For two of the children, a fluency duration of 10 sec (that is, 10 sec of continuous talking without stuttering) was selected, while 5 sec of continuous fluency was the target behavior for the third child. During the baseline session, the number of targeted fluent utterances that occurred was counted for each child. After instructions regarding the reinforcement system and the desired nonstuttered behavior, sessions involved the clinician presenting a positive reinforcer every time the child spoke without stuttering for the required amount of time. Fluent utterances increased substantially (and thus stuttering decreased) for all subjects in comparison to baseline. In the third session, the contingencies were reversed and moments of stuttering, rather than fluency, were reinforced. The data for all three subjects indicated that stuttering increased to baseline levels (thus fluent utterances decreased in number) during this condition.

It is reasonable to ask why one would want to reinforce stuttering. However, this procedure is valuable for two reasons. First, the observation that changes in the frequency of fluent utterances and stuttering coincide with the introduction and removal of the reinforcement contingency indicates that those changes were a function of the experimental manipulation of the independent variable, reinforcement. That is, behavior did not change by accident or for some unknown reason. It is most likely that fluency increased in the first place because it was being reinforced, and that it subsequently returned to baseline levels because it was no longer being reinforced. Further, these data suggest that fluency may be just a "plain old response" like any other operant behavior. When it was reinforced, it increased in frequency of occurrence; and when an incompatible response was reinforced (in this case, stuttering), it decreased. These data might lead us to believe that we need no special principles of behavior to describe and understand fluency and stuttering. The principles already well known in behavioral psychology serve quite adequately.

In the fourth session Shaw and Shrum once again reinforced nonstuttered utterances, and once again these increased (while stuttering reciprocally decreased). The effects of the contingencies observed in the second session were replicated, giving us yet more confidence in the findings. Thus, Shaw and Shrum demonstrated that reinforcement for fluency (at least when the reinforcement contingencies were combined with instructions) produced clinically significant changes in fluent and stuttered talking in children.

A similar study was conducted by Peters (1977) with two 8-year-old male stutterers in a public school setting. When a predetermined number of tokens had been earned for fluent utterances of a particular length, the child was allowed to bring a friend to the next session (the child-selected reinforcer). The data indicated that stuttering was essentially eliminated in the clinic setting within a time span of 3½ to 4 months.

A variation of the reinforcement-for-fluency strategy was described by Johnson (1980), who taught parents of seven young stuttering children to treat their children's stuttering themselves, in the home setting. Parents were taught to ignore children's talking when it contained moments of stuttering, and to reinforce with attention and interaction those utterances that were not stuttered. She also asked parents to speak more slowly to their children. The data from this study tend to indicate that children's fluency improved over time with this parent-administered treatment. However, no data on parent behavior were obtained, so whether parents actually applied the extinction and reinforcement techniques, or slowed their speaking rates when communicating with their children, cannot be verified. Parents' anecdotal reports indicated that they felt the selective attention for fluency was the more powerful of the two procedures.

The addition of punishment of stuttering

Punishment studies have centered their attention on the stuttering moment, although most of these studies have combined punishment for stuttering with reinforcement for fluency. When one is using the term as part of the technical terminology of behavioral psychology, punishment simply means attaching a consequence to behavior which results in a decrease in the frequency of occurrence of that behavior. It does not mean using a shock stick on children who stutter. It does not mean yelling at a child every time a moment of stuttering occurs. It just means following a moment of stuttering with some kind of feedback—a consequence—that produces a reduction in that behavior. It may be a seemingly neutral consequence. It may be saying "No!" It may be taking a token away. It may be frowning. It may be asking the child to stop talking for a moment, or to slow down, or to repeat the utterance. It may be innocuous, or it may be intense. The nature of the "punishing" stimulus depends upon the child and what is functionally effective for that particular child.

Some of the stuttering literature would lead us to believe that if stuttering is punished, it increases (e.g., Brutten & Shoemaker, 1967). It does not. If a moment of stuttering occurs and is followed swiftly by an effective punishing consequence, the frequency of stuttering will decrease. The early research that first demonstrated this finding and a comprehensive discussion of punishment issues is provided in an excellent article by Siegel (1970).

The first study to bravely forge ahead and test the use of punishment contingencies with young children who stuttered was conducted by Martin, Kuhl, and Haroldson (1972). (It was pretty daring to attempt to punish stuttering in young children in 1972 because the theories of Wendell Johnson were still hovering over stuttering theory and practice.) Their two subjects were male stutterers aged 3;6 and 4;6. Each child was engaged in conversation with a puppet named Suzibelle. During baseline sessions, Suzibelle and the child conversed while the experimenters measured the child's rate of stuttering until it was stable over time. Then the experimental treatment was introduced, and each time the child stuttered the puppet would stop talking to the child and go limp, and the lights illuminating Suzibelle would go out briefly. As long as the child was talking fluently, he could maintain Suzibelle's attention (reinforcement for fluency); but as soon as a moment of stuttering occurred, punishment was delivered through the immediate removal of this positive reinforcer. For both children, this condition produced an impressive drop in the frequency of stuttering so that their speech was essentially stutter-free. After several sessions of this condition, the baseline condition was reinstated by withdrawing the punishment contingency for several more sessions. For both children, stuttering remained at the low rate it had attained during the punishment condition. Furthermore, the reduction of stuttering was also observed to generalize to each child's conversations with a stranger outside of the clinic room and to each child's conversations with his mother at home. These changes were also observed to be maintained at the time of a 1-year follow-up.

Reed and Godden (1977) conducted a study that was similar in design. However, their punishment procedure consisted of saying "slow down" to the subject each time a moment of stuttering occurred. For two children, a 5;10-year-old male and a 3;9-year-old female, this contingency led to decreases in stuttering that generalized beyond the experimental treatment setting. (Whether these decreases were a direct result of the contingencies or a byproduct of the slower speech induced by these contingencies was not evaluated.)

Another demonstration of the effectiveness of a combination of positive reinforcement for fluent utterances and punishment for stuttering was described in a clinical report by Johnson, Coleman, and Rasmussen (1978). Their subject was a 6-year-old male stutterer who received treatment in which progressively longer nonstuttered utterances were reinforced by the clinician's attention and praise. The consequence for a moment of stuttering was having the child repeat after the clinician any word that had been stuttered, and then the entire sentence or phrase that contained the word. Johnson et al. reported that not only did stuttering decrease substantially during their use of this treatment method, but the form of stuttering also changed so that at the end of the study those infrequent moments of stuttering that still occurred were generally whole-word repetitions. No prolongations, and only a few part-word repetitions, remained. The authors also commented that this young child's awareness or concern about his stuttering did not appear to increase as a byproduct of this direct approach to modifying his speaking behavior.

Other well-documented demonstrations of the effectiveness of combining reinforcement for fluency and punishment for stuttering in modifying the speech of stuttering children of all ages can be found in the excellent clinical reports of Ryan (1971, 1974).

Two summary statements could be interjected at this point. First, based on my knowledge of the data in the literature, my own research (Costello, 1975; Costello & Ferrer, 1976), and my own clinical experience, I am of the opinion that the most effective treatment provides *both* reinforcement for nonstuttered responses and feedback (punishment) for occurrences of stuttering in the speech of young children. When punishment contingencies are included, children do not cringe or cry or hate the clinician. They simply figure out much faster what it is that they are supposed to do.

Second, I have been impressed by the experimental data and some of my own clinical experience regarding the speed of the effectiveness of this direct approach to stuttering with young children. Although the degree to which fluent speech was established and the nature and requirements of each treatment method differed in the above-described research, it is interesting to review the amount of time each child participated in direct treatment to establish nonstuttered speech within the clinic environment. The least time spent in effective treatment was Shaw and Shrum's (1972) 1 hour and 20 minutes per subject, while the longest treatment duration (Johnson et al., 1978) was only 21 hours. The message here, for clinicians and researchers alike, is that fluency and stuttering in young children may be a relatively malleable set of responses.

THE BASICS OF BEHAVIORAL TREATMENT OF STUTTERING

As all clinicians know, before one begins treatment a careful assessment of the behavior of interest is demanded. Since this has been described in detail elsewhere in this volume (chap. 15) and in other places (Costello, 1981; Ingham & Costello, 1984), there is no need to reiterate here beyond saying that it is important to have a clear description of a child's stuttering behavior, its frequency of occurrence in connected speech samples and in tasks to be used during treatment, and to have data regarding the child's speaking rate as well. All of these (as well as other) aspects of the child's behavior are likely to change during treatment, and one must appreciate their status before treatment in order to evaluate improvement during and at the end of treatment.

After one has obtained assessment data regarding the child's talking performance, a treatment program can be designed. There are many ways to go about this. I am not one who advocates the use of a single, commercially or clinician-prepared treatment method for all children who stutter. The assessment data that have been gathered give the clinician relevant information regarding the type of individualized treatment design that might be effective for a given client. Nonetheless, varieties of behavioral treatments are based upon common principles of treatment design. These principles are the principles of learning as applied through operant conditioning and programmed instruction described elsewhere in this volume (chap. 10) and in other places (e.g., Costello, 1977; 1980; 1982). A basic premise that I advocate and practice, however, is the following. Treatment for stuttering in young children should begin with the basics—with the most simplistic and uncomplicated treatment format. The clinician can then allow the treatment data to provide guidance for the alteration of treatment variables, *only* if such alteration is demonstrated to be necessary (Ingham & Costello, 1984).

What is meant by "the basics" is arranging differential consequences for the occurrence of fluent utterances and moments of stuttering. That is about as simple as one can get, yet we have reliable clinical-experimental data that say this is an effective treatment strategy for young children who stutter. Why, then, should we make the task more difficult for ourselves and the child by attempting to do more than this if, in fact, this is enough to produce fluent-sounding speech that is used consistently by the child in the natural environment?

In the appendix of Costello (1983) is a complete, detailed version of the Extended Length of Utterances (ELU) program (Costello, 1980), one version of the basic treatment we use with young stuttering children.[1]

---

[1] It is advisable for clinicians interested in trying this program with stuttering clients to review this complete version of the program and the more detailed description of it published in Costello (1983).

This program is similar in principle and form to what Ryan (1974) has described as GILCU (Gradual Increase in Length and Complexity of Utterance). This treatment program is often a good starting place for applying the basics and is offered as an illustration of one way to design such treatment.

Briefly, the ELU program moves gradually from evoking short, simple nonstuttered utterances to evoking fluent utterances that are progressively longer, more linguistically complex, and more naturalistic. For example, Step 1 requires that the child produce only a one-syllable word without stuttering. When that behavior is consistently correct, Step 2 evokes two-syllable utterances (e.g., *house, car; mother; red rose*). By the time Step 9, for example, is reached, the child is formulating connected speech utterances in monologue for a specified length or duration (10 sec in Step 9). The program simply continues to move the child's fluent behavior in this manner, bit by bit, until the last step in the program is passed and the child is able to speak in spontaneous conversation in the clinic with the clinician for 5 minutes without stuttering.

The child's behavior is moved through the treatment program with the systematic use of reinforcement and punishment contingencies. For positive reinforcement of nonstuttered responses, a token system of positive reinforcers combined with social reinforcement is utilized. Reinforcers are initially given for every nonstuttered response. As the program continues, the token system is gradually faded out and the reinforcement schedule is gradually made more intermittent so that by the end of the program the child is no longer relying on continuous social and token reinforcers in order to be fluent.

Punishment contingencies are included for stuttering. For most of the steps of this program, stuttered responses are followed by the clinician saying "stop" to the child *as soon as* a moment of stuttering is recognized—even before the child has completed the attempted word. At this time the child refrains from continuing the utterance until the next trial is initiated. Only on later steps of the program is the delivery of punishment delayed (until the entire 4- or 5-minute nonstuttered talking response is completed). As is well known, the power of attaching consequences to behavior is strongest when those consequences immediately follow the behavior of interest. However, by the end of the establishment phase of treatment, one does not want the client to be dependent upon such feedback or upon artificial reinforcers and punishers not likely to occur in the natural environment. Hence, contingencies are faded gradually so that clients learn to maintain their newly acquired behavior without artificial or immediate feedback.

In our experience it has not been necessary (nor believed helpful or appropriate) to explain to young children the treatment strategies. We simply provide reinforcers for nonstuttered utterances and some other kind of feedback for moments of stuttering. We do not explain what the child must do to earn a reinforcer (although some of our social reinforcers are comments such as, "That's really good talking"); nor do we explain what is the matter with his or her speech when we say "stop," or remove a token reinforcer, or ask that an utterance be repeated. Explanations may actually confuse young children rather than provide help. If the proper reinforcers and punishers are selected and administered contingently and immediately, the contingencies usually function quite well on their own. Some children figure out the nature of their responses that produce reinforcers or punishers and verbalize this to the clinician. We have even known children who, having been on a program where a token is removed following each moment of stuttering, give back a token each time they catch themselves stuttering. Intuitively, it seems to be a good sign if a child understands the goals of treatment and correctly monitors his or her own behavior. However, where very young children are concerned, at least, it appears that such awareness is not a prerequisite to the success of treatment. It would be interesting to study the role of such signs of awareness as a predictor of the speed and magnitude of treatment effects. Lacking such data, however, we do not bother children with the rationales underlying their treatment.

Another reason to encourage clinicians not to provide elaborate explanations of the tasks presented, or the nature of the response required, or the rules for earning reinforcers or punishers, is because clinicians should be encouraged to talk as little as possible during sessions. In most clinical settings, available treatment time is all too short and infrequent as it is. And if a substantial part of treatment time is used as clinician talking time, less talking time is left for the child. Fluency and stuttering are, first and foremost, motor behaviors; and motor behaviors are learned through repeated practice. One learns motor behavior by emitting a great deal of it (practice) and by receiving differential feedback for correct and incorrect responses. The more opportunities the child has to produce nonstuttered responses, the more rapidly this form of talking becomes automatic in his or her repertoire.

ADDITIVES

What if simple reinforcement of fluent utterances and punishment of moments of stuttering does not work, or produces a less-than-satisfactory change in the child's manner of talking? Figure 18-1

Figure 18-1. A schematic illustration of basic treatment supplemented progressively by the addition of other variables to the treatment method.

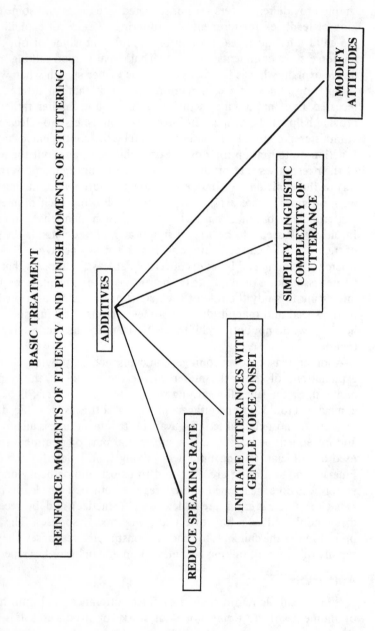

BASIC TREATMENT

REINFORCE MOMENTS OF FLUENCY AND PUNISH MOMENTS OF STUTTERING

ADDITIVES

REDUCE SPEAKING RATE

INITIATE UTTERANCES WITH GENTLE VOICE ONSET

SIMPLIFY LINGUISTIC COMPLEXITY OF UTTERANCE

MODIFY ATTITUDES

illustrates what could be called "additives"—additions to the "basics" that are appropriate supplements to treatment for some stuttering children. (Many researcher–clinicians would advocate incorporating one or more of these additives from the beginning of treatment for adults who stutter because their behavior may be more difficult to change otherwise [e.g., Ingham & Andrews, 1973; Perkins, 1973a, 1973b; Perkins, Rudas, Johnson, Michael, & Curlee, 1974]. In my opinion, too many persons writing about the treatment of stuttering in young children operate in the same fashion, designing treatment that includes some of these variations before they find out whether the simple "basics" are sufficient to produce meaningful changes in a child's speech.)

Rate control

Probably the method of first choice is some kind of rate control, especially if assessment and treatment data indicate that the child speaks rapidly. To find this out, one must measure not overall speaking rate (the average number of syllables per minute when all syllables spoken, including stuttered ones, are counted), but *articulatory rate* (Costello, 1981; Perkins, 1975: the average number of syllables produced per minute in segments of nonstuttered speech). This is a more appropriate measure of how rapidly the child is actually talking. (For a complete discussion of this issue and instructions regarding how to measure articulatory rate, see chap. 15 in this volume or Costello, 1981.) When articulatory rate is above 180 or 200 syllables per minute, children's speaking rates are probably too fast to allow them to learn to produce fluent speech. However, there is little research on optimum speaking rates for children, stutterers or not, so it is difficult to specify what rates are appropriate and what rates are too fast. It may turn out that stuttering children, in order to be fluent, must speak more slowly than the above-proposed 180 to 200 syllables per minute, or it may turn out that speaking rate is not an important variable where the development of fluency is concerned. (It does appear, however, to be important in the treatment of adults.)

At any rate (no pun intended), if the clinician suspects that a child's speaking rate is too fast, then the basic program can be modified to require that responses not only be fluent, but be produced within certain rate limits. The best-known rate control methods are those that have used delayed auditory feedback (DAF) so that speakers slow their speaking rate through prolongation of continuants and vowels in order to better cope with the disruptive effects of DAF (Perkins et al., 1979; Perkins, Rudas, Johnson, & Bell, 1976). The work of Ryan (1971; 1974) and Shames and Florance (1980) exemplifies the use of DAF and slow, prolonged speaking rates to establish fluency in the speech of stuttering children. It is my opinion, however, that it is generally unnecessary to go to such extremes to modify speaking rate in young children, and Adams (1980) points out what we have also observed—that young children do not like DAF and have difficulty using extremely prolonged speech and maintaining it for any significant period. Further, if one were successful in teaching a child to use this kind of speech (and it does produce speech that does not contain stuttering), then one would be faced with the problem of shaping this unusual pattern of speech to one that sounds normal while keeping the fluency it has generated at the same time. This is not easy to do with adults, and there is no reason to believe that it would be any easier with children.

There are other less extreme but effective ways of reducing speaking rate in the speech of young children. For example, simply instructing the child to slow down and then reinforcing, at each step of the program, only responses that are both fluent and within a prescribed speaking rate limit, has been effective in our clinic. Sometimes we model the desired speaking rate for the child, and sometimes we have them add a tiny bit of prolongation to their speech in order to slow it down and make phonetic transitions more continuous. Once again, though, any additions of this kind are more difficult to teach the child and are more difficult to get rid of later on. We have found that it is not necessary to slow a child's speaking rate below about 120 syllables per minute, and then we let the rate move gradually back up to a maximum of 180 syllables per minute.

During this treatment it is important that the clinician do two additional activities. First, along with measuring the frequency of stuttered and nonstuttered responses, as she would do during administration of the basic program, she must also measure speaking rate on each (or frequent) trial to be sure that this additive is being utilized. Further, the clinician needs to develop a system for evaluating whether the use of the additive (rate of speech in this example) is producing the desired behavior change. The introduction of within session ABAB manipulations (Hersen & Barlow, 1976) advocated by Costello (1979) is a simple and convenient method for providing such information. For example, blocks of trials could be conducted in which control of speaking rate was alternately required or not required. Then, one could look at the data and see if slower responses contained less stuttering than faster responses.

Gentle onset

Another additive that some people use is to teach the stutterer to initiate utterances with a gentle onset of voice. This is essentially synonomous with airflow types of treatment and treatments that discuss management of the breathstream. Adams (1980) and Adams and Runyan (1981) describe such treatment with children and appear to use it regularly. Shine (1980) has children whisper their responses during early steps of his treatment program, and then gradually use a louder voice while maintaining fluency until they are talking, eventually, at a conversational level of vocal intensity. Children whose speech contains acute moments of articulatory closure (often described as hard contacts or silent prolongations) and whose initiation of vocalization is abrupt and frequently contains glottal stops might be signaling the appropriateness of a treatment tactic that would smooth out those interruptions in the flow of air past the vocal folds. This kind of speech is generally initiated with a bit of breathiness which is later faded out so that normal speech is attained. Once again, getting this response variation into the child's repertoire in the first place can be a bit difficult, and getting it out again may be difficult as well, so one would not want to use this additive technique unless the data clearly indicated that the basics were not sufficient for a given child. Further, one would want to include measurement of gentle onset for each trial and also test the effectiveness of the technique (by making ABAB manipulations as described above for speaking rate alterations) to be sure that changes in fluency and stuttering were clearly due to the addition of gentle onset techniques. (It has been my observation that use of gentle onset usually precipitates a decrease in speaking rate, so it may be difficult to assess which component, slowed speaking rate or gentle initiation of voicing, is responsible for observed treatment effects.)

Linguistic simplification

Many persons conducting research these days hypothesize a language component to the stuttering child's problems. For example, Gregory and Hill (1980) state that 55% of 52 children they studied demonstrated problems of word retrieval (although these data have not been published for the scrutiny of others). Adams (1980) apparently believes there is a substantial subgroup of such children. He described his treatment requiring slowed speech and gradually increasing utterance lengths as being well suited to the stuttering child with language problems, because it gives the child time to organize central language processing functions. Among a myriad of studies investigating the role of language in the problems of stuttering are two recent articles with similar findings (Bernstein, 1981; Wall, Starkweather, & Cairns, 1981). Using different methodologies with young stuttering subjects, both studies found that moments of stuttering were most likely to occur at clause boundaries. Since both studies were interested in the role of syntax in the stuttered speech of young children, both suggested that the child's ability to plan and/or process syntactic strings might be related to stuttering. However, one could offer an alternative hypothesis to account for these findings. Clause boundaries often occur at the place in utterances where the talker is motorically initiating a new utterance. Therefore, one could argue that motor planning deficits, rather than syntax planning problems, are related to the unusually high occurrence of moments of stuttering at these loci. In fact, in Wall, Starkweather, and Cairns (1981), it was found that stuttering occurred most often on words that were preceded by a pause (juncture) and that began with a voiced phoneme, thereby providing more evidence for the thesis espoused by some that stuttering could be a phonetic transition defect (e.g., Adams, 1981; Van Riper, 1975; Wingate, 1969). Further, children appear to stutter more on longer utterances. Whether this is because such utterances are more complex linguistically, or more complex motorically, is still a question for study. The separation of language and motor issues is a matter yet to be resolved by research.

Just as was mentioned regarding other additives, one should not assume that language variables such as vocabulary selection, semantic relations, syntactic rules, or pragmatic functions are potential targets for manipulation in a stuttering child's treatment program *unless* one has data that indicate a child has deficiencies in one or more of these areas. (It is perfectly possible, as well, that a given child could have a language disorder and a stuttering disorder that are completely independent of one another.)

Attitudes

A last look at Figure 18-1 illustrates another additive that has been considered in the treatment of children who stutter: the modification of their attitudes about communication and about themselves as communicators. There are some serious questions about the role of attitudes in the precipitation and maintenance of stuttering. Even in adults, it is not clear whether adult stutterers' pessimistic attitudes negatively influence the outcome of treatment—or even whether attitudes can be measured with validity or reliability (Guitar, 1976, 1979, 1981; Guitar & Bass, 1978; Ingham, 1979; Ulliana & Ingham, 1984; Young, 1981). Research by Andrews and Cutler (1974) with adult stutterers showed that measures of attitude changed in a positive direction without attitudinal treatment when direct treatment for stuttering produced reductions in stuttering. There is essentially no literature that demonstrates that children who go through stuttering treatment have attitudinal problems beforehand or afterward. Turnbaugh and Guitar (1981) described a public school treatment program that incorporated attitudinal treatment as a significant component in the overall treatment plan. Although the authors appear to assume that an initial stage of attitude treatment is necessary for the success of the direct (DAF) treatment component of their program, this assumption was not demonstrated (or tested) by their research.

We have all observed stuttering children who were reticent and who seemed to be shy or embarrassed, presumably because of the difficulty in talking their stuttering provoked. And we have all seen many of those same children turn into little chatterboxes as their treatment progressed and they became fluent. We have no standardized and validated measures of attitudes in children yet, and it is probably not helpful to engage in idle, clinical speculation. Until and unless there is some reason to suspect a crucial role for problems of communicative attitude in a given child, my suggestion is to stick with the basics when designing treatment.

GENERALIZATION, TRANSFER, AND MAINTENANCE

The above-described basic treatment program is designed to *establish* nonstuttered speech in the clinic environment. This fluent speech may or may not spontaneously generalize beyond the clinic setting. There are some data to indicate that young children may produce their newly acquired nonstuttered speech in the natural environment without the necessity of additional treatment to produce transfer and maintenance (Martin et al., 1972; Reed & Godden, 1977; Ryan, 1971, 1974; Shaw & Shrum, 1972). The older the client, however, the more intractible stuttering may become. If the clinician's extraclinic measures do not indicate that the fluent speech observed in the clinic has also carried over to the child's natural environment, then, of course, treatment designed to promote such generalization would be next on the agenda— but that is another topic (e.g., Boberg, 1981; Hanna & Owen, 1977; chap. 21, in this volume).

SUMMARY

The purpose of this chapter has been twofold. One purpose was to describe the behavioral literature on the direct treatment of stuttering in young children and to provide a systematic, data-based model illustrating one way a clinician can go about applying such treatment. The second purpose was to express the view that young children who stutter should be enrolled in this kind of treatment and to prod clinicians into believing that they can provide successful treatment for such children.

REFERENCES

Adams, M. R. The young stutterer: Diagnosis, treatment, and assessment of progress. In W. H. Perkins (Ed.), *Strategies in stuttering therapy. Seminars in Speech, Language and Hearing,* 1980, *1,* 289-300, New York: Thieme-Stratton.

Adams, M. R. The speech production abilities of stutterers: Recent, ongoing, and future research. *Journal of Fluency Disorders,* 1981, *6,* 311-326.

Adams, M. R., & Runyan, C. M. Stuttering and fluency: Exclusive events or points on a continuum? *Journal of Fluency Disorders,* 1981, *6,* 197-218.

Ainsworth, S. *Stuttering: What it is and what to do about it.* Lincoln, NE: Cliff Notes, 1975.

Ainsworth, S., & Fraser-Gruss, J. *If your child stutters—A guide for parents* (3rd printing). Speech Foundation of America, 1981.

Andrews, G., & Cutler, J. Stuttering therapy: The relation between changes in symptom level and attitudes. *Journal of Speech and Hearing Disorders,* 1974, *39,* 312-319.

Bar, A. The shaping of fluency not the modification of stuttering. *Journal of Communication Disorders,* 1971, *4,* 1-8.

Bernstein, N. E. Are there constraints on childhood disfluency? *Journal of Fluency Disorders,* 1981, *6,* 341-350.

Boberg, E. *Maintenance of fluency.* New York: Elsevier, 1981.

Brutten, E. J., & Shoemaker, D. J. *The modification of stuttering.* Englewood Cliffs, NJ: Prentice-Hall, 1967.

Cooper, E. B. *Clinician attitudes toward stuttering: A study of bigotry?* A paper presented at the convention of American Speech and Hearing Association, Washington, D.C., 1975.

Cooper, E. B. *Understanding stuttering: Information for parents.* Chicago: National Easter Seal Society for Crippled Children and Adults, 1979.

Costello, J. M. The establishment of fluency with timeout procedures: Three case studies. *Journal of Speech and Hearing Disorders,* 1975, *40,* 216-231.

Costello, J. M. Programmed instruction. *Journal of Speech and Hearing Disorders,* 1977, *43,* 3-28.

Costello, J. M. Clinicians and researchers: A necessary dichotomy? *Journal of the National Student Speech and Hearing Association,* 1979, *7,* 6-26.

Costello, J. M. Operant conditioning and the treatment of stuttering. In W. H. Perkins (Ed.), *Strategies in stuttering therapy. Seminars in Speech, Language and Hearing,* 1980, *1,* 311-327, New York: Thieme-Stratton.

Costello, J. M. Pretreatment assessment of stuttering in young children. *Communicative disorders: An audio journal for continuing education* (Vol. 6). New York: Grune & Stratton, December, 1981.

Costello, J. M. Techniques of therapy based on operant conditioning. In W. H. Perkins (Ed.), *Current therapy of communication disorders: General principles of therapy.* New York: Thieme-Stratton, 1982.

Costello, J. M. Current behavioral treatments for children. In D. Prins & R. J. Ingham (Eds.), *Stuttering in early childhood: Treatment methods and issues.* San Diego: College-Hill Press, 1983.

Costello, J. M., & Ferrer, J. Punishment contingencies for the reduction of correct responses during articulation instruction. *Journal of Communication Disorders,* 1976, *9,* 43-61.

Egolf, D., Shames, G., Johnson, P., & Kasprisin-Burrelli, A. The use of parent–child interaction patterns in therapy for young stutterers. *Journal of Speech and Hearing Disorders,* 1972, *37,* 222-232.

Few, L., & Lingwall, J. A further analysis of fluency within stuttered speech. *Journal of Speech and Hearing Research*, 1972, *15*, 356–363.

Gregory, H. H., & Hill, D. Stuttering therapy for children. In W. H. Perkins (Ed.), *Strategies in stuttering therapy. Seminars in Speech, Language and Hearing*, 1980, *1*, 351–364, New York: Thieme-Stratton.

Guitar, B. E. Pretreatment factors associated with the outcome of stuttering therapy. *Journal of Speech and Hearing Research*, 1976, *19*, 590–600.

Guitar, B. E. A response to Ingham's critique (Letter to the Editor). *Journal of Speech and Hearing Disorders*, 1979, *44*, 400–403.

Guitar, B. E. A correction to "A Response to Ingham's critique" (Letter to the editor). *Journal of Speech and Hearing Disorders*, 1981, *46*, 440.

Guitar, B. E., & Bass, C. Stuttering therapy: The relation between attitude change and long-term outcome. *Journal of Speech and Hearing Disorders*, 1978, *43*, 392–400.

Hanna, R., & Owen, N. Facilitating transfer and maintenance of fluency in stuttering therapy. *Journal of Speech and Hearing Disorders*, 1977, *42*, 65–76.

Hegde, M. N. Fluency and fluency disorders: Their definition, measurement and modification. *Journal of Fluency Disorders*, 1978, *3*, 51–71.

Hersen, M., & Barlow, D. H. *Single case experimental designs*. New York: Pergamon Press, 1976.

Ingham, R. J. Comment on "Stuttering therapy: The relation between attitude change and long-term outcome" (Letter to the editor). *Journal of Speech and Hearing Disorders*, 1979, *44*, 397–400.

Ingham, R. J., & Andrews, G. An analysis of a token economy in stuttering therapy. *Journal of Applied Behavior Analysis*, 1973, *6*, 219–229.

Ingham, R. J., & Carroll, P. J. Listener judgment of differences in stutterers' nonstuttered speech during chorus- and nonchorus-reading conditions. *Journal of Speech and Hearing Research*, 1977, *20*, 293–302.

Ingham, R. J., & Costello, J. M. Stuttering treatment outcome evaluation. In J. M. Costello (Ed.), *Speech disorders in children: Recent advances*. San Diego: College-Hill Press, 1984.

Ingham, R. J., & Packman, A. C. Perceptual assessment of normalcy of speech following stuttering therapy. *Journal of Speech and Hearing Research*, 1978, *21*, 63–73.

Johnson, G. F., Coleman, K., & Rasmussen, K. Multidays: Multidimensional approach for the young stutterer. *Language, Speech and Hearing Services in Schools*, 1978, *9*, 129–132.

Johnson, L. J. Facilitating parental involvement in therapy of the disfluent child. In W. H. Perkins (Ed.), *Strategies in stuttering therapy. Seminars in Speech, Language and Hearing*, 1980, *1*, 301–310, New York: Thieme-Stratton.

Johnson, W. An open letter to the mother of a stuttering child. In W. Johnson & D. Moeller (Eds.), *Speech handicapped school children* (3rd ed., pp. 543–544). New York: Harper & Row, 1967.

Kasprisin-Burrelli, A., Egolf, D., & Shames, G. A comparison of parental verbal behavior with stuttering and nonstuttering children. *Journal of Communication Disorders*, 1972, *5*, 335–346.

Martin, R., Kuhl, P., & Haroldson, S. An experimental treatment with two preschool stuttering children. *Journal of Speech and Hearing Research*, 1972, *15*, 743–752.

Metz, D. E., Conture, E. G., & Caruso, A. Voice onset time, frication, and aspiration during stutterers' fluent speech. *Journal of Speech and Hearing Research*, 1979, *22*, 649–656.

Perkins, W. H. Replacement of stuttering with normal speech: I. Rationale. *Journal of Speech and Hearing Disorders*, 1973, *38*, 283-294.(a)

Perkins, W. H. Replacement of stuttering with normal speech: II. Clinical procedures. *Journal of Speech and Hearing Disorders*, 1973, *38*, 295-303.(b)

Perkins, W. H. Articulatory rate in the evaluation of stuttering treatments. *Journal of Speech and Hearing Disorders*, 1975, *40*, 277-278.

Perkins, W. H., Bell, J., & Johnson, L. Phone rate and the effective planning time hypothesis of stuttering. *Journal of Speech and Hearing Research*, 1979, *22*, 747-755.

Perkins, W. H., Rudas, J., Johnson, L., & Bell, J. Stuttering: Discoordination of phonation with articulation and respiration. *Journal of Speech and Hearing Research*, 1976, *19*, 502-522.

Perkins, W. H., Rudas, J., Johnson, L., Michael, W. B., & Curlee, R. F. Replacement of stuttering with normal speech: III. Clinical effectiveness. *Journal of Speech and Hearing Disorders*, 1974, *39*, 416-428.

Peters, A. D. The effect of positive reinforcement on fluency: Two case studies. *Language, Speech and Hearing Services in Schools*, 1977, *8*, 15-22.

Prins, D., & Ingham, R. J. (Eds.). *Treatment of stuttering in early childhood. Methods and issues.* San Diego: College-Hill Press, 1983.

Reed, C. G., & Godden, A. L. An experimental treatment using verbal punishment with two preschool stutterers. *Journal of Fluency Disorders*, 1977, *2*, 225-233.

Rickard, H., & Mundy, M. Direct manipulation of stuttering behavior: An experimental-clinical approach. In L. Ullman & L. Krasner (Eds.), *Case studies in behavior modification.* New York: Holt, Rinehart & Winston, 1965.

Ryan, B. Operant procedures applied to stuttering therapy for children. *Journal of Speech and Hearing Disorders*, 1971, *36*, 264-280.

Ryan, B. *Programmed therapy for stuttering in children and adults.* Springfield, IL: Thomas, 1974.

St. Louis, K. O., & Lass, N. J. A survey of communicative disorders students' attitudes toward stuttering. *Journal of Fluency Disorders*, 1981, *6*, 49-79.

Shames, G. H., & Florance, C. L. *Stutter-free speech: A goal for therapy.* Columbus, OH: Merrill, 1980.

Shaw, C. K., & Shrum, W. F. The effects of response-contingent reward on the connected speech of children who stutter. *Journal of Speech and Hearing Disorders*, 1972, *37*, 75-88.

Shine R. E. Direct management of the beginning stutterer. In W. H. Perkins (Ed.), *Strategies in stuttering therapy. Seminars in Speech, Language and Hearing*, 1980, *1*, 339-350, New York: Thieme-Stratton.

Siegel, G. M. Punishment, stuttering and disfluency. *Journal of Speech and Hearing Research*, 1970, *13*, 677-714.

Starkweather, C. W., & Myers, M. Duration of subsegments within the intervocalic interval in stutterers and nonstutterers. *Journal of Fluency Disorders*, 1979, *3*, 205-214.

Stephen, S. C. G., & Haggard, M. P. Acoustic properties of masking/delayed feedback in the fluency of stutterers and controls. *Journal of Speech and Hearing Research*, 1980, *23*, 527-538.

Turnbaugh, K. R., & Guitar, B. E. Short-term intensive stuttering treatment in a public school setting. *Language, Speech and Hearing Services in Schools*, 1981, *12*, 107-114.

Ulliana, L., & Ingham, R. J. Behavioral and nonbehavioral variables in the measurement of stutterers' communication attitudes. *Journal of Speech and Hearing Disorders*, 1984, *49*, 83-93.

Van Riper, C. The Ablauf problem in stuttering. *Journal of Fluency Disorders,* 1975, *1,* (1), 2-9.

Wall, M. J., Starkweather, C. W., & Cairns, H. S. Syntactic influences on stuttering in young child stutterers. *Journal of Fluency Disorders,* 1981, *6,* 283-298.

Wall, M. J., Starkweather, C. W., & Harris, K. S. The influence of voicing adjustments on the location of stuttering in the spontaneous speech of young child stutterers. *Journal of Fluency Disorders,* 1981, *6,* 299-310.

Wendahl, R. W., & Cole, J. Identification of stuttering during relatively fluent speech. *Journal of Speech and Hearing Research,* 1961, *4,* 281-286.

Wingate, M. E. Stuttering as a phonetic transition defect. *Journal of Speech and Hearing Disorders,* 1969, *34,* 107-108.

Wingate, M. E. The fear of stuttering. *Asha,* 1971, *13,* 3-5.

Young, M. A. A reanalysis of "Stuttering therapy: The relation between attitude change and long-term outcome" (Letter to the editor). *Journal of Speech and Hearing Disorders,* 1978, *43,* 392-400.

Zimmerman, G. Articulatory dynamics of fluent utterances of stutterers and nonstutterers. *Journal of Speech and Hearing Research,* 1980, *23,* 95-107.

Chapter 19

Treatment of Adults: Managing Stuttering

David Prins

BACKGROUND

"The development of principles and procedures of behavioral change is largely determined by the model of causality to which one subscribes" (Bandura, 1969, p. 1). The approach to treatment, called in this chapter "managing stuttering," developed precisely in this way. It is based fundamentally on the notion that the "moment of stuttering" embodies the dynamics that developed and maintain the disorder, and that "the moment" is therefore the principal target of therapy. Before examining the elements of this approach, however, we should understand something about its evolution.

The cornerstone was laid by hypotheses introduced and research undertaken during the 1930s at the University of Iowa. Wendell Johnson and Charles Van Riper were the primary architects, but each had a quite different principal contribution to make. Johnson focused chiefly on the nature of the stuttering response; Van Riper, after completing early experiments dealing with the nature of stuttering, devoted most of his attention to the development, description, and clinical evaluation of treatment procedures and programs.

In 1933 and in subsequent papers Johnson (1933, 1936b; Johnson & Knott, 1936c) developed the concept of the moment of stuttering. His ideas helped to spawn an enormous number of studies in which variations in the occurrence of overt stuttering episodes were tabulated in a variety of different speaking and reading conditions. Table 19-1 lists the principal studies that (1) grew from Johnson's early work and (2) pertain to managing stuttering in the older child and adult. It is interesting to note the chronology of this work, the large number of studies done at the University of Iowa, and the relative paucity of studies

TABLE 19-1. Principal article and chapter references pertaining to the "moment of stuttering" and to "managing stuttering" in older children and adults.*

Nature and Definitions of Stuttering	Studies Pertaining to Stuttering's Nature	Therapy Techniques & Program Descriptions	Technique Effect Studies	Program Outcome Studies	Historic Reviews & Interpretation
Johnson (1933)	Johnson (1935)	Bryngelson (1935)	Van Riper (1938)	Van Riper (1958)	Williams (1968)
Van Riper (1937c)	Johnson (1936b)	Johnson (1936a)	Sheehan (1951)	Gregory (1969)	Van Riper (1970a)
Wischner (1948)	Johnson (1936c)	Van Riper (1937e)	Chotolas (1955)	Prins (1970)	Starkweather (1973)
Wischner (1950)	Steer (1936)	Johnson (1939)	Oxtoby (1955)	Gregory (1972)	Van Riper (1974b)
Sheehan (1953)	Van Riper (1936)	Hahn (1943)	Sheehan (1957)	Prins (1974)	Boberg (1979)
Sheehan (1954a)	Johnson (1937a)	Johnson (1955b)	Frick (1965)	Prins (1976)	Gregory (1979)
Johnson (1955a)	Johnson (1937b)	Van Riper (1957)	Shames (1969)		Sheehan (1979)
Johnson (1955c)	Johnson (1937c)	Gregory (1968)			Williams (1979)
Williams (1957)	Johnson (1937d)	Ryan (1970)			Bloodstein (1981)
Bloodstein (1975)	Johnson (1937e)	Shames (1970)			Williams (1982)
	Johnson (1937f)	Van Riper (1970b)			
	Van Riper (1937a)	Van Riper (1971)			
	Van Riper (1937b)	Van Riper (1973)			
	Van Riper (1937d)	Van Riper (1974a)			
	Johnson (1938)	Van Riper (1974c)			
	Wischner (1952a)	Sheehan (1975)			
	Wischner (1952b)	Boberg (1976)			
	Sheehan (1954b)	Shames (1976)			
	Berwick (1955)	Maxwell (1982)			
	Connett (1955)				
	Dixon (1955)				
	Donohue (1955)				
	Downton (1955)				
	Jones (1955)				
	Shulman (1955)				
	Tanberg (1955)				
	Van Riper (1955)				
	Luper (1956)				
	Sheehan (1962)				
	Wingate (1966a)				
	Wingate (1966b)				
	Sheehan (1967)				
	Wingate (1975)				
	Prins (1980)				

* References are shown chronologically in the category of principal contribution. Only first authors' names are listed, and alphabetic notation in the reference list is adapted accordingly.

in recent years pertaining to the nature of stuttering, the effects of treatment techniques, and program outcome.

Referring in 1955 to the results of the prodigious research effort at Iowa throughout the 1930s and 1940s, Johnson (Johnson & Leutenegger, 1955) summarized the essential change in thinking that had occurred and that formed the basis for the stuttering management approach:

> Neither of the traditional theories of stuttering—that one which attributed it to a physical fault and the other which viewed it as a symptom of an unstable or turbulent personality—was based on sufficient information about the ways in which stuttering behaves. If they explained stuttering, they did not account for the stutterer's nonstuttered speech, and they did not explain the variations in stuttering frequency or severity in response to particular cues and conditions now known to be associated with these variations. The kinds of data presented. . . prompt one to regard stuttering as learned behavior, and to investigate it, theorize about it, and treat it clinically, as such. (p. 18)

What had happened was that the research being done at Iowa concerning the phenomena of stuttering and their variations had come under the influence of the work on conditioning and learning theory of Clark Hull and Kenneth Spence. As a consequence, Johnson, Van Riper, and others turned away from the view that stuttering was a neurophysiological disorder (i.e., evidence of a breakdown in coordination of the speech musculature) and toward the view that stuttering was a lawful, predictable reaction; governed to a marked degree by circumstantial events associated with the act of speaking.

The moment of stuttering had become the window through which the essence of the disorder could be seen. It was therefore a logical focal point for both theory and treatment. In a paper written in 1935–1936 Johnson (Johnson & Leutenegger, 1955) described what he believed were the essential characteristics of the stuttering response (the moment of stuttering):

> A stutterer in a situation calling for communication will have two tendencies: one will be to speak; the other will be to avoid stuttering. . . . The positive charge, or valence, surrounds the perception of the desirability of speaking. The negative valence surrounds the perception of the desirability of not stuttering. Thus the positive valence is facilitory; the negative, inhibitory. . . . It is the duality of the perception, calling for both progressing and retreating behavior, which causes the partially inhibitory behavior called stuttering. The total response is made up of two response tendencies, one positive and one negative. A conflict between the two is the obvious result. (p. 27)[1]

Johnson's definition (1948) of the reactive sequence involved in the stuttering episode also encapsulates nicely the beliefs that were developing in the 1930s among the Iowa group: "Stuttering is an anticipatory, apprehensive, hypertonic, avoidance reaction" (p. 182).

These early ideas about the moment of stuttering were modified and elaborated extensively. If the stuttering response was in fact learned, then an explanation of the reinforcing events was required. A major refinement in this regard was provided in the late 1940s and early 1950s by George Wischner (1948, 1950, 1952a, 1952b) who proposed that anxiety was the primary motivational ingredient in stuttering, and that anxiety reduction at the termination of the moment was the principal reinforcing mechanism that maintained the stuttering reaction. Later, however, when independent measures of anxiety could not be reliably associated with stutterers or with the stuttering response, anxiety fell into disrepute as an essential feature of the disorder.

Currently, stuttering can no longer be looked upon reasonably as an "anxiety motivated avoidance response." What, then, is the contemporary view that supports the stuttering management approach? Bloodstein (1981) provides a succinct definition: "Stuttering is an anticipatory struggle reaction. In its clinical form it represents a relatively severe degree of tensions and fragmentations that are a common occurrence in the speech of young children" (p. 336). Bloodstein goes on to say that, in its inception, stuttering does not require an avoidance reaction, per se, but rather struggle responses associated with the threat of, or the experience of, failures in performing the complex motor acts of speech. According to Bloodstein, uncertainty about speaking, which can arise from many different internal and external sources, leads to tension and fragmentation reactions during speech. These reactions, in turn, produce prolongations and repetitions in the surface structure of speech. Through learning, these responses by the stutterer become differentially associated with words, sounds, vocal tract postures, and other physical events associated with speaking. Likewise, the severe struggle components that often become superimposed on the basic stuttering response are added over time through the dynamics that govern learned behavior.

Prins (1976) has explained it somewhat differently by accentuating the defensive nature of the stuttering reaction, at least in its developed form:

> Much of what is abnormal in the confirmed stutterer's speech results from his attempts to cope desperately with expected or perceived interruptions in speech flow. . . . Developed out of frustration and desperation, the coping reactions of the stutterer are essentially self-protective. They are what he does to save himself in an emergency. (p. 462)

From the earlier notions that required anxiety motivation and avoidance, to the current ideas of anticipatory struggle and defensive reactions, explanations of the moment of stuttering (as a basis for clinical management) are essentially those of social learning theory (Bandura, 1977b). In this scheme, defensive behavior is activated in the face of a perceived threat. Although anxiety may be a coeffect of this threat, it is not causally linked to the defensive reaction (Bandura, 1977a). The defensive response, extraordinarily difficult to extinguish, comes to be reinforced in two ways: (1) It postpones (or even avoids) the potential aversive consequence; and (2) it escapes the now aversive signal that foretells of the impending difficulty.

The essence of the stuttering response can be depicted by analogy to the novice's emergency defensive reactions during skiing. They are anticipatory in nature, have potentially debilitating consequences, and are very resistant to extinction. When catching an outside ski edge while negotiating a turn, the novice usually responds to this signal by tensing, bearing down on the ski, and, in many cases, leaning back. (It is worth noting, too, that these reactions may be accompanied by significant autonomic nervous system arousal (negative emotion) and rather unpleasant cognitive images of the dreaded consequence.) These neuromuscular reactions, instinctively self-protective, are also maladaptive in the sense that they inhibit the flow of skiing movements and serve to increase, rather than decrease, the chance of disaster. In spite of this debilitating characteristic, however, the novice finds these reactions extraordinarily difficult to give up. Applying this analogy to the stutterer, an early anticipatory signal could be a speaking situation or a given word (the skier looking down a steep hill or at a large mogul). More important, however, is the later (proximal) anticipatory signal that warns of the immediate emergency (the skier sensing that the outside edge of the ski is caught). For the stutterer, this signal can be delivered by a postural set of the articulatory musculature, a degree of muscle tension in the vocal tract, a timing delay in the onset of phonation, and so on. This is the immediate stimulus, the triggering mechanism, for the defensive reactions of stuttering. Its proximity to the stuttering response is so close, and the stuttering reaction to it so automatically implemented, that modification of that reaction in the chronic stutterer is usually a difficult process.

TREATMENT PRINCIPLES AND PROCEDURES

The overall objective of all symptomatic therapies for adults who stutter, whether the focus is on "managing fluency" or "managing stuttering, " should be the same: to help the person who stutters learn to *speak as fluently as he is able*, and has the *will* and the *motivation*, to do. This objective is at apparent odds with the principle Van Riper championed (1939) of helping a person to stutter in a more acceptable, controlled way. In his own words, "Teach the case to stutter in a fashion tolerable to both society and himself" (Van Riper, 1957, p. 880) and later: "We establish and strengthen a new fluent way of stuttering" (Van Riper, 1973, p. 210). Over time, this objective has come under considerable fire and, I believe, rightly so. Nonetheless, its authority has been sufficiently pervasive that Starkweather (1973), for example, felt compelled to state that: "The ultimate goal, *which the therapist keeps to himself*, is fluent speech" (p. 287, italics added). It is almost as if there is a sense of guilt (making it necessary to hide the real objective of treatment) about the possible repudiation of the dictum that stuttering is an avoidance response and that therefore an explicit therapy goal of fluent speech (i.e., the ultimate avoidance of stuttering) is doomed to failure.

The strength of the idea that the objective of managing stuttering is to help the person to "stutter fluently, " has led, during the last decade or longer, to an unnecessary decline in credibility of this approach. On the other hand, there is no reason to avoid stating explicitly to the stutterer that the ultimate goal in treatment is to help him "speak as fluently as he is able and has the will and motivation to do. " A lesser objective will have limited appeal to the stutterer and will not be embraced as reasonable by most clinicians. In fact, if stuttering in the adult is primarily an anticipatory struggle, a defensive reaction, then the words "fluent stuttering" are contradictory. If a person stutters, by definition he engages in inhibitory reactions that are not fluent. If, on the other hand, he responds fluently to the signals that used to trigger stuttering reactions, then he is not stuttering. Recently, this same issue was considered from a somewhat different point of view by Williams (1979).

The material that follows provides a review of the major components of a stuttering management approach. Each component is discussed in terms of (1) objectives, (2) historic contributions of major figures, (3) procedures and techniques, (4) landmarks for client achievement and for moving forward in treatment, and (5) evaluation from the viewpoint of contemporary social learning theory and cognitive behavioral therapy. Concerning evaluation (5), Bandura's article (1977a) is used as a principal reference.

Confrontation: Exploring, understanding, and accepting responsibility for behavior

The overall objective and the essence of the first phase of treatment is to help the stutterer get in touch with what he is doing *while* speaking and stuttering, that is, to experience speaking and stuttering as resulting from his own actions. You are helping to make known and voluntary the details of behavior that have been unknown and seemingly involuntary; you are developing a level of ongoing consciousness that will help to make manageable, responses that have been unmanageable.

This component of treatment owes its origins to Wendell Johnson. The ideas are fundamentally rooted in general semantics and its view that internalized belief systems and inferences are important in governing behavior and one's perceptions thereof. Johnson (Johnson & Leutenegger, 1955) gave two basic principles: (1) the descriptional principle; (2) the principle of static analysis. The former, Johnson defined as "translating inferences into their descriptive equivalence, of keeping discussion and instruction on a descriptive level" (p. 435). The latter, in essence a procedure that serves the purposes of description, requires the use of "slow motion" analysis of one's behavior.

These approaches were refined by Williams (1957) and are best understood by reviewing his own explanation: "*the stutterer is asked to describe* what he does as he talks that normal speakers both do and do not do. If, when he is talking, he starts tensing his throat and jaw muscles and hence begins to interfere with the forward flow of speech, it must be recognized that there is no mysterious entity inside of him that is beginning to stop him from talking. Nothing is happening! He is simply beginning to tense his throat and jaw muscles.[2] Moreover, he will stop talking when, for example, he tenses them sufficiently. The things he does which interfere with normal speech production are the things he does that are labeled 'stuttering' " (p. 394).

Sheehan (1970, chap. 7) also has contributed fundamentally to this aspect of treatment through what he terms "role therapy" in which the stutterer learns to accept, rather than deny, his behavior as a speaker and to assume responsibility for changing it.

Procedures and techniques. Videotape and mirror evaluation are useful activities for this component of treatment. Before such sessions with a client, the clinician should study carefully the client's videotape (presumably made on an earlier occasion) and have a thorough understanding of fluent speech and stuttering characteristics. The clinician should be able to imitate stuttering responses accurately. The initial session may begin with a statement such as, "I want to be able to understand, and help you to understand as clearly as possible, what you do when you speak and when you stutter. " The tape is played and replayed as appropriate, accompanied by (1) observations, descriptions, and imitations of the observable expectancy responses and struggle/release reactions that are a part of stuttering, and (2) discussions of their function and associated feelings and attitudes. In each case the clinician should begin by imitating the behavior of the stutterer, by illustrating how he (the clinician) would go about doing the same things, and by commenting on their functions and his own feelings about them.

After post hoc evaluations of stuttering with videotape, mirror evaluations provide an even more important on-line activity, an opportunity to interrupt and describe behavior while it is happening. The clinician starts by looking into the mirror while the client observes. As he talks, the clinician describes the movements he is making, his awareness of them, and how he feels about what he is doing. He asks the client to do some of the same things. He shows the client how to freeze at a signal, and he (the clinician) describes what he observes the client doing at that point. The clinician then assumes the talking role again and asks the client to signal him to freeze at the point when stutterings are introduced in his (the clinician's) speech. At that point the client describes what he observes. Next, the client describes his own behavior when the clinician signals him to freeze: what he is doing, how it feels to do these things, why he believes he is doing them, and how he feels about them and about observing them. Throughout these activities the emphasis is on describing physical actions that result from things the speaker does. The objective is to develop awarenesses that are typified by such comments as, "I didn't realize I was doing that"; "I notice how I am pushing my lips out, and that has nothing to do with what I'm trying to say."

From the beginning of therapy the client must spend major amounts of time in *self-therapy* activities that are designed cooperatively by him and the clinician. The principles and therapeutic functions of self-therapy are considered in a separate section of this chapter; however, useful activities are suggested as each treatment component is described. During the confrontation/exploration phase, the client should begin keeping a log of outside speaking situations with specific targets for observing and reporting various aspects of his behavior, the behavior of his listeners, and the circumstances. Similarly, he should make and evaluate audio- and videotapes (if feasible) of himself, and do mirror observations with analysis. Both taping and mirror observations of telephone conversations can be useful. With regard to activities of this type, however, it is essential that the clinician demonstrate and role play them before asking the client to do so.

What achievements associated with this phase of treatment suggest that a client is ready to move forward? First of all, it is important to note that phases of therapy are not discrete; they overlap and serve to reinforce each other. For example, self-awareness with regard to talking and stuttering will presumably develop throughout the course of treatment (and perhaps even throughout life). Also, client achievements associated with this phase of treatment are less objective than those associated with later phases. Nonetheless, before moving ahead, the client should clearly demonstrate, by what he says and does, that he can describe his behavior concretely and specifically, what he does when he stutters and when he expects to stutter, and how this directly affects his speaking behavior. More explicitly, the client should bring evidence from self-therapy that demonstrates clearly that he is entering different types of speaking situations and becoming descriptive about himself. Perhaps the best statement of the ultimate objective of this aspect of treatment is provided by Williams (1982):

> Our fundamental goal in therapy should be to help the stutterer learn problem solving; learn that what he does as he prepares to talk and as he talks affect his manner of speaking. This opens up alternatives for change. Studying the cause/effect relationship between what he wants to do and what he is doing will help him learn most importantly that there is cause and effect involved. Then, he is free to learn that he has a choice as to the way he talks. (p. 168)

The confrontation phase is concerned principally with (1) establishing a new cognitive set as a basis for change and for future self-reinforcement of change and (2) kindling the client's motivation to work in the face of adversity toward accomplishing realistic objectives. From Johnson's point of view, stutterers needed to gain new beliefs about their behavior and themselves through semantic reevaluation. It is interesting to compare Johnson's belief with Bandura's (1977a) summary concerning current approaches to cognitive behavior therapy: "It has now been amply documented that cognitive processes play a prominent role in the acquisition and retention of new behavior patterns. Transitory experiences leave lasting effects by being coded and retained in symbols for memory representation" (p. 192). Similarly, the ability to understand current events and to see and evaluate them in relation to goals and anticipated outcomes is a primary source of motivation. This idea is fundamental in cognitive behavior therapy (Bandura, 1977a), and the problem of establishing and revitalizing motivation in the adult stutterer is one of the keys to successful treatment (Van Riper, 1973, chap. 9).

Calming the stutterer and stuttering

The principal aim of this treatment component is to reduce the intensity of reactions *during* stuttering. The essence of the stutterer's objective is to be able to remain calm while stuttering in terms of internal "feelings" (i.e., negative emotion) and overt motor behavior. A diagram (Figure 19-1) helps to portray this concept.

Figure 19-1. *A.* Triggering mechanism for stuttering (e. g., a degree of phonatory mistiming) leading to the perception of fluency failure. *B.* Struggle reactions (e. g., increased muscular tension, sound/silence prolongations, rapid sound repetitions, tremor-type facial movements, other facial/bodily movements). Dotted line: Reduced stuttering intensity—both arousal and motor aspects.

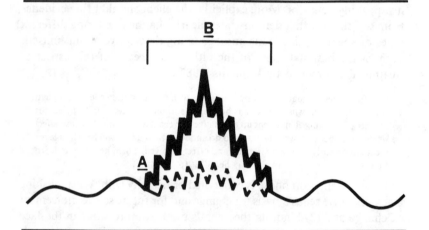

After the intensity of stuttering reactions is reduced, they can be replaced by responses that lead to fluent speech production. On the other hand, if the reactions are not deintensified, if they remain at the extremes exemplified by the dark lines in Figure 19-1, then it will be difficult, if not impossible, to replace them with new, nondefensive responses. To help understand this aspect of treatment, the stutterer may ask himself, "Can I get to the point where stuttering is dull, even boring?"

As a part of this treatment component, attention should also be directed toward giving up "expectancy" responses (devices such as vocalized pauses and word substitutions) and maintaining eye contact with the listener during stuttering. The challenge for the stutterer is to (1) seek out (rather than postpone or avoid) stuttering moments, and (2) face the listener, thereby experiencing the calming influence such behavior can have.

Van Riper (1973, 1974a), more than anyone else, has been responsible for conceiving the importance of this aspect of treatment and for developing procedures associated with it. It is not only the foundation for replacing stuttering reactions with new actions that lead to fluent speech, but, when accomplished effectively, it is one of the best insurance policies against post-therapy relapse.

Procedures and techniques. After the concept and rationale for this phase of treatment are discussed with the client, the clinician demonstrates extremes of stuttering episode intensity from high to low (in terms of motor behavior), while discussing also the extremes of internal arousal that may accompany these episodes. He asks the client to respond orally, and together they begin to rate the motor intensity of each moment of stuttering by signaling their perceptions of the episode's intensity from the stutterer's highest (5) to his lowest (1). The level of accompanying internal arousal is also signaled by the stutterer.[3]

The clinician emphasizes the importance of confronting the moments of stuttering—of not avoiding or postponing them—because they are the targets, the challenge. When the range (high to low) of emotional arousal and motor intensity during stuttering moments has been demonstrated and evaluated, the clinician explains the objective of reducing the high end of the range so that all (or nearly all) instances of stuttering fall at the low end in both arousal and motor intensity. Accompanied by the clinician's encouragement, reassurance, and explanations, the client practices signaling (with no verbal comment) the level of arousal and motor intensity that characterize each stuttering moment until there is a decided, consecutive pattern of low-level responses. This can be assured by the supportive responses of the clinician and, if necessary, simplifying verbal content to repeated one-word utterances. All of these activities serve to *demonstrate* the procedures and their rationale, the expected outcomes, and their potential for problem elimination.

The client should next be ready to *establish* new low-level stuttering reactions in a variety of carefully sequenced activities in which a success rate criterion is specified and the client moves forward by virtue of having met that criterion. In other words, techniques of behavior modification should be used at this point to help establish behavior change. Sequenced activities are selected for the individual by taking into account his sensitivity to the problem, its severity and variability. Appendix 19-1 provides a sample activity sequence that moves from one-word responses to printed sentences read orally, one-sentence answers and short answers to questions, and dialogue. For each activity a criterion response rate should be met (usually 80-90% of all stuttering episodes at the low-intensity range) and reinforced verbally by the clinician at a decreasing frequency rate.

Transfer of response change to other speaking circumstances is brought into therapy early. With the same success criterion, selected establishment activities are undertaken with other persons in the therapy room, in other building locations, in outside situations, and with the telephone. Initially, the clinician should be present during these activities. In those outside the building and with the telephone, the clinician should first demonstrate, in the actual activity, calm overt stuttering, with listener eye contact as appropriate. For the clinician, these situations are a challenge of similar magnitude to that required by the client. Both clinician and client should understand this, and the clinician should meet the success criterion, by both his own and the client's evaluation, before the client is asked to attempt the situations.

Self-therapy during this phase of treatment uses adaptations of the activities used during clinician/client treatment and transfer sessions. Essentially, self-therapy activities are part of a transfer program with the client assuming responsibility for collecting data on, and evaluating, his performance. Self-therapy may take place in clinic rooms designed for that purpose, as well as at home and in other outside situations. Video (when feasible) and audio tape recorders should be used to collect samples that are evaluated by the client to verify that success criteria have been met. The samples should be reviewed by the clinician and, periodically, by the client and clinician together at the outset of treatment sessions.

It will be evident from the client's progression through establishment and transfer activities that progress is being made. The time to move on to the next phase of treatment will vary with the individual client. Before moving forward, the client should have success in complex (dialogue) transfer activities. Some of the surest signs that a client is ready to move forward are successes in self-therapy activities; that is, clear evidence that episodes of stuttering are becoming a challenge rather than a threat and that they can be experienced consistently at low intensity levels. It is unrealistic this early in the program, however, to expect the stutterer to maintain criterion success rates in all types of speaking situations. In fact, there will usually be situations that are so difficult that this treatment component will continue in parallel with later phases. Ultimate success in remaining calm while stuttering may, therefore, be partially dependent on progress made in later treatment activities.

The importance of this component to the ultimate outcome of treatment is grounded in the hypothesis that undergirds the stuttering management approach: Stuttering episodes in the adult are habitual, defensive, self-protective reactions—triggered by certain physical events during speaking. Current models of treatment for behavior of this type recommend the reduction of internal arousal and of the strength of stimuli that signal it. Clinician modeling, tasks of sequential difficulty and aversiveness, joint clinician/client participation, client modeling and direct encounters, and cognitive appraisal of these activities and their effects are all basic ingredients in the successful management of defensive reactions (Bandura, 1977a). Bandura's summary statement is instructive in this regard:

> Individuals who come to believe that they are less vulnerable than they previously assumed are less prone to generate frightening thoughts in threatening situations. Those whose fears are relatively weak may reduce their self-doubts and debilitating self-arousal to the point where they perform successfully. (p. 200)

Replacing stuttering reactions with actions that produce fluent speech

The stutterer's ultimate objective is to respond with new responses (that result in fluent production of the syllable or word) to stimuli that formerly triggered anticipatory struggle reactions. A somewhat removed, but applicable, analogy captures the objective of this and preceding phases of treatment: A professional driver had just driven his car through a disastrous multiple-car accident on the track ahead of him and was asked how he could possibly have done it without hitting other vehicles and people. His response was that he stayed acutely sensitive to the physical details of driving the car; the elements of what he was doing and of what needed to be done to move the vehicle forward through the flames, wrecked cars, and injured drivers. He further explained that a novice could not have done it, for he would have flinched, tensed up, jerked the wheel, hit the brake, or otherwise reacted so as to assure further disaster. The driver was essentially explaining how, in an emergency, he could replace instinctive defensive reactions (ones that literally would have prevented him from driving the car) with specific purposeful actions. And so it is with the person who stutters. He must learn, when he perceives the now-weakened signal for old emergency reactions, to attend to and respond with the physical gestures needed to produce fluent speech. An addition to the earlier diagram (Figure 19-2) will help illustrate this point.

The principles and procedures of this treatment component have evolved primarily from the contributions of Van Riper, although Bryngelson's (1935) "voluntary stuttering" technique was the forerunner. In a landmark chapter on symptomatic therapy Van Riper (1957) described the basic techniques for this aspect of treatment and supported each from the viewpoint of learning theory and psychotherapeutic principles. He recommended a three-stage sequence for implementing the replacement response depicted in Figure 19-2: (1) *after* the stuttering

Figure 19-2. *A*. Triggering mechanism for stuttering. B. Struggle reactions. Dotted line: Reduced stuttering intensity. Dark arrow: New responses that replace the residual stuttering reaction.

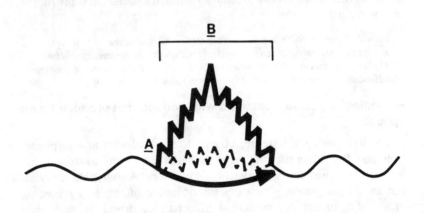

instance has been completed, the stutterer stops and reproduces the stuttered word/syllable using the new response (cancellation); (2) the new response is implemented *during* the old stuttering reaction (pullout); and (3) the new response is implemented just *before* the old stuttering reaction (preparatory set). Van Riper did not specify a detailed sequential program of reinforcement strategies for these procedures. Rather, he implemented them, and other therapeutic techniques, in a highly individualistic way, using his own unique insights and personality as a clinician and his perceptions of the client's strengths, weaknesses, and needs (see Van Riper, Therapy in Action, undated). Nonetheless, according to Franks' (1969) definition, Van Riper (1939, p. 374–392; 1957) had pioneered the development of a behavior therapy for replacing stuttering reactions:

> If behavior is defined in terms of response, the behavior therapy becomes a matter of response modification involving the application of some S(timulus) R(esponse) type of learning theory. More explicitly, behavior therapy may then be defined as the beneficial modification of behavior in accordance with experimentally validated principles based upon SR concepts of learning and the biophysical properties of the organism. (Franks, 1969, p. 2)

Van Riper's mode of implementation was so highly individualistic, however, that it is often considered too technically casual to be embraced by many present-day behavior therapists.

Procedures and techniques. The procedural sequence suggested in this chapter specifies small step programming, achievement criteria as a basis for moving forward in treatment, and the use of reinforcement. Others have also suggested ways of superimposing such techniques on stuttering management approaches (Ryan, 1970; Shames, Egolf, & Rhodes, 1969; Shames, 1970). In fact, though seldom acknowledged or cited, Hahn (1943) described, very early in the game, a rather explicit "program" for stuttering's management.

The reader should also note that the procedures suggested here will depart from the "cancellation, pullout, preparatory set" sequence developed by Van Riper. In fact, when actions to replace stuttering are introduced, they are initiated at the point Van Riper referred to as preparatory set.

Before beginning to replace residual stuttering reactions, an intermediate level of accomplishment is important for the stutterer. He must be able, consistently, to detect moments of stuttering in ongoing speech. As a part of activities to establish his ability to do so, it is important also to give him experience in varying his responses during stuttering instances (Van Riper, 1973). The outline below illustrates a series of detection/variation activities.

Activity	Target Response	Success Criterion
1. Reading	*Clinician* signals stuttering instances	90% accuracy
2. Spontaneous Speech	*Clinician* signals stuttering instances	90% accuracy
3. Reading	*Client* signals stuttering instances	90% accuracy
4. Spontaneous Speech	*Client* signals stuttering instances	90% accuracy
5,6. Repeat 3 and 4	*Client* introduces variations into residual stuttering reactions	90% accuracy

The complexity of the reading and speaking activities varies with client and problem severity. If stuttering is frequent in reading and spontaneous speech, initial activities will probably be of single-sentence length or even shorter. The number of activity repetitions is adapted to the individual client. Note that the clinician is responsible at first for accurate detection of stuttering instances (Activities 1 and 2). The signaling device can be a counter of some kind and, if verification of accuracy is in question, one that emits a sound as it counts. After the clinician has achieved at least 90% accuracy in detecting stuttering instances during reading and speaking activities, it becomes the client's responsibility to achieve the same success criterion (Activities 3 and 4). In order to do so, he must be able to identify and count each instance of stuttering as it happens. After establishing this ability reliably during spontaneous speech, the client should be given some opportunities to vary his actions during stuttering instances (Activities 5 and 6). The kinds of variations will depend upon the individual. They can include slowing and speeding up sound repetition patterns, changing volume, and so on. Usually, a prescribed success criterion is not used for variation activities. Their purpose, following successful establishment of detection ability, is to allow the stutterer to demonstrate to himself that he can begin voluntarily to change his responses during stuttering; that he is ready to move forward to replace what remains of old stuttering reactions.

Three principal target activities are used in sequence to establish a replacement response: (1) preselected single words; (2) nonstuttered words in contextual speech; (3) stuttered words in contextual speech. The nature of the response itself may be adapted to the individual stutterer; however, certain rules of thumb concerning its characteristics follow principles of motor learning and are important for client motivation and cognitive set (Marteniuk, 1976).

The replacement response should be:
  Directed toward normal actions required to utter a syllable/word;
  More appealing than stuttering reactions;
  Specific, composed of clearly identifiable elements;
  Simple;
  Used to move forward, not to postpone or avoid;
  Clearly contrastive to stuttering reactions *and* to what the client would
    have done had he simply uttered the syllable/word without stuttering.

Using these as a guide, the basic actions of the replacement response are:
  Assume the appropriate articulatory posture for the intended sound of the
    syllable/word;
  Sustain the sound (or vowel following a stop consonant) briefly;
  Make an exaggerated movement and transition to the subsequent sound;
  Complete the transition and the syllable smoothly without using any
    struggle reactions.

This response will be used by the stutterer when he perceives physical signals during speech that formerly triggered stuttering reactions.

The audible effect of the response just described is a brief sound prolongation (somewhat under 1 sec) that blends deliberately and noticeably with the following sound. The physical actions usually feel, and their outcomes sound, awkward to the stutterer at first, and likewise to the clinician as he performs them for the first time. Consequently, it is important that the clinician practice this response until he can do it smoothly and effortlessly in ongoing speech, so that the response does not interrupt movement continuity or the prosodic features of speech. Considerable practice is required in order that appropriate modeling can be done for the client. As with any new motor actions that are to become part of patterned movements, elements of the response will at first be done slowly and with concentrated attention and effort. However, it must be demonstrated and understood from the outset that with practice the response can become smooth, effortless, and automatic. Analogies from sport skills instruction are pertinent: e.g., learning to make christy turns in skiing and learning to pivot in basketball. In each case, the actions are taught in discrete, sequential steps that, done slowly and awkwardly at first, eventually become smooth automatic movement patterns.

Appendix 19-2 illustrates an activity program for demonstrating and establishing a stuttering replacement response. As in other phases of treatment, the number of successful repetitions of an activity before moving forward should be adapted individually to each client. Verbal reinforcement of successful responses during demonstration and establishment activities should be planned in terms of frequency and content. In addition to praise and encouragement, the rationale of a procedure should be repeated periodically as a part of reinforcement.

The need to use a replacement response on non-stuttered words requires special emphasis. By doing this, a client establishes his ability to change in a non-emergency circumstance. He practices the response so as to make it nearly automatic, loses his sensitivity to the feeling and sound of the response and to the anticipation of listeners' reactions, and establishes an active, rather than a passive, mode of responding during speech. These changes are necessary if the client is to be able to use the new response effectively to replace residual stuttering reactions. The replacement response must become so automatic that it can be invoked instantly, with little or no conscious attention, whenever physical triggers for stuttering reactions are perceived. The use of the new response on an established percentage of nonstuttered words in contextual speech will help to assure that this is possible.

Transfer and self-therapy activities follow those used in clinician/client sessions, with specific target responses, success criteria, and the use of recording equipment for evaluation and verification. Landmarks of successful achievement for this phase of treatment are associated with criteria for terminating therapy which will be considered under the Special Concerns section of this chapter.

In order to replace defensive reactions, the signals that trigger them must lose as much of their aversive character as possible, and the more successful alternative responses to these signals must be reinforced (Bandura, 1969, chap. 6). The replacement response procedures just described are designed to help accomplish these objectives. Bandura (1977a) describes this approach to eliminating defensive behavior as follows:

> The participant modeling approach to the elimination of defensive behavior utilizes successful performance as the primary vehicle of psychological change. . . . In implementing participant modeling, therapists therefore structure the environment so that clients can perform successfully despite their incapacities. This is achieved by enlisting a variety of response induction aids, including preliminary modeling of threatening activities, graduated tasks, enactment over graduated temporal intervals, joint performance with the therapist, protective aids to reduce the likelihood of feared consequences, and variation in the severity of the threat itself. As treatment progresses, the supplementary aids are withdrawn so that clients cope effectively unassisted. Self-directed mastery experiences are then arranged to reinforce a sense of personal efficacy. (p. 196-197)

Van Riper (1973) added a stabilization phase to his stuttering management program. Although it will not be described in this chapter, its focus is on procedures to sustain changes made in earlier phases and to produce a more naturally fluent overall speech pattern. The techniques associated with this aspect of treatment are more akin to those used for "managing fluency" than those used for "managing stuttering," per se. Moreover, they have not been highly developed as features of stuttering management programs. Readers may wish to become familiar with these procedures by reading Van Riper (1970b, 1973).

Special concerns

Therapeutic groups. Whenever possible, therapeutic groups should be an integral part of a stuttering management program. Van Riper (1957, 1973) and Sheehan (1970) have particularly emphasized the importance of group work and the kinds of activities that may be undertaken. Group structure and functions vary with the specific nature of the program and the beliefs and competencies of the clinician. A major purpose of group therapy, in a program for managing stuttering, is the provision of so-called "vicarious experience. " By observing others perform successfully in threatening activities, the stutterer adds importantly to his self-efficacy expectations and thereby to his motivation to persist in the difficult tasks of therapy and to successfully achieve its hoped-for outcomes (Bandura, 1977a). Later in such programs, groups also provide a controlled transfer situation in which new responses are positively reinforced by group recognition and approval.

Self-therapy. Successful treatment outcomes depend greatly on the effectiveness of the self-therapy program. It begins at the outset of treatment and provides the framework for self-reinforcement and for the client's active participation in challenging experiences. After clinician/client treatment has been terminated, self-therapy is the foundation for helping offset regression to former defensive behavior patterns (Bandura, 1969, 1977a).

Self-therapy should be as thoroughly planned as the activities that take place during clinician/client sessions. Whenever possible, self-therapy should be undertaken in clinical laboratory rooms set up for that purpose as well as in situations outside the clinic. Audio and (in the clinic) video recorders should be available to provide samples for evaluation and verification. Clinician/client sessions should be matched in participation time by client self-therapy. The activities selected should be mutually agreed upon and should be adaptations of those modeled and/or performed successfully during sessions with the clinician. Activities should have clearly identified target responses and success criteria. In-clinic self-therapy should generally precede self-therapy activities outside the clinic. All activities should be self-motivating, challenging, and achievement oriented and should yield data that can be reported and evaluated. Treatment failure is virtually assured unless self-therapy is practiced effectively.

Termination and outcome. The questions of when and how to terminate the clinician/client therapy program have never had definitive answers. In reference to *when* to terminate treatment, programs that "manage stuttering" do not use the kind of numeric criteria that commonly are used for "fluency management" programs; for example, less than 2% stuttering frequency in most speaking situations. Rather, the decision to terminate a stuttering management program is based on the client's ability to respond effectively and confidently as a speaker. Criteria for reaching this decision include the following, which are similar to Van Riper's (1957):

> The client is speaking in most outside situations with little-to-no word or situation fears;
> Speech avoidances relative to words, situations, and people are reduced to zero;

The client responds fluently, that is, without tension and struggle, to cues that formerly triggered stuttering reactions;[4]

Speaking ability is no longer perceived as a barrier to communication;

The client is comfortable about and confident in his speaking ability.

The matter of *how* to terminate direct therapy is presumed to be very important in offsetting stuttering's persistent tendency, in adults, to recur after treatment. Boberg, Howie, and Woods (1979) have presented an interesting review of this literature. The gradual phasing out of clinician/client treatment sessions, clients assuming more and more responsibility for stabilizing behavior change, active self-therapy programs with verifiable reporting, and clients' cognitive awareness of the nature of the problem and recovery process, appear to be important factors in helping to offset post-treatment relapse.

Assessment of ultimate treatment outcome for the adult and older child who stutter is a difficult process, and to date it has not been done satisfactorily (Ingham, 1981). Using criteria of the type described above, Van Riper (1957) reported anecdotal accounts of group therapy outcomes over a 20-year period. Using similar criteria, Prins collected questionnaire data (1970, 1974) and tape-recorded follow-up samples (1976) to describe client post-treatment improvement and regression. Gregory (1969, 1972) and others (see Table 19-1) have also assessed post-treatment status of clients following a stuttering management program. These and other follow-up accounts of treatment outcomes, whether for stuttering management or fluency management programs, contain multiple sources of error including, but not limited to, the outcome criteria used, sampling and measurement procedures, and experimenter bias. In general, the sum total of outcome studies provides evidence that (1) treatment programs of the type described above, and of other types as well, have substantial positive effects on the speaking ability and personal adjustment of individuals who stutter; and (2) post-treatment regression of speaking performance is a common problem. Andrews, Guitar, and Howie (1980) state a similar opinion, noting, however, that "relapse over time is slow" (p. 305).

Within the embrace of these statements concerning outcome, stand the individual stutterers. Many have been greatly helped by what appear to be substantially different types of programs. Others have experienced little-to-no permanent success in spite of repeated participation in programs of different types. It is possible that these wide variations result from the accident of client–program mismatches, but this is doubtful. A more plausible explanation is that stuttering, after being an integral part of a person's speaking behavior for 10 or more years, is complexly woven into the unique fabric of the individual's physical and mental abilities, personal characteristics, and needs. This makes the problem extraordinarily difficult for the person who stutters, and for the clinician, to resolve with assurance. There is no reason to believe that a preplanned program of treatment, no matter how carefully devised, will assure total, permanent success for all, or nearly all, participants. There is every reason to believe, however, that a thoughtful program of treatment, based on a thorough understanding of human behavior, and adapted intelligently to the needs of an individual client and the talents of the clinician, has a very good chance of helping many adults who stutter to resolve their speaking difficulties.

APPENDIX 19-1. Calming the Stutterer and Stuttering

Sample case: Severe stutterer with stuttering instances that occur repeatedly on one-word responses.

Demonstration

Clinician explains concept and rationale.
Clinician illustrates, using client's pattern, two extremes of stuttering moments.
    Score the severe: a 5 in motor intensity level.
    Score the mild: a 1 in motor intensity level.
    Describe and discuss the levels of motor intensity and of emotional arousal.
    Illustrate again, and have the stutterer practice scoring the levels.
Ask the client questions with one-word responses—Both client and clinician rate the
    severity of struggle/arousal intensity: 5, most intense; 1, least intense. (Focus
    chiefly on arousal and observe how motor intensity usually follows.)
Illustrate by stuttering adaptation the difference between high and low intensity.
Practice on a series of one-word ratings until both clinician and client feel com-
    fortable with the activity and the client can respond more-or-less routinely at
    a 1–2 level in both motor and arousal intensity. (Use mirror for feedback as
    appropriate.)

Establishment

Activity*	Reinforcement
1. One-word responses to questions.[a]	Verbal w/explanation
2. Printed sentences read orally.	"
3. Sentence responses to questions.	End of activity
4. Short answers to questions/topics.	"
5. Sustained dialogue.	"

Transfer

Activity*	Reinforcement
1. 1 above w/outside person.[a]	End of activity
2.–4. Activities (3-5) above w/ a) outside person/ b) in various building locations.	"
5. Store dialogue (demonstrate 1st).	"
6. Phone situations (demonstrate 1st).	"

Self-Therapy

Activity	Reinforcement
1. Make up hierarchy of situations.	
2. Rate severity range in selected situations.	
3. Controlled conversations.[a]	Record/Evaluate
4. Telephone hierarchy.	"
5. Other ranked situations.	"

* The number of activity repetitions is adapted to the individual client.
[a] Criteria are 80–90% at about the 1–2 level.

APPENDIX 19-2. Stuttering Replacement Response

Demonstration

Explain concept and rationale for replacement of stuttering.

Explain and demonstrate elements of the replacement response.

Model the response on a selected group of words that are printed on cards.

Have client practice the response on the selected words until both clinician and client are satisfied that the response, although somewhat awkwardly produced, contains the component elements.

Discuss moving on to the level of establishment where success will depend on a 90% rate of correct use of the replacement response in relation to each use opportunity.

To illustrate the goal, model use of replacement response on 10–20% of words in contextual speech.

Establishment

Replacement Response

Task	Activity[a]	Target Response
Preselected single words:	Words read aloud from cards.	Response on each word.
	Sentences with single underlined words, read aloud from cards.	Response only on underlined words.
Nonstuttered words in contextual speech:*	Sentences with multiple underlined words, read aloud from cards.	Response only on underlined words.
	Sentences without underlined words, read aloud from cards.	Response on nonstuttered words at an established frequency rate (±20%).*
	Paragraphs without underlined words, read aloud from cards.	"
	Short answers to questions.	"
	Dialogue.	"
Nonstuttered and stuttered words in contextual speech:	Sentences read aloud from cards.	Response on nonstuttered words at established rate (10–20%) of words spoken, *and* on all stuttered words.**
	Paragraphs read aloud from cards.	"
	Short answers to questions.	"
	Dialogue.	"

* At this level, the replacement response is not expected on stuttered words.
** At this level, the client continues the established rate of replacement response use on nonstuttered words, but also uses the response on stuttered words as well.
a Criterion of success is 90% of all instances for each activity.

NOTES

[1] This description of stuttering as an inhibitory, avoidance reaction during speech is clearly the forerunner of Sheehan's application of approach/avoidance conflict theory to stuttering (Sheehan, 1953).

[2] It should be pointed out that many contemporary theorists and clinicians would disagree with Williams on this point, and argue that some degree of "tensing" and "blocking" (that serves to interrupt fluency) occurs in stutterers as a result of involuntary, reflexive reactions. Even if true, however, that would not invalidate Williams' approach for most of the behavioral components of the stuttering reaction.

[3] A useful mechanism for signaling is simply to raise the appropriate number of fingers on one hand. Later, during establishment activities (when no verbal comments are needed), this method of rating is particularly effective.

[4] Van Riper (1957), it should be noted, stated a rather demanding fluency goal: "First of all, the stutterer must be speaking better than this author in all situations" (p. 390).

REFERENCES

Andrews, G., Guitar, B., & Howie, P. Meta-analysis of stuttering treatment outcome studies. *Journal of Speech and Hearing Disorders,* 1980, *45,* 287–307.

Bandura, A. *Principles of behavior modification.* New York: Holt, Rinehart & Winston, 1969.

Bandura, A. Self-efficacy: Toward a unifying theory of behavioral change. *Psychological Review,* 1977, *84,* 191–215(a).

Bandura, A. *Social learning theory.* Englewood Cliffs, NJ: Prentice–Hall, 1977. (b)

Berwick, N. Stuttering in response to photographs of selected listeners. In W. Johnson & R. Leutenegger (Eds.), *Stuttering in children and adults.* Minneapolis: University of Minnesota Press, 1955.

Bloodstein, O. Stuttering as tension and fragmentation. In J. Eisenson (Ed.), *Stuttering, a second symposium.* New York: Harper & Row, 1975.

Bloodstein, O. *A handbook on stuttering.* Chicago: National Easter Seal Society, 1981.

Boberg, E. Intensive group therapy program for stutterers. *Human Communication,* 1976, *1,* 29–41.

Boberg, E., Howie, P., & Woods, L. Maintenance of fluency: A review. *Journal of Fluency Disorders,* 1979, *4,* 93–117.

Bryngelson, B. A method of stuttering. *Journal of Abnormal Psychology,* 1935, *30,* 194–198.

Chotolas, J. Covariation in frequency of types of stuttering reactions. In W. Johnson & R. Leutenegger (Eds.), *Stuttering in children and adults.* Minneapolis: University of Minnesota Press, 1955.

Connett, M. Experimentally induced changes in the relative frequency of stuttering on a specified speech sound. In W. Johnson & R. Leutenegger (Eds.), *Stuttering in children and adults.* Minneapolis: University of Minnesota Press, 1955.

Dixon, E. Stuttering adaptation in relation to assumed level of anxiety. In W. Johnson & R. Leutenegger (Eds.), *Stuttering in children and adults.* Minneapolis: University of Minnesota Press, 1955.

Donohue, I. Stuttering adaptation during three hours of continuous oral reading. In W. Johnson & R. Leutenegger (Eds.), *Stuttering in children and adults.* Minneapolis: University of Minnesota Press, 1955.

Downton, W. The effect of instructions concerning mode of stuttering on the breathing of stutterers. In W. Johnson & R. Leutenegger (Eds.), *Stuttering in children and adults.* Minneapolis: University of Minnesota Press, 1955.

Franks, C. (Ed.), *Behavior therapy: Appraisal and status.* New York: McGraw–Hill, 1969.

Frick, J. *Evaluation of motor planning techniques for the treatment of stuttering.* Unpublished report, Pennsylvania State University, Speech and Hearing Clinic, 1965.

Gregory, H. Applications of learning theory concepts in the management of stuttering. In H. Gregory (Ed.), *Learning theory and stuttering therapy.* Evanston, IL: Northwestern University Press, 1968.

Gregory, H. An assessment of the results of stuttering therapy. Final report, SRS Project 1725-S. Evanston, IL: Department of Communicative Disorders, Northwestern University, 1969.

Gregory, H. An assessment of the results of stuttering therapy. *Journal of Communication Disorders,* 1972, *5,* 320–334.

Gregory, H. Controversial issues: Statement and review of the literature. In H. Gregory (Ed.), *Controversies about stuttering therapy.* Baltimore: University Park Press, 1979.

Hahn, E. Procedures in a clinic for stutterers. *Stuttering: Significant theories and therapies.* Stanford, CA: Stanford University Press, 1943.

Ingham, R. Evaluation and maintenance in stuttering treatment: A search for ecstasy with nothing but agony. In E. Boberg (Ed.), *Maintenance of fluency.* New York: Elsevier/North Holland, 1981.

Johnson, W. A course of treatment for stutterers. In H. Koepp-Baker (Ed.), *Handbook of clinical speech.* Ann Arbor, MI: Edwards, 1936. (a)

Johnson, W. Stuttering: Research findings and their therapeutic implications. *Journal of the Iowa Medical Society,* 1936, *26,* 464–469. (b)

Johnson, W. A systematic approach to the psychology of stuttering. In W. Johnson & R. Leutenegger (Eds.), *Stuttering in children and adults.* Minneapolis: University of Minnesota Press, 1955. (a)

Johnson, W. The descriptive principle and the principle of static analysis. In W. Johnson & R. Leutenegger (Eds.), *Stuttering in children and adults.* Minneapolis: University of Minnesota Press, 1955. (b)

Johnson, W. The time, the place and the problem. In W. Johnson & R. Leutenegger (Eds.), *Stuttering in children and adults.* Minneapolis: University of Minnesota Press, 1955. (c)

Johnson, W. An interpretation of stuttering. *Quarterly Journal of Speech,* 1933, *19,* 70–77.

Johnson, W. The treatment of stuttering. *Journal of Speech Disorders,* 1939, *4,* 170–172.

Johnson, W., & Ainsworth, S. Studies in the psychology of stuttering: X. Constancy of loci of expectancy of stuttering. *Journal of Speech Disorders,* 1938, *3,* 101–104.

Johnson, W., & Brown, S. Stuttering in relation to various speech sounds. *Quarterly Journal of Speech,* 1935, *21,* 481–496.

Johnson, W., & Knott, J. Studies in the psychology of stuttering: I. The distribution of moments of stuttering in successive readings of the same material. *Journal of Speech Disorders,* 1937, *2,* 17–19. (a)

Johnson, W., & Knott, J. The moment of stuttering. *Journal of Genetic Psychology,* 1936, *48,* 473–479. (c)

Johnson, W., Larson, R. P., & Knott, J. Studies in the psychology of stuttering: III. Certain objective cues related to the precipitation of the moment of stuttering during oral reading. *Journal of Speech Disorders,* 1937, *2,* 23–25. (b)

Johnson, W., & Leutenegger, R. (Eds.) *Stuttering in children and adults.* Minneapolis: University of Minnesota Press, 1955.

Johnson, W., & Millsapps, L. Studies in the psychology of stuttering: VI. The role of cues representative of stuttering moments during oral reading. *Journal of Speech Disorders,* 1937, *2,* 101–104. (c)

Johnson, W., & Rosen, L. Studies in the psychology of stuttering: VII. Effect of certain changes in speech pattern upon frequency of stuttering. *Journal of Speech Disorders,* 1937, *2,* 105–109. (d)

Johnson, W., & Sinn, A. Studies in the psychology of stuttering: V. Frequency of stuttering with expectation of stuttering controlled. *Journal of Speech Disorders,* 1937, *2,* 98–100. (e)

Johnson, W., & Solomon, A. Studies in the psychology of stuttering: IV. A quantitative study of expectation of stuttering as a process involving a low degree of consciousness. *Journal of Speech Disorders,* 1937, *2,* 95–97. (f)

Johnson, W. *Speech handicapped school children.* New York: Harper, 1948.

Jones, E. Explorations of experimental extinction and spontaneous recovery in stuttering. In W. Johnson & R. Leutenegger (Eds.), *Stuttering in children and adults.* Minneapolis: University of Minnesota Press, 1955.

Luper, H. Consistency of stuttering in relation to the goal gradient hypothesis. *Journal of Speech and Hearing Disorders,* 1956, *21,* 336–342.

Marteniuk, R. *Information processing in motor skills.* New York: Holt, Rinehart & Winston, 1976.

Maxwell, D. Cognitive and behavioral self control strategies: Applications for the clinical management of adult stutterers, *Journal of Fluency Disorders,* 1982, *7,* 403–433.

Oxtoby, E. Frequency of stuttering in relation to induced modifications following expectancy of stuttering. In W. Johnson & R. Leutenegger (Eds.), *Stuttering in children and adults.* Minneapolis: University of Minnesota Press, 1955.

Prins, D. Improvement and regression in stutterers following short-term intensive therapy. *Journal of Speech and Hearing Disorders,* 1970, *32,* 123–135.

Prins, D., & Beaudet, R. Defense preference and stutterers' speech disfluencies: Implications for the nature of the disorder. *Journal of Speech and Hearing Research,* 1980, *23,* 757–768.

Prins, D., & Miller, M. Client impressions of the effectiveness of stuttering therapy—A comparison of two programs. *British Journal of Disorders of Communication,* 1974, *9,* 123–133.

Prins, D., & Nichols, A. Stutterers' perceptions of therapy improvement and of post-therapy regression: Effects of certain program modifications. *Journal of Speech and Hearing Disorders,* 1976, *41,* 452–464.

Ryan, B. An illustration of operant conditioning therapy for stuttering. In *Conditioning in stuttering therapy.* Memphis, TN: Speech Foundation of America, 1970.

Shames, G. Operant conditioning and therapy for stuttering. In *Conditioning in stuttering therapy.* Memphis, TN: Speech Foundation of America, 1970.

Shames, G., & Egolf, D. Evaluation and therapy for adults. In G. Shames & D. Egolf (Eds.), *Operant conditioning and the management of stuttering.* Englewood Cliffs, NJ: Prentice–Hall, 1976.

Shames, G., Egolf, D., & Rhodes, R. Experimental programs in stuttering therapy. *Journal of Speech and Hearing Disorders,* 1969, *34,* 30–47.

Sheehan, J. Conflict theory and avoidance-reduction therapy. In J. Eisenson (Ed.), *Stuttering: A second symposium.* New York: Harper & Row, 1975.

Sheehan, J. Current issues on stuttering and recovery. In H. Gregory (Ed.), *Controversies about stuttering therapy.* Baltimore: University Park Press, 1979.

Sheehan, J. Modification of stuttering through non reinforcement. *Journal of Abnormal Psychology,* 1951, *46,* 51–63.

Sheehan, J. Theory and treatment of stuttering as an approach avoidance conflict. *Journal of Psychology,* 1953, *36,* 27–49.

Sheehan, J. An interpretation of psychotherapy and speech therapy through a conflict theory of stuttering. *Journal of Speech and Hearing Disorders,* 1954, *19,* 474–482. (a)

Sheehan, J. Stuttering as conflict: Comparison of therapy techniques involving approach and avoidance. *Journal of Speech and Hearing Disorders,* 1957, *22,* 714–723.

Sheehan, J. *Stuttering: Research and therapy:* New York: Harper & Row, 1970.

Sheehan, J., Cortese, P., & Hadley, R. Guilt, shame, and tension in graphic projection of stuttering. *Journal of Speech and Hearing Disorders,* 1962, *27,* 129–139.

Sheehan, J., Hadley, R., & Gould, E. Impact of authority on stuttering. *Journal of Abnormal Psychology,* 1967, *72,* 290–293.

Sheehan, J., & Voas, R. Tension patterns during stuttering in relation to conflict, anxiety-binding, and reinforcement. *Speech Monographs,* 1954, *21,* 272–279. (b)

Shulman, E. Factors influencing the variability of stuttering. In W. Johnson & R. Leutenegger (Eds.), *Stuttering in children and adults.* Minneapolis: University of Minnesota Press, 1955.

Starkweather, W. A behavioral analysis of Van Riperian therapy for stuttering. *Journal of Communication Disorders,* 1973, *6,* 273–291.

Steer, M., & Johnson, W. An objective study of the relationship between psychological factors and the severity of stuttering. *Journal of Abnormal and Social Psychology,* 1936, *31,* 36–46.

Tanberg, M. A study of the role of inhibition in the moment of stuttering. In W. Johnson & R. Leutenegger (Eds.), *Stuttering in children and adults.* Minneapolis: University of Minnesota Press, 1955.

Van Riper, C. The *Ablauf* problem in stuttering. *Journal of Fluency Disorders,* 1974, *1,* 2–10. (c)

Van Riper, C. The effect of penalty upon the frequency of stuttering. *Journal of Genetic Psychology,* 1937, *50,* 193–195. (a)

Van Riper, C. The effects of devices for minimizing stuttering on the creation of symptoms. *Journal of Abnormal and Social Psychology,* 1937, *32,* 185–192. (b)

Van Riper, C. Experiments in stuttering therapy. In J. Eisenson (Ed.), *Stuttering, a symposium.* New York: Harper & Row, 1958.

Van Riper, C. The growth of the stuttering spasm. *Quarterly Journal of Speech,* 1937, *23,* 70–73. (c)

Van Riper, C. Historical approaches. In J. Sheehan (Ed.), *Stuttering: Research and therapy.* New York: Harper & Row, 1970. (a)

Van Riper, C. The influence of empathic response on frequency of stuttering. *Psychological Monographs,* 1937, *49,* 244–246. (d)

Van Riper, C. Identification; desensitization: the reduction of negative emotion; modification; stabilization. In C. Van Riper, *The treatment of stuttering.* Englewood Cliffs, NJ: Prentice-Hall, 1973.

Van Riper, C. Modification of behavior. In *Therapy for stutterers.* Memphis, TN: Speech Foundation of America, 1974. (a)

Van Riper, C. The preparatory set in stuttering. *Journal of Speech Disorders,* 1937, *2,* 149–154. (e)

Van Riper, C. *Speech correction.* New York: Prentice-Hall, 1939.

Van Riper, C. A study of thoracic breathing of stutterers during expectancy and occurrence of stuttering spasms. *Journal of Speech Disorders,* 1936, *1,* 61–72.

Van Riper, C. Stuttering: Where and whither. *Asha,* 1974, *16,* 483–487. (b)

Van Riper, C. A study of the stutterer's ability to interrupt the stuttering spasm. *Journal of Speech Disorders,* 1938, *3,* 117–119.

Van Riper, C. Symptomatic therapy for stuttering. In L. Travis (Ed.), *Handbook of speech pathology.* New York: Appleton–Century–Crofts, 1957.

Van Riper, C. Symptomatic therapy for stuttering. In L. Travis (Ed.), *Handbook of speech pathology and audiology.* Englewood Cliffs, NJ: Prentice–Hall, 1971.

Van Riper, C. *Therapy in action* (8 video tapes). Memphis, TN: Speech Foundation of America, undated.

Van Riper, C. The use of DAF in stuttering therapy. *British Journal of Disorders of Communication,* 1970, *5,* 40–45. (b)

Van Riper, C., & Hull, C. The quantitative measurement of the effect of certain situations on stuttering. In W. Johnson & R. Leutenegger (Eds.), *Stuttering in children and adults.* Minneapolis: University of Minnesota Press, 1955.

Williams, D. A perspective on approaches to stuttering therapy. In H. Gregory (Ed.), *Controversies about stuttering therapy.* Baltimore: University Park Press, 1979.

Williams, D. A point of view about "stuttering." *Journal of Speech and Hearing Disorders,* 1957, *22,* 390–397.

Williams, D. Stuttering therapy: An overview. In H. Gregory (Ed.), *Learning theory and stuttering therapy.* Evanston, IL: Northwestern University Press, 1968.

Williams, D. Stuttering therapy: Where are we going and why? *Journal of Fluency Disorders,* 1982, *7,* 159–170.

Wingate, M. Expectancy as basically a short-term process. *Journal of Speech and Hearing Research,* 1975, *18,* 31–42.

Wingate, M. Stuttering adaptation and learning. I. The relevance of adaptation studies to stuttering as learned behavior. *Journal of Speech and Hearing Disorders,* 1966, *31,* 148–156. (a)

Wingate, M. Stuttering adaptation and learning. II. The adequacy of learning principles in the interpretation of stuttering. *Journal of Speech and Hearing Disorders,* 1966, *31,* 211–218. (b)

Wischner, G. An experimental approach to expectancy and anxiety in stuttering behavior. *Journal of Speech and Hearing Disorders,* 1952, *17,* 139–154. (a)

Wischner, G. Anxiety-reduction as reinforcement in maladaptive behavior: Evidence in stutterers' representations of the moment of difficulty. *Journal of Abnormal and Social Psychology,* 1952, *47,* 566–571. (b)

Wischner, G. An experimental approach to stuttering as learned behavior. *American Psychologist,* 1948, *3,* 278–279.

Wischner, G. Stuttering behavior and learning: A preliminary theoretical formulation. *Journal of Speech and Hearing Disorders,* 1950, *15,* 324–335.

Chapter 20

Treatment of Adult Stutterers: Managing Fluency

Pauline Howie and Gavin Andrews

Recent developments in the treatment of stuttering have involved a shift from earlier therapeutic emphases in which clinicians aimed to modify the form of clients' stuttering and to minimize its disruptive effects—what Gregory (1979) calls the "stutter more fluently" approach. This traditional approach contrasts markedly with the "speak more fluently" approaches. These newer therapies focus on what traditional therapies might regard as the impossible aim of eliminating stuttering by training the client in speaking techniques that are incompatible with stuttering and that should, therefore, ensure continued fluency. The techniques used often involve distortion of some aspect of speech or some interference with the speech process. But it is assumed that once fluency is established, in however distorted a form, it can be shaped to approximate normal sounding speech. In a recent metanalysis of stuttering treatments for which outcome data are available in the literature (Andrews, Guitar, & Howie, 1980), some of these fluency management therapies emerged as extremely effective, in both the short- and long-term gains they offered to stutterers. It is with these kinds of therapies and their application in the treatment of adult stutterers that this chapter is concerned.

The first part of this chapter describes various fluency management treatment programs: those using prolonged speech with or without the use of delayed auditory feedback as espoused by ourselves and by Perkins, Ingham, or Ryan; the closely related precision fluency shaping technique of Webster; Brady's application of rhythmic speech; the airflow techniques associated with Azrin and Nunn and with Schwartz, and finally Lanyon's use of EMG-controlled relaxation. We have not dealt with any treatments, however promising, for which no objective outcome data are available.

The training techniques used in fluency management therapies generally spring from behavioral psychology and fulfil many of the criteria of behavior therapy: The target behaviors of therapy are usually specified and measurable, the procedures explicit and replicable, the results of therapy are evaluated, and many of the specifics of treatment have been developed on an empirical basis. The treatments typically involve a similar framework: Fluency is instated in some exaggerated or distorted form, then is shaped until it sounds essentially normal, and finally generalized to situations which are less and less under clinic control. Structured maintenance programs are also common.

We shall see that many of these techniques produce comparable results: Stuttering is virtually eliminated in the short term, and the average client is able to speak at normal rates and not be handicapped by his stutter in the long term. Some of the apparently less effective techniques might prove to be as effective if they were applied with the intensity, duration, and structure that is characteristic of the more successful therapies.

The quality of outcome evaluation for the fluency management therapies is uneven. As one of us has argued elsewhere (Andrews, in press), there are certain minimal requirements of a stuttering treatment outcome evaluation study. They are first, the inclusion of reliable measures of stuttering frequency, speech rate, and extent of handicap (avoidance of speech and negative self concept). Second, these measures should be taken at first contact, immediately before and after fluency instatement, after generalization, and 3, 6, and 9 months after completion of treatment (defined as the point of maximal improvement). Not all of the fluency management outcome studies fulfil these requirements which may misrepresent the success of a particular program. Therefore, we provide cautions where necessary. In addition, to facilitate comparison between treatments, we use conversion formulas provided by Ryan (1981) to standardize all stuttering frequency measures to percent stuttered syllables (% SS) and all speech rate measures to syllables per minute (SPM).

The second part of this chapter deals with the problems of critically evaluating fluency management treatments in order to select the most effective procedures. We review the various sources of research evidence and the results of our metanalysis of the stuttering treatment literature. We outline those issues that still need to be resolved before we can identify what aspects of these treatments are primarily responsible for their efficacy: The importance of intensive versus spaced treatment, of individual versus group treatment, of highly structured generalization procedures, of attitude modification, and of self-evaluation training. We will not discuss transfer and maintenance issues in detail since these are dealt with in chapter 21.

PROLONGED SPEECH TECHNIQUES

In this section we describe a group of related treatment programs which have developed over the last 10 to 15 years and which have reported dramatic improvements in stutterers' speech, both in the short and long term. In most cases, the originators of the technique have taken care to evaluate objectively the outcome of their treatments; therefore, we have evidence of their effectiveness.

There are two hallmarks of the prolonged speech therapies: The unique speech skills which they train and the specific training procedures which they use. The prolonged speech procedures involve the instatement, shaping, generalization, and maintenance of fluent, prolonged speech. The speech skill—prolonged speech—originally referred to the slowing of speech by prolonging vowels, a pattern which usually occurs during artificially delayed auditory feedback of speech (DAF) at about a quarter of a second delay. However, over the years, the term prolonged speech has embraced various combinations of gentle onsets of words, soft articulatory contacts, smooth transitions between sounds, and exaggerated continuity of speech.

In the early 60s, Goldiamond, a behavioral psychologist, had discovered that under DAF some stutterers spontaneously used a prolonged style of speech in order to counteract the disruptive effects of DAF. This had the unexpected effect of reducing stuttering, and Goldiamond began to use DAF-induced prolonged speech as a direct means of inducing a slow prolonged speech pattern that was incompatible with stuttering (Goldiamond, 1965).

Curlee and Perkins: Conversational rate control therapy and breathstream management therapy

Curlee and Perkins (1969, 1973) saw the potential of Goldiamond's findings and developed the approach further in their conversational rate control therapy. They took advantage of the fact that the duration of auditory feedback delay determines the rate of the resulting speech. This made it possible to use DAF to elicit slow prolonged speech, and then gradually increase stutterers' speech rate to normal by stepwise decreases in feedback delay, while requiring clients to demonstrate zero stuttering at each step. Once the delay was eliminated, the client gradually extended his new, fluent speech pattern into the real world in increasingly demanding situations.

Data reported by Curlee and Perkins (1973) showed dramatic reductions in stuttering frequency when measured overtly outside the clinic immediately after treatment: The mean stuttering frequency decreased from 16% SS before treatment to 1.3% SS immediately after. But the authors suspected that clients' unrecorded speech was less fluent than the recorded samples suggested. Furthermore, the authors noted that the speech of their treated clients often sounded abnormally slow and monotonous. This led to the development of the breathstream management techniques currently used by Perkins and his colleagues (Perkins, 1973; Perkins, in press). This treatment retains the original rate control procedures, but emphasizes, in addition, the achievement of normal sounding speech, via the management of breathstream, phrasing, and prosody.

Perkins' broadened approach did seem to produce improved long-term results, both in terms of a greater reduction in stuttering frequency and more normal speech rates (Perkins, Rudas, Johnson, Michael, & Curlee, 1974). But the determination of Perkins and his colleagues to grapple with the rather elusive quality of normal prosody meant that they had to depart somewhat from strict, behavioral criteria for progression through their program. The treatment as it now stands involves the consecutive acquisition of seven skills (slow rate, phrasing, easy voice onset, soft contacts, breathy voice, blended words, and normal stress), with mastery of each required before progression to the next is permitted. But the mastery of these skills is largely based on subjective judgments which, Perkins argues, are best made by the clinician (Perkins, 1981). This underlines one of the problems of behavioral therapies: The conflict between which behaviors require treatment and which are amenable to objective measurement and, therefore, systematic modification.

Andrews and Ingham: Intensive token economy therapy

In Australia in 1970, Ingham and Andrews, who at that time were conducting a highly structured, token reinforced rhythmic speech program, learned of DAF-induced prolonged speech and substituted it for rhythmic speech in their program (Ingham & Andrews, 1973a, 1973b). As in the Curlee and Perkins procedures, this program instated prolonged speech at slow rates using DAF, although like Perkins, the Australians found that instruction and modeling of prolonged speech were as effective as DAF. Speech was then gradually shaped to normal rates in structured group conversations. A unique feature of this treatment was that clients could be required to speak at quite specific rates at each step in therapy, because clinicians were trained to carry out on-line measurement of rate, and individual display units provided clients with constant feedback on their stuttering and speech rate. This contrasts with Perkins' use of DAF to regulate speech rate. (We do not know whether this difference affects outcome, but it may be quite fundamental: DAF controls speech rate externally, whereas the Andrews–Ingham technique demands voluntary control from the client.)

The original Ingham and Andrews program aimed for total stimulus control over fluency during the entire speaking day. At every step in the program, zero stuttering was the criterion for progress. Clients were hospitalized for 3 weeks of intensive treatment, and a full token economy was used, with penalties for stuttering and rewards for achieving fluency and speech rate targets. Transfer and maintenance phases were carefully programmed and rewarded also. Yet, in spite of this rigorous approach, the entire treatment was carried out in a conversational context: Treatment took place during group conversations around a circular table with six clients and the clinician, who rated the speech from a central console. Transfer assignments were carried out in the real world with the aid of concealed, portable tape recorders and were evaluated later in the clinic. Maintenance was structured, with decreasingly frequent contact for clients who met speech target criteria. Immediately after this treatment, stutterers showed virtually zero stuttering and normal speech rate. In the longer term, there was evidence of slight relapse to a mean of about 2% SS and perhaps slightly slower speech rate but still within the normal range (Andrews & Ingham, 1972; Ingham, 1975a; Guitar, 1976).

Since the original Ingham–Andrews treatment program was published, it has undergone various modifications by the two authors working independently in different centers, and detailed manuals are available (Ingham, 1980; Andrews, Craig, & Feyer, 1983). Ingham's modifications are notable for their further development of more structured maintenance procedures (see chapter 21) and their incorporation of self-evaluation training. We examine the Andrews et al. (1983) modifications in more detail below.

Recently there has been some debate over the extent to which the success of programs such as these depends upon the powerful controls exerted by constant monitoring of speech and token rewards (Howie & Woods, 1982; Ingham, Note 1; Howie, Note 2). It seems likely that token rewards are not crucial to rapid progress in this treatment (Howie & Woods, 1982), and in recent modifications of the program, token economy rewards have not been used (Ingham, 1980; Andrews et al., 1983).

Ryan: Operant DAF therapy

Another prolonged speech program, which has held firmly to the classical behavioral approach, was developed by Ryan and Van Kirk. Their operant DAF therapy uses simple, replicable criteria for progress through treatment (5 minutes of stutter-free speech at each stage), detailed record keeping, clearly specified branch programs at certain points in treatment if speech targets are not met, together with a carefully planned hierarchy of increasingly difficult transfer assignments, each requiring 5 minutes of stutter-free speech. Dramatic decreases in stuttering frequency and the achievement of normal speech rates have been reported both immediately after treatment (Ryan, 1974; Ryan & Van Kirk, 1974) and in the long term (Ryan, 1981). But since these data are based on in-clinic conversations with the clinician, we do not know the extent to which treatment gains generalize beyond the clinic, and so we cannot make a direct comparison between the results of these rigorous behavioral procedures and the broader approach of Perkins and his colleagues.

Webster: Precision fluency shaping program

Another example of a strict behaviorist approach to prolonged speech therapy is the precision fluency shaping program which Webster developed in the early 70s (Webster, 1974, 1975a, 1975b). The approach is based on the premise that stutterers' articulatory and phonatory gestures are distorted and require reconstruction through intensive overlearning of appropriate speech targets. Webster attempted to dissect the required speech pattern into specific components and to develop methods of quantifying and evaluating them objectively. The targets are stretched syllables, smooth transitions between syllables, slow change within syllables, diaphragmatic breathing, and gentle onsets. Clients work individually through a work manual which guides intensive practice of these speech targets, first in single syllables, then longer words and phrases. Feedback on the major two speech targets is objective: Prolongation ("stretched syllables") is checked with a stop watch, and gentle onsets and continuity are acquired with the aid of feedback from a computerized voice onset monitor (VOM) which monitors voice amplitude at the beginning of an utterance and its rate of increase. For further details on the VOM see Webster (1980).

In Webster's program, the strict behavioral approach is largely restricted to the overlearning of the stretched syllable, gentle onset, and continuity targets. The other targets are not quantified, speech rate increase is not systematically programmed as it is in the DAF therapies, and the transfer and maintenance phases of treatment are much less rigorously programmed than the intensive target practice phase. However, the program appears to be effective, with many clients demonstrating minimal stuttering as long as 2 years after treatment (Webster, 1974, 1980). No data on speech rate are given, which is regrettable, since we need to be assured that normal speech rate can be achieved in a program that does not systematically program speech rate increase. One application of Webster's procedures has reported very slow post-treatment speech rates (Mallard & Kelley, 1982).

Andrews, Craig, and Feyer: The Prince Henry program

We finish this discussion of prolonged speech treatments for adult stutterers with a detailed description of the current Prince Henry Hospital program (Andrews et al., 1983). There is, of course, no substitute for hands-on experience of treatment as a means of acquiring therapy skills. But we consider it important to give the reader some details of the specifics of at least one treatment program. The Prince Henry program represents the cumulative developments of treating some 50 adult stutterers each year since 1971. It has repeatedly produced objective, reliable evidence of its efficacy, based on a range of speaking situations both immediately after treatment and 1 to 2 years later, with covert checks on the validity of overt measures. The procedures have proved replicable; when employed in various parts of the world, comparable outcomes have been reported.

The Prince Henry program grew out of the original Andrews–Ingham program and is still based on systematic acquisition and generalization of a prolonged speech pattern. On the other hand, it has eliminated some of the more rigorous aspects of the earlier program, in exchange for features which provide more realistic speech training conditions. It still involves treatment of groups of six stutterers during 3 weeks of intensive treatment for 12 hours daily, although weekend attendance is no longer required. Clients are hospitalized during the instatement of fluency phase (but no longer during the transfer phase). Compulsory, tape-recorded homework assignments are required in order to maintain some control over speech during out-of-clinic hours.

Currently, the speech pattern taught is labeled smooth motion speech. The characteristics of this pattern are gentle onset of phonation, continuous airflow, continuous movement of articulators throughout each utterance, soft contacts, and extension of vowel and consonant duration. Smooth motion speech retains voiceless sounds rather than using the more distorted continuous vocalization, which is sometimes associated with prolonged speech at slow rates.

Smooth-motion nonstuttered speech is instated during the first week. The required speech pattern is trained, using instruction and modeling (not DAF), at a speech rate of 50 SPM, which is approximately a quarter of normal rate. At this rate, stuttering is virtually impossible if the correct speech pattern is used, and secondary symptoms of stuttering disappear automatically. Speech rate is then gradually shaped to normal rate over the course of the week, in gradual increments of 5 SPM. This is done in a series of 45-minute rating sessions in which each stutterer's speech is rated on-line by the clinician, and constant feedback on fluency and speech rate is provided on individual display units. At each step the client must display zero stuttering, correct speech rate (within 20 SPM of target), and a specified minimum number of syllables spoken, all within the 45-minute rating session. The use of virtually imperceptible increases in speech rate during shaping avoids the daunting prospect of sudden, large (30 SPM) increases, as was the case in the original Ingham–Andrews program. Conversational speech is required in the rating sessions in the interest of realism, and the rating equipment is designed so that each group member's contribution to a rapid conversational exchange can be rated.

As we have already noted, the original token reward system has been abandoned. However, clients now earn a small monetary reward if they achieve the targets in each rating session (as well, of course, as the reward of progress to the next stage of treatment).

Self-evaluation training has also been incorporated into the program. In the instatement phase, there are two sessions daily in which monetary rewards are paid for accurate self-assessment rather than for the usual targets of fluency and speech rate. A 1-minute monologue is video-recorded for each client, who then evaluates his speech for acceptable continuity, gentle onsets (acceptability being defined as less than three errors in each case), and speech rate (within 20 SPM of target). If his assessment agrees with the clinician's, he is rewarded. He is also rewarded at the end of the session for accurate assessments of other clients. Later three other characteristics are evaluated also: Intonation, presentation (assessment of overall acceptability in each case), and appropriate pauses (less than 3 inappropriate pauses).

By the end of the first week, the majority of clients are stutter-free in the clinic and are speaking at normal rates. Clients transfer these skills to the real world during the second and third weeks of treatment. They complete a graded hierarchy of 25 speech assignments, each recorded on cassette tapes (for example, phone calls, shopping, public speech, call-in radio). There are 15 standard assignments which must be completed by all clients, and 15 "personal assignments," which clients plan individually to cover many aspects of their speaking life. Each assignment must contain at least 1,400 consecutive syllables of stutter-free speech at 200 ± 40 SPM; otherwise it must be repeated. Clients must evaluate their speech quality and rate in each assignment before submitting it for the clinician's evaluation. One dollar rewards are earned for each standard assignment. Each day of the transfer phase begins and ends with a 2-hour session of smooth speech practice at 100, 150, 180, 200, and 220 SPM.

The maintenance phase in this program is less structured than in the original program. In our experience, compliance in the more rigid maintenance program was low, and a more realistic approach has evolved. At 3, 6, and 9 weeks and at 6 months after intensive treatment in this program, clients are required to attend a follow-up clinic which involves participation in rating sessions and planning of maintenance activities. If they cannot complete the rating sessions without stuttering, or if they report dissatisfaction with their progress, they are asked to continue attendance at follow-up clinics until reliably fluent. Clients are strongly encouraged to carry out formal practice and generalization assignments daily for at least 9 weeks after completion of intensive treatment, and to attend weekly self-help meetings of former clients. Booster treatment programs are also available.

At the end of intensive treatment in the Prince Henry program, clients, who are stuttering on an average of 14% SS and speaking at 140 SPM, demonstrate virtually zero stuttering and speech rate within normal range (Howie, Tanner, & Andrews, 1981; Howie, Woods, & Andrews, 1982). A year or more later, average stuttering is still dramatically reduced. Clients treated before 1978 were achieving means of 3.9% SS and 207 SPM a year after treatment, but those treated in a more recent modification of the program show lower means of 1 to 2% SS (Andrews & Craig, 1982). The most recent evaluations presently being conducted in our clinic confirm this result. Outcome is similar whether covert or overt measures are used. In general, while some clients are never heard to stutter, most still regard themselves as stutterers who are now able to speak fluently, and some have relapsed and are again in need of treatment (Howie et al., 1981).

Summary

In summary, what can be said of the prolonged speech treatments for adult stutterers? The weight of evidence suggests that they are effective both in short and long term. The available data are not always complete: The representativeness of the speech measures reported is sometimes less than satisfactory, and speech rate and normalcy of speech are not always evaluated. But in general the picture is a consistent one. Regardless of the specifics of treatment, on average, as long as a year after treatment, stutterers can be expected to demonstrate fluency at less than 2% SS with normal speech rate (between 160 and 240 SPM). Any new therapies would need to equal or better this outcome.

Although prolonged speech treated stutterers rarely stutter and do not speak excessively slowly, we shall see later that their speech can be distinguished from nonstutterers' speech, although it is not clear on what basis. If the basis of this discriminability can be established, then it may be possible to improve the outcome of prolonged speech treatments.

The effectiveness of these treatments does not appear to depend on whether they are intensive or spaced, group or individual, molar or molecular in emphasis. We discuss some of these issues later. Similarly, the particular aspects of "prolonged speech" that are emphasized in training do not appear to be critical to the success of treatment, although we suspect that slowed articulation rate is more effective than simply increasing pausing, and that continuity and soft attacks are important. It may be that a major value of prolonged speech treatments is that they force a client to slow his speech sufficiently to allow him to pay attention to what he does when he is fluent and to reprogram his articulators accordingly.

We do not know why the prolonged speech therapies work. Some of the recent evidence of aberrant laryngeal behavior, speech pattern and breath characteristics and abnormalities in speech motor control among stutterers suggests that the modification of these aspects of speech is a proper concern of stuttering treatment. Beyond that, the basis for the potency of these techniques remains a mystery.

AIRFLOW THERAPIES

Of the fluency management therapies, prolonged speech techniques have been the most painstakingly developed and researched. But there are other fluency management techniques which may prove valuable when acceptable outcome data are available and when carefully structured programs are available. Among these are airflow management therapies. For example, the regulated breathing method of Azrin and his colleagues (Azrin & Nunn, 1974; Azrin, Nunn, & Frantz, 1979) trains stutterers to control a wide range of aspects of airflow: Smooth breathing, exhalation prior to speech, blending words into the exhalation pattern, continued exhalation after the last sound of the utterance, pausing at natural juncturing points, and smooth inhalation during the prespeech pause, as well as formulation of general speech content. The rationale is that stuttering is a habitual disorder of the initiation and maintenance of airflow, and should be eliminated if the stutterer emits speech behaviors that are incompatible with these airflow anomalies. The treatment is brief: One or two sessions, each of 2 to 3 hours. In a recent treatment description (Azrin et al., 1979), breath management skills are practiced first in reading, then in spontaneous speech, gradually decreasing the frequency of pauses. Structured generalization of skills is minimal and restricted to the clinic and its environs.

Azrin and his colleagues have reported impressive results, but these are based on clients' self-recorded "stuttering episodes," which we would expect to be highly unreliable. Two independent studies, based on objective speech measures, have reported consistent data suggesting that immediately after this treatment, stuttering frequency is about 5% SS, but deteriorates to 8% SS 2 to 3 months later with speech rate probably slow (Andrews & Tanner, 1982a; Ladouceur, Cote, Leblond, & Bouchard, 1982). This outcome is distinctly inferior to the prolonged speech therapies. However, it is interesting to speculate whether outcome would improve if treatment were longer, generalization procedures were expanded and structured, and shaping to normal speech rates were more systematic.

Schwartz's (1976) "flow and slow" techniques also raise some interesting possibilities for fluency management treatment via airflow, but since Schwartz has presented no objective outcome data, the power of the treatment is still open to question. The technique is based on the assumption that stuttering is the result of excessive tensing of the vocal folds before speech, producing feedback that triggers conditioned struggle behaviors, but no details of supportive empirical evidence are given. To counteract this presumed malfunction, stutterers are trained to initiate passive airflow prior to speech and to slow the first syllable of each utterance. Treatment involves 5 days of intensive practice of the flow and slow skills in increasingly long and complex utterances, and finally in generalization tasks. For a year after the intensive treatment, daily home assignments are carried out and audiotape samples are mailed to the clinic.

Reports by Schwartz (1976) and Lee (1976) of "symptom free" speech in large numbers of stutterers at long-term follow-up are inspiring but require better quantitative backup. The only objective data available for these procedures (Andrews & Tanner, 1982b) suggest that the immediate outcome of the 5 intensive days of treatment (means of 2.8% SS and 184 SPM) is less impressive than the prolonged speech therapies. Until hard data on long-term outcome is available, we can say nothing of the lasting effects of this technique. But there is no doubt that the manipulation of airflow can reduce stuttering dramatically in the short term, and it may be that airflow techniques may prove powerful in more structured programs, or as an adjunct to other techniques.

RHYTHMIC SPEECH

It has long been known that pacing words or syllables to a rhythmic stimulus reduces or eliminates stuttering. As we noted earlier, Andrews and Ingham were achieving good short-term outcomes in the late 60s with a highly structured, operant treatment program in which slowed, syllable-timed speech was gradually shaped to normal rates, then generalized in a hierarchy of assignments (Ingham, Andrews, & Winkler, 1972). However, these researchers dispensed with rhythmic speech in favor of prolonged speech on the basis of research which suggested that although the two treatments produced similarly low stuttering frequencies (means of less than 1% SS), the fluent speech of syllable-time-treated stutterers was more restricted in rate than prolonged speech treated stutterers. Furthermore, when stuttering did occur following syllable-timed treatment, it was more likely to be "secondary" disabling stuttering than following prolonged speech treatment (Ingham & Andrews, 1971).

A program developed by Brady (1971) includes procedures which might be expected to improve the efficacy of rhythmic speech treatments. In this program, after speech has been shaped to normal rates, longer and longer units of speech are paced to each metronome beat, and unit lengths are varied to allow more normal speech cadence and juncturing. Brady also devised a portable hearing aid-like metronome, which is worn by clients while they complete a hierarchy of transfer assignments. The assignments are then repeated without the metronome, although some stutterers find this impossible. Short-term outcome is similar to the airflow treatments: A mean of 2.5% SS was observed in the clinic. Brady provides no speech rate data, but a report by Ost, Gotestam, and Melin (1976) suggests that Brady's clients may have experienced difficulties similar to those of Ingham and Andrews' in maintaining normal speech rates without stuttering. In addition, since there are no hard data on speech outside the clinic or long-term performance, the potency of Brady's treatment has yet to be determined.

BIOFEEDBACK

There has been some interest in the use of biofeedback techniques to train stutterers to minimize muscle tension associated with speaking. Such treatments are based on the assumption that stuttering is associated with (if not actually caused by) excessive tension in speech muscles, which interferes with speech production. This assumption is supported by evidence of excessive EMG levels in speech-related muscles in stutterers, of high EMG activity prior to stuttered speech, and of reduced EMG accompanying reduced stuttering frequency (see a recent review by Craig & Cleary (1982) for further details).

The EMG treatment literature tends to be restricted to reports of single cases; large outcome studies are conspicuous by their absence. Details of treatment procedures, as well as outcome data on four stutterers, have been presented by Lanyon (1978). In this program, clients are trained using biofeedback to reduce masseter muscle tension to a maximum of 5 mV. Then masseter tension is reduced before and during utterances of increasing length, first in reading and then in spontaneous speech. Ninety-five percent fluency is required at each step before progress is permitted. This hierarchy is completed first with direct EMG feedback and then with "indirect" feedback from the clinician. The skills are then generalized in a hierarchy of speech tasks. Two of the clients in Lanyon's report completed the generalization tasks in the clinic environs, accompanied by the clinician who gave indirect feedback. The others completed the generalization tasks as part of their everyday activities, using portable feedback machines.

Objective speech measures presented by Lanyon suggest that, for some stutterers, these techniques may produce short- and long-term results comparable with the prolonged speech treatments. But Lanyon's subjects received different variations of this treatment, and, on the basis of the existing evidence, it is impossible to determine what are the powerful features of this technique. The variability of outcome in the individual stutterers reported by Lanyon suggest that the techniques may be appropriate for a subgroup of stutterers only, for example, those with marked speech muscle tension symptoms. Different electrode sites might be appropriate for different stutterers (Guitar, 1975). We also need data on the question of whether muscle tension reduction is necessary during as well as before speech, and whether it is necessary only when stuttering is anticipated, or regardless of the anticipation of stuttering.

THE PURSUIT OF NORMAL SPEECH

We have now examined the major approaches used in fluency management treatment of adult stutterers. Because most of these involve deliberate distortion of speech in order to instate fluency, they have sometimes been charged with leaving stutterers with grossly distorted speech after treatment. Most researchers have tackled the problem simply by asking whether treated stutterers can be distinguished from normal speakers. Runyan and his colleagues (Runyan & Adams, 1978, 1979) collected recordings of the speech of clients treated in six stuttering treatment programs, and then paired them with recordings of nonstutterers. They found that for four of the six treatments, naive subjects were able to pick the stutterer of each pair at better than chance levels, and when speech pathologists made the judgments, none of the treated stutterers were reliably taken for nonstutterers. These results were similar to those obtained when speakers were presented singly rather than in pairs (Runyan, Hames, & Prosek, 1982).

As a comparison of different treatments, this research is seriously flawed, since stutterers selected by each treatment may not have been representative of that treatment, and it is unlikely that stutterers from different treatments were matched for severity of symptoms, and so forth. But the data are intriguing in suggesting that treated stutterers usually sound different. What is the basis for this difference? There is no obvious answer. For example, Ingham and Packman (1978) have reported that, even though naive listeners could distinguish between nonstutterers and stutterers treated in their prolonged speech program, they did not rate treated stutterers and nonstutterers any differently on scales of prosody, rate, fluency, nor on a natural/unnatural dichotomy. Graduates of Perkins' breathstream management program were actually rated as more fluent (though slower) than nonstutterers immediately after treatment (Perkins et al., 1974). Apparently, something is different about the speech of stutterers treated in fluency management programs, but we do not know whether it should be classed as "abnormal." Treated stutterers sometimes report a feeling of artificiality, which may simply be the experience of deliberate control which is necessary to maintain fluency.

SELECTING TREATMENT PROCEDURES: ISOLATING CRITICAL FEATURES OF TREATMENT

On what basis can decisions be made when selecting or designing a fluency management program for stuttering adults? Most of the fluency management therapies involve a cluster of different components, and it is difficult to determine which are crucial to effective treatment. The classical means of determining the value of a component of therapy is to include it in an experimental treatment and compare the outcome with that produced by treatment without the component. This approach strikes problems, however, when applied to treatments in which outcome is already impressive. In such a situation, the addition of a single component is unlikely to produce a large improvement in outcome, and thus impossibly large sample sizes are necessary to provide the experimenter with the power to detect any difference, making research a time-consuming and costly enterprise.

A second possible means of identifying crucial features of treatments is via single-case research, using reversal or multiple baseline methods (Hersen & Barlow, 1976). But these methods cannot evaluate the long-term effects of procedures, and they presume that the subject is able or willing to stop using a speech skill which has been effective in reducing stuttering (see Falkowski, Guilford, & Sandler (1982) for a contrary example).

Metanalysis is a third way of isolating critical features of treatment (Andrews et al., 1980). This statistical technique allows us to make direct comparisons of the outcomes of very different treatments, with very different outcome measures. Outcome can be expressed as a standardized "outcome effect size," that is, the difference between pre- and post-treatment means, divided by the pretreatment standard deviation. Then, if data from sufficient studies are available, those treatment features associated with good outcome (large effect sizes) can be isolated. In the Andrews et al. (1980) metanalysis, of the principal treatment types, prolonged speech was the major predictor of outcome effect size (accounting for 15% of the variance), then rhythm (accounting for a further 4.8%), and finally attitude therapy (1.3%). The critical components of treatment were (in order of the amount of outcome variance explained) reinforcement, then slow speech, transfer activities, maintenance activities, and finally social support. Of the treatment format features examined, only hours of treatment was critical, with longer treatments producing larger outcome effect sizes. Intensity of treatment did not predict outcome, although this may have been because it was confounded with hours of treatment, longer duration being invariably associated with intensive procedures.

The clinician wishing to apply fluency management techniques is faced with the task of selecting or designing effective treatment procedures which can be expected to produce outcomes comparable with those already reported in the research literature. The clinician then has a responsibility to carry out regular outcome measurements. Failure to produce an acceptable outcome means that the program should be modified or abandoned. As we have seen, there are several existing fluency management programs of proven efficacy, especially among those using prolonged speech, which can be applied without modification. But if the clinician wishes to design his or her own therapy, the decision about whether to include a particular procedure can be difficult, since some procedures (for example, systematic shaping of speech rate) are present in some highly effective treatments and absent in others. The decision to include a component in treatment involves a combination of various considerations: The results of laboratory or metanalytic research, the clinician's preferred style of operation or theoretical stance, and the resources available to the clinician. In the following discussion we consider issues relevant to some of the as yet unresolved aspects of fluency management treatments.

Intensive versus spaced treatment

The nature of fluency management treatments allows them to be used intensively or to be spread over time. We have seen that, in the metanalysis, intensiveness of treatment did not predict treatment outcome, but this may have been confounded by hours of treatment. Perkins et al. (1974) reported no difference in fluency outcome between intensively and nonintensively treated stutterers, although intensively treated stutterers did complete treatment in fewer hours. Theoretically speaking, continuously reinforced behaviors have the fastest acquisition rate but also the fastest extinction rate, whereas behaviors which are reinforced at variable intervals have a slower acquisition and extinction rate (Shames, 1975). Ingham (1975b) argues that without the continuous control and feedback provided by intensive treatment, the critical speech skills are unlikely to be maintained beyond treatment. Whether or not this is so, the rapid acquisition of fluency in intensive treatment is very rewarding and probably encourages clients to persevere with a demanding treatment. The choice of intensive or nonintensive treatment may simply depend upon the client's availability and his capacity to persist under conditions of massed practice, as well as the practical considerations of clinic scheduling.

Individual versus group therapy

There are some obvious advantages of group therapy: The efficient use of clinician time, the beneficial effect on client morale, and the provision of a conversational setting for speech practice. On the other hand, individual treatment may be more economical in time if treatment can be tailored to the needs of a particular client. But the main issue here is whether standardized fluency management procedures applied to groups can cater to the individual needs of each stutterer. In the case of prolonged speech treatments, at least, group treatment seems justified since the techniques work with the great majority of stutterers. A reasonable compromise seems to be standardized group treatment in which there is some flexibility. For example, branching procedures may operate if clients fail to reach criteria within a specified time (Ingham, 1980; Ryan, 1974). The transfer phase of treatment may include individual personal assignments as well as standard assignments

(Andrews et al., 1983). Or a program may simply allow for different amounts of time to be spent by different clients at different stages in treatment (Webster, 1980).

Importance of generalization during transfer phase

We have seen that some fluency management programs do not include carefully structured generalization of speech skills to the real world. Limiting generalization activities to the clinic and its environs is unlikely to result in successful post-treatment maintenance of fluency. Even if speech skills are practiced in the real world, the presence of a clinician or tape recorder may interfere with generalization, because the speaking situation is too unnatural. Yet, some form of monitoring of generalization activities is needed to assess the client's performance. It may, therefore, be valuable to use FM remote microphones, and to vary assignments in the degree of monitoring present (for example, taped versus untaped, accompanied by an observer versus unaccompanied). Alternatively, the clinician may refuse to accept assignments which sound "staged" (Andrews et al., 1983), or insist on evidence of the "realness" of the conversation by requiring parts of the other side of the conversation to be recorded (Ingham, 1980).

Modification of attitudes and self-concepts

Does manipulation of attitudes to speech improve the outcome of stuttering therapy? In the metanalysis, attitude modification made only a very minor contribution to treatment outcome. On the other hand, in prolonged speech treatments, long-term prognosis may be poorer for clients who begin treatment with highly negative attitudes to speech (Guitar, 1976) or with external locus of personal control (Craig, Franklin, & Andrews, in press). Negative attitudes may not cause stuttering, but in some individuals, at least, the attitudinal consequences of stuttering may interfere with treatment. On the other hand, the experience of achieving fluency may automatically produce change in attitudes and self-concept to bring them into congruence with the new behavior. If we can develop valid measures of attitude which predict outcome, then the clinician may be able to select for special attention any clients whose pre- or post-treatment attitudes put them at risk of relapse.

Self-evaluation and reinforcement

A relatively new development in fluency management techniques is the inclusion of structured training in self-monitoring, self-management, and sometimes self-reinforcement (Ingham, 1980; Andrews et al., 1983).

Specific training in self-control may be particularly important in intensive programs that maintain strict stimulus control over behavior. Without systematic weaning from clinician control, the client cannot be expected to take responsibility for his own behavior after treatment ends.

The evidence available on self-control in stuttering therapy is still limited. Self-monitoring of stuttering can reduce stuttering (La Croix, 1973; Unterman, Note 3), but in some individuals it may increase stuttering (Ingham, Adams, & Reynolds, 1978; James, 1981). It may prove more beneficial to train stutterers to self-monitor fluency or fluency-producing skills, rather than stuttering.

Conclusion

It remains to be seen whether the apparent superiority of prolonged speech treatments will be sustained when other treatments refine their techniques, program their procedures more systematically, and evaluate their outcomes more thoroughly. For the time being, however, the clinician's choice is clear if he or she wishes to maximize treatment outcome. Some of the specifics of treatment, such as its intensiveness, group versus individual setting, and details of generalization, attitude modification, and self-control training may, at present, be left to the clinician's preference, but prolonged speech treatment is the most effective of the fluency management treatments of adult stutterers. Fluency management treatments can be effective and rewarding, provided the clinician has expertise and self-discipline, and the stutterer works hard to gain and maintain the speech skills associated with fluency.

NOTES

[1] Ingham, R. J. *On token reinforcement and stuttering therapy. Another view on findings reported by Howie and Woods.* Manuscript submitted for publication, 1982.

[2] Howie, P. M. *A response to "On token reinforcement and stuttering therapy. Another view on findings reported by Howie and Woods.* Manuscript submitted for publication, 1982.

[3] Unterman, R. M. *The effect of self-evaluation on dysfluencies of stutterers.* Paper presented at the annual convention of the American Speech, Language and Hearing Association, Atlanta, GA, 1979.

REFERENCES

Andrews, G. Stuttering: Evaluation of the benefits of treatment. In W. H. Perkins, (Ed.), *Current therapy in communication disorders: Stuttering disorders.* New York: Thieme-Stratton, 1984.

Andrews, G., & Craig, A. Stuttering: Overt and covert measurement of the speech of treated subjects. *Journal of Speech and Hearing Disorders,* 1982, 47, 96–99.

Andrews, G., Craig, A., & Feyer. A. M. *Therapist's manual for the stuttering treatment programme.* Sidney: Division of Communication Disorders, The Prince Henry Hospital, 1983.

Andrews, G., Guitar, B., & Howie, P. Metanalysis of the effects of stuttering treatment. *Journal of Speech and Hearing Disorders,* 1980, *45,* 287-307.

Andrews, G., & Ingham, R. J. An approach to the evaluation of stuttering therapy. *Journal of Speech and Hearing Research,* 1972, *15,* 296-302.

Andrews, G., & Tanner, S. Stuttering treatment: An attempt to replicate the regulated-breathing method. *Journal of Speech and Hearing Disorders,* 1982, *47,* 138-140.(a)

Andrews, G., & Tanner, S. Stuttering: The results of five days treatment with an airflow technique. *Journal of Speech and Hearing Disorders,* 1982, *47,* 427-429.(b)

Azrin, N. H., & Nunn, R. G. A rapid method of elimination of stuttering by a regulated breathing approach. *Behaviour Research and Therapy,* 1974, *12,* 279-286.

Azrin, N. H., Nunn, R. G., & Frantz, S. E. Comparison of regulated-breathing vs abbreviated desensitization on reported stuttering episodes. *Journal of Speech and Hearing Disorders,* 1979, *44,* 331-339.

Brady, J. P. Metronome-conditioned speech retraining for stuttering. *Behavior Therapy,* 1971, *2,* 129-150.

Craig, A., & Cleary, P. J. Reduction of stuttering by young male stutterers using EMG feedback. *Biofeedback and Self-Regulation,* 1982, *7,* 241-255.

Craig, A., Franklin, J., & Andrews, G. A scale to measure the locus of control of behaviour. *British Journal of Medical Psychology,* in press.

Curlee, R. F., & Perkins, W. H. Conversational rate control therapy for stuttering. *Journal of Speech and Hearing Disorders,* 1969, *34,* 245-250.

Curlee, R. F., & Perkins, W. H. Effectiveness of a DAF conditioning program for adolescent and adult stutterers. *Behaviour Research and Therapy,* 1973, *11,* 395-401.

Falkowski, G. L., Guilford, A. M., & Sandler, J. Effectiveness of a modified version of airflow therapy: Case studies. *Journal of Speech and Hearing Disorders,* 1982, *47,* 160-164.

Goldiamond, I. Stuttering and fluency as manipulable operant response classes. In L. Krasner & L. P. Ullman (Eds.), *Research in behavior modification.* New York: Holt, Rinehart & Winston, 1965.

Gregory, H. H. Controversial issues: Statement and review of the literature. In H. H. Gregory, (Ed.), *Controversies about stuttering therapy.* Baltimore: University Park Press, 1979.

Guitar, B. Reduction of stuttering frequency using analog electromyographic feedback. *Journal of Speech and Hearing Research,* 1975, *18,* 672-685.

Guitar, B. Pretreatment factors associated with the outcome of stuttering therapy. *Journal of Speech and Hearing Research,* 1976, *19,* 590-600.

Hersen, M., & Barlow, D. H. *The use of single-case experimental designs.* Englewood Cliffs, NJ: Prentice-Hall, 1976.

Howie, P. M., Tanner, S., & Andrews, G. Short- and long-term outcome in an intensive treatment program for adult stutterers. *Journal of Speech and Hearing Disorders,* 1981, *46,* 104-109.

Howie, P. M., & Woods, C. L. Token reinforcement during the instatement and shaping of fluency in the treatment of stuttering. *Journal of Applied Behavior Analysis,* 1982, *15,* 55-64.

Howie, P. M., Woods, C. L., & Andrews, G. Relationship between covert and overt speech measures immediately before and immediately after stuttering treatment. *Journal of Speech and Hearing Disorders,* 1982, *47,* 419-426.

Ingham, R. J. A comparison of covert and overt assessment procedures in stuttering therapy outcome evaluation. *Journal of Speech and Hearing Research,* 1975, *18,* 346–354.(a)

Ingham, R. J. Operant methodology in stuttering therapy. In J. Eisenson (Ed.), *Stuttering: A second symposium.* New York: Harper & Row, 1975.(b)

Ingham, R. J. *Stuttering therapy manual: Hierarchy control schedule. A clinician's guide.* Sydney: School of Communication Disorders, Cumberland College of Health Sciences, 1980.

Ingham, R. J., Adams, S., & Reynolds, G. The effects on stuttering of self-recording the frequency of stuttering or the word "the." *Journal of Speech and Hearing Research,* 1978, *21,* 459–469.

Ingham, R., & Andrews, G. Stuttering: The quality of fluency after treatment. *Journal of Communication Disorders,* 1971, *4,* 279–288.

Ingham, R. J., & Andrews, G. Details of a token economy stuttering therapy programme for adults. *Australian Journal of Human Communication Disorders,* 1973, *1,* 13–20.(a)

Ingham, R. J., & Andrews, G. An analysis of a token economy in stuttering therapy. *Journal of Applied Behavior Analysis,* 1973, *6,* 219–229.(b)

Ingham, R. J., Andrews, G., & Winkler, R. Stuttering: A comparative evaluation of the short-term effectiveness of four treatment techniques. *Journal of Communication Disorders,* 1972, *5,* 91–117.

Ingham, R. J., & Packman, A. C. Perceptual assessment of normalcy of speech following stuttering therapy. *Journal of Speech and Hearing Research,* 1978, *21,* 63–73.

James, J. E. Self-monitoring of stuttering: Reactivity and accuracy. *Behaviour Research and Therapy,* 1981, *19,* 291–296.

La Croix, Z. E. Management of disfluent speech through self-recording procedures. *Journal of Speech and Hearing Disorders,* 1973, *38,* 272–274.

Ladouceur, R., Cote, C., Leblond, G., & Bouchard, L. Evaluation of regulated-breathing method and awareness training in the treatment of stuttering. *Journal of Speech and Hearing Disorders,* 1982, *47,* 419–422.

Lanyon, R. I. Behavioral approaches to stuttering. In M. Herson, R. M. Eisler, & P. M. Miller (Eds.), *Progress in behavior modification* (Vol. 6). New York: Academic Press, 1978.

Lee, J. Application of Martin Schwartz's airflow technique in the treatment of stuttering. *Journal of Speech and Hearing Disorders,* 1976, *41,* 133–138.

Mallard, A. R., & Kelley, J. S. The precision fluency shaping program: Replication and evaluation. *Journal of Fluency Disorders,* 1982, *7,* 287–294.

Ost, L., Gotestam, G., & Melin, L. A controlled study of two behavioral methods in the treatment of stuttering. *Behavior Therapy,* 1976, *7,* 587–592.

Perkins, W. H. Replacement of stuttering with normal speech: II. Clinical procedures. *Journal of Speech and Hearing Disorders,* 1973, *38,* 295–303.

Perkins, W. H. Measurement and maintenance of fluency. In E. Boberg (Ed.), *The maintenance of fluency.* New York: Elsevier, 1981.

Perkins, W. H. Techniques for establishing fluency. In W. H. Perkins (Ed.), *Current therapy in communication disorders: Stuttering disorders.* (pp 173–181). New York: Thieme-Stratton, 1984.

Perkins, W. H., Rudas, J., Johnson, L., Michael, W. B., & Curlee, R. F. Replacement of stuttering with normal speech: III. Clinical effectiveness. *Journal of Speech and Hearing Disorders,* 1974, *39,* 416–428.

Runyan, C. M., & Adams, M. R. Perceptual study of the speech of 'successfully therapeutized' stutterers. *Journal of Fluency Disorders,* 1978, *3,* 25–39.

Runyan, C. M., & Adams, M. R. Unsophisticated judges' perceptual evaluations of the speech of 'successfully treated' stutterers. *Journal of Fluency Disorders,* 1979, *4,* 29–38.

Runyan, C. M., Hames, P. E., & Prosek, R. A. A perceptual comparison between paired stimulus and single stimulus methods of presentation of the fluent utterances of stutterers. *Journal of Fluency Disorders,* 1982, *7,* 71–77.

Ryan, B. P. *Programmed therapy for stuttering in children and adults.* Springfield, IL: Thomas, 1974.

Ryan, B. P. Maintenance programs in progress—II. In E. Boberg (Ed.), *Maintenance of fluency.* New York: Elsevier, 1981.

Ryan, B. P., & Van Kirk, B. The establishment, transfer, and maintenance of fluent speech in 50 stutterers using delayed auditory feedback and operant procedures. *Journal of Speech and Hearing Disorders,* 1974, *39,* 3–10.

Schwartz, M. F. *Stuttering solved.* Philadelphia: Lippincott, 1976.

Shames, G. H. Operant conditioning and stuttering. In J. Eisenson (Ed.), *Stuttering: A second symposium.* New York: Harper & Row, 1975.

Webster, R. L. A behavioral analysis of stuttering: Treatment and theory. In K. S. Calhoun, H. L. Adams, & K. M. Mitchell (Eds.), *Innovative treatment methods in psychopathology.* New York: Wiley, 1974.

Webster, R. L. *The precision fluency shaping program: Speech reconstruction for stutterers.* Roanoke, VA: Communications Development Corp., 1975.(a)

Webster, R. L. *The precision fluency shaping program: Speech reconstruction for stutterers. Clinician's program guide.* Roanoke, VA: Communications Development Corp., 1975.(b)

Webster, R. L. Evolution of a target-based behavioral therapy for stuttering. *Journal of Fluency Disorders,* 1980, *5,* 303–320.

Chapter 21

Generalization and Maintenance of Treatment

Roger J. Ingham

Despite promising advances in stuttering therapy over the past decade, few have diminished concern about the durability of therapy benefits (Boberg, 1981; Boberg, Howie & Woods, 1979; Gregory, 1979; Ingham, 1984). It is a concern fueled by the questionable quality of stuttering therapy outcome evaluations (Ingham & Costello, 1984) and an astonishing shortage of research on procedures that might assist generalization and maintenance. This problem is not unique to stuttering therapy (Goldstein & Kanfer, 1979; Karoly & Steffen, 1980). Recently, however, there has emerged a body of research specific to generalization and maintenance, which is also beginning to benefit stuttering treatment. The purpose of this chapter is to review the contribution to stuttering therapy of these emerging approaches to generalization and maintenance.

The infant state of research in this area is probably one reason why there is still uncertainty about its terminology (Ingham, 1981). In essence, this topic area is concerned with therapy procedures that enhance outcome by improving the probability of *carryover, transfer, generalization,* and *maintenance*. These terms usually refer to treatment benefits that endure in beyond-clinic and/or post-treatment conditions. But they are often used interchangeably without regard to some important differences among their meanings. One reason for this is that the terms not only describe different therapy effects, but they also describe certain therapy procedures.

Stokes and Baer (1977) endeavored to improve the clarity of this terminology by describing all of its aspects as part of *generalization*. Their frequently cited definition reads as follows:

> The occurrence of relevant behavior under different nontraining conditions (i.e., across subjects, settings, people, behaviors, and/or time) without the scheduling

of the same events in those conditions as had been scheduled in the training conditions. Thus, generalization may be claimed when no extratraining manipulations are needed for extra training changes; or may be claimed when some extra manipulations are necessary, but their cost or extent is clearly less than that of the direct intervention. Generalization will not be claimed when similar events are necessary for similar effects across conditions. (1977, p. 350)

Terms such as "cost" or "extent" in this definition might cause debate, but it simply relates a claim for generalization to the relationship between data trends and treatment operations. Thus, it has kinship with principles used in applied behavior analysis (Baer, Wolf, & Risley, 1968)—It only draws upon evidence of where and when behavior is measured relative to treatment intervention in order to identify generalization (of course, this means a treatment's claim for generalization would actually stem from a systematic investigation of the relationship between specifiable operations and behavior). Perhaps the only drawback in Stokes and Baer's definition is that it bypasses reference to *maintenance* which is a well-entrenched description of sustained behavior change following treatment.

In general, there seems to be much merit in defining *generalization*, as Stokes and Baer have done, while retaining *maintenance* for treatment benefits sustained over time. It is important however, to distinguish between *active* and *passive* generalization/maintenance. There are obvious differences between generalization/maintenance that is supported by certain continuing procedures, and generalization/maintenance that occurs in the absence of such procedures. Also (and for this chapter) the term *transfer* usually embraces the concept of *generalization*. *Transfer* cannot be easily dispensed with since numerous therapy programs employ *transfer stages* within their formats. The function of these stages is to increase the probability that therapy gains will emerge in different settings or, in other words, will generalize.

METHODOLOGICAL ISSUES IN GENERALIZATION/MAINTENANCE RESEARCH

There are substantial difficulties involved in determining a treatment's contributions to generalization/maintenance. Such difficulties range from problems of measurement through to the unique impediments to generalization/maintenance research. The difficulties of measuring speech in pertinent circumstances have been greatly relieved, however, by the availability of miniature recorders—a simple technology which has made generalization/maintenance evaluation (even measurement-based treatment) possible. But convincing generalization/maintenance studies require evaluations across diverse settings and over periods ranging between 6 months and 5 years after treatment (Silverman, 1981). For this reason alone it is difficult to ascertain the extent to which a treatment is responsible for a *maintained* behavior change. For example, many therapies recommend a variety of practices (speech practice, enrollment in speaking clubs, changes in employment, parent control, etc.), which may help sustain post-treatment performance during periods when generalization and maintenance are determined. Furthermore, treatment outcome research may also involve time spans that clash with the constraints operating in many research settings (time available for the completion of theses, time provided by grant support, etc.). Despite all of these difficulties it is still possible to discern a growing and effective "technology of generalization" (Stokes & Baer, 1977) within stuttering therapy.

It is challenging to try to specify the criteria that must be met to show that stuttering therapy has produced generalization/maintenance. Doubtless, one desired therapy goal is normally fluent speech,[1] with no evidence of stuttering in any situation and speech that remains indistinguishable from the speech of normal speakers. But a brief reflection on how to determine such outcomes highlights several major difficulties: What situations are sufficiently representative; for how long should the client's speech be measured; and, of course, what measures should be employed? Furthermore, this ultimate outcome is but one depiction of generalization/maintenance— and an extreme one at that. Beneficial therapy may also produce only partial generalization and/or maintenance. But such partial gains should also have clinical worth. Consequently, useful criteria should somehow reflect a "clinically significant" change. Needless to say, the constituents of these criteria are yet to be agreed upon, although some of the measurement operations that will help identify these constituents *are* becoming evident.

The long debate concerning appropriate speech measures in stuttering therapy is yielding some areas of agreement (Bloodstein, 1981; Ingham & Costello, 1984). There is some consensus that audibly measured frequency counts of stuttering (rather than disfluencies or dysfluencies) are the most basic datum, although they should be combined with speech rate measures to ensure that stuttering frequency changes are not offset by unusual speaking rates. These measures may be aided by data on the duration of stutterings. There is also some agreement that measures of stuttering should be supplemented by measures of speech normalcy or naturalness. Several attempts to use listener judgments to measure speech quality have been described in recent years (Ingham & Packman,

---

[1] Some data reported by Silverman (1980) suggest that some clinicians are still not satisfied that this is the ultimate goal of stuttering therapy.

1978; Jones & Azrin, 1969; Perkins, Rudas, Johnson, Michael, & Curlee, 1974). Among these the approach used by Martin, Haroldson, and Triden (1984) to investigate naturalness ratings appears to be the most promising. Some clinicians have recommended that these measures be accompanied by questionnaire assessment of a client's reactions and attitudes to speaking (Andrews & Cutler, 1974; Erickson, 1969; Johnson, Darley, & Spriestersbach, 1963), speaking time in different speaking situations (Johnson et al., 1963), or time spent monitoring speech in order to sustain improvement (Perkins, 1981; Webster, 1974b). But there is still no evidence that such measures, especially questionnaires, supplement or improve the validity of speech performance data.

The methods used to measure a stutterer's speech performance may also be a source of variability. There is some evidence that the very act of measuring stuttering may influence that behavior (Ingham, 1975b, 1980, 1981), but it is difficult to predict the extent of this influence. It is also evident that, across populations of stutterers, speech performance differences have been related to whether speech is assessed auditorily or audiovisually (Luper, 1956; Martin, 1965), or during either oral reading, monologue, or conversational speech (Ryan, 1974)—differences that are also unpredictable.

The growing complexity of measurement methodology undoubtedly has improved therapy evaluation. But it has also brought into question any claims for generalization/maintenance not based on multidimensional speech performance measures. For example, when only stuttering frequency data are reported, it is impossible to determine if a therapy's "benefits" depend on slow or unusual sounding speech.

One final consideration concerns identification of the variability of stuttering behavior. Because there is little evidence that a stutterer's speech behavior can be predicted across situations, or even across assessments in the same situation, one cannot assume that data gathered on one occasion necessarily predicts performance on another. For this reason there is increasing recognition that procedures used to achieve generalization/maintenance should be assessed within time-series therapy evaluation designs (Hersen & Barlow, 1976; Ingham & Costello, 1984).

INVESTIGATIONS OF GENERALIZATION/MAINTENANCE IN STUTTERING TREATMENT

The virtual certainty that many stuttering treatment benefits will fade activated the search for supplementary procedures to prevent this effect. That seemingly shaped the structure of many stuttering therapies, for these procedures are invariably "tacked" to the end of treatment formats

(Ingham, 1984). Typically, most treatments begin with a reliable method for reducing stuttering—normally in a clinic setting. *Transfer* strategies are then used to extend this improvement in typical beyond-clinic speaking conditions. Thereafter some strategy(s) is usually introduced to maintain that improved beyond-clinic performance. What follows in this chapter, therefore, is largely a review of *add-on* therapy strategies.

The generalization/maintenance strategies used in stuttering treatments can be described in various ways. One useful approach is to adopt the nine categories that Stokes and Baer (1977) used to describe an emerging "technology of generalization" among behavior therapies. These categories are: (1) Train and Hope, (2) Sequential Modification, (3) Introduce to Natural Maintaining Contingencies, (4) Train Sufficient Exemplars, (5) Train Loosely, (6) Use Indiscriminable Contingencies, (7) Program Common Stimuli, (8) Mediate Generalization, and (9) Train "To Generalize."

Train and Hope

The Train and Hope label characterizes therapies that *do not* use procedures specifically designed for generalization/maintenance. As Stokes and Baer state, "It is usually hoped that some generalization (and maintenance) may occur, which will be welcomed yet not explicitly programmed" (1977, p. 351).

There are few reports of treatments that have not used additional manipulations to achieve generalization and maintenance. The most obvious use of Train and Hope occurs in therapies that employ a relatively unchanging treatment. Thus, some pertinent findings should emerge from reports about portable treatment devices, such as earpiece metronome or masking units. Silverman (1976), for example, gave a dataless account of his own 12–18 hour per day use of the earpiece metronome unit known as the Pacemaster (Brady, 1971); he claimed that the unit's initial benefits "wore off" after 3 years. Another example is Trotter and Lesch's (1967) account of the senior author's experience in lecturing with the aid of various portable masking units. Over the course of 360 fifty-minute lectures he reported that his normal 80 blocks per lecture were reduced by about 75% while wearing a unit; however, no within-lecture maintenance effects were reported. In view of the widespread use of such devices, it would be intriguing to learn whether these are representative accounts.

Yet another method of obtaining beyond-clinic treatment control was Shelton's (1975) use of self-managed shadowing treatment for a 21-year-old stutterer. This subject was simply given homework assignments to shadow recorded passages containing difficult words. But only self-counts supported claims that reduced daily stuttering frequencies generalized and were maintained a month after treatment ceased.

Response contingent therapy procedures have also employed Train and Hope procedures with mixed results. Leach (1969) used monetary reinforcement for intervals of disfluency-free oral reading by a 12-year-old stutterer. His data, from an untreated part of each session, show that session-to-session treatment gains were maintained—although the absence of speech rate, reliability, and treatment condition data limits the study's clinical value. It was also limited because 2 months after treatment ceased there was "a partial return of dysfluent behavior" (p. 123). More promising data have resulted from the use of contingencies for stuttering. Martin, Kuhl, and Haroldson (1972) used time out from talking to a puppet, contingent on stuttering, in treating two young male stutterers (3.5 and 4.5 years). Over the course of weekly 20-minute sessions, the children were also intermittently recorded speaking in another setting with either a clinician or the child's mother. Both children reduced stuttering (from approximately 6% and 2.5% words stuttered) to near zero during treatment and subsequent nontreatment sessions. Parallel improvements were evident in concurrent nontreatment sessions. Post-treatment covert recordings of each child conversing with family members also showed virtually no stuttering, and this was also true during follow-up recordings made a year after treatment. These data certainly suggest that generalization/maintenance can occur without additional treatment manipulations. A related result was obtained by Reed and Godden (1977) who treated two children (3.9 and 5 years) in twice-weekly 20-minute clinic sessions using the verbal contingency "slow down." Intermittent home recordings throughout treatment revealed substantial generalization of reduced stuttering which was sustained 8 months after treatment ceased.

The initial DAF/"Prolonged Speech" treatments also sought generalization/maintenance mainly through Train and Hope practices. Goldiamond (1965) reported establishing virtually stutter-free oral reading at "normal and supernormal" rates among eight adult stutterers and claimed (without data) that only one subject failed to show generalization in beyond-clinic speaking conditions. Self-control procedures were taught to these subjects at the end of the establishment phase, but without information on their efficacy. A similar within-clinic treatment procedure was used with eight adult stutterers by Webster (1970) in his first report on the Hollins Program. At the end of treatment, subjects were instructed to use their new speech pattern in their home environment. With this limited assistance it was claimed that the treatment gains "persisted in all eight up to the time of this report, that is, approximately ten months" (1970, p. 158).

The uncertain level of generalization/maintenance from the initial DAF treatments, however, stimulated many developments with this therapy procedure (Ingham, 1984). Indeed, almost all generalization/maintenance research on stuttering therapy has involved therapies that use variants of Goldiamond's procedure. Nevertheless, relatively few studies have demonstrated failed generalization/maintenance. One exception is Boberg and Sawyer's (1977) report on a follow-up "refresher weekend" of treatment. These sessions, which may be more aptly described as "Retrain and Hope" technology, used a telescoped and "loosely structured" version of the original treatment. Approximately 12 months after their original treatment, subjects showed a mean 22% relapse in their percentage of disfluent syllables. Five stutterers were then enrolled in refresher weekends, which occurred every 3 months, and over a 6-month period all had reversed "the trend toward relapse."

Perhaps the most surprising feature of Train and Hope procedures is that, in some instances, they *do* appear to yield generalized and maintained therapy gains—particularly the response contingent treatments of young children. Only a few successful cases are reported, but their findings suggest that this age group may evidence beyond-clinic benefits from Train and Hope practices.

Sequential Modification

The Sequential Modification category refers to the sequential introduction of treatment to settings where generalization or maintenance is absent or deficient. One might assume that this procedure would have been tried frequently in treating a disorder that is known to vary markedly between settings. Unhappily, few studies have collected multiple baseline data across speaking situations, and fewer still report the effects of introducing treatments to these situations.

Many current therapies use procedures that move from the clinic to beyond-clinic settings (Boberg, 1976, 1980; Curlee & Perkins, 1969; Howie, Tanner, & Andrews, 1981; Ingham & Andrews, 1973a; Mowrer, 1975; Perkins, 1973; Ryan, 1974), although few report data which permit generalization/maintenance to be clearly attributed to this type of intervention. An example of this approach is Ryan's (1970, 1971, 1974) therapy program which uses a variety of establishment procedures (programmed traditional, GILCU, DAF, and punishment) to achieve within-clinic target levels of speaking performance. His transfer procedure requires the clinician to accompany the client in various beyond-clinic settings, wherein the client is instructed to speak fluently and negotiate graduated tasks within each setting by speaking without stuttering for 5 to 10 minutes. A subsequent maintenance phase involves decreasingly frequent clinic visits over a minimum of 21 months. The transfer schedule's effects on beyond-clinic performance were determined (Ryan, 1979) from assessments made over the course of this treatment. These assessments included a within-clinic "Criterion Interview" (5 minutes of oral reading, monologue, and conversation), a "Fluency Interview" (14 or 20 speaking tasks which include speaking with others and on the telephone), and a "Natural Speech Sample" (from recordings made in home and school settings). The group data, reproduced in Table 21-1, indicate that the fluency interview and natural speech sample (or essentially beyond-clinic) data resembled the criterion test, or within-clinic data, only after the transfer schedule was completed (although subject attrition may have also contributed to this tendency).

Only a handful of studies have reported using Sequential Modifications along with repeated assessments of speech performance. Guitar (1975) investigated the use of EMG biofeedback in treating a 32-year-old male stutterer. Base rate conversational and telephone call data showed that his mean percentages of syllables stuttered (% SS) in these settings were, respectively, 17 and 19%. The subject's chin was selected as an optimal site for reducing muscle action potentials via audiofeedback. Following training, stuttering in conversations was reduced to near zero over three treatment sessions, but daily recordings of telephone conversations showed that stuttering continued at approximately 22% SS. After instructions to use muscle tension reduction skills during all telephone conversations, stuttering in this setting quickly reduced to virtually zero over a 12-day period. A video recording of a conversation with a stranger made 5 weeks later also revealed no stuttering; this was true also during a conversation and telephone call recording made 9 months later (his speech rate was then stated to be normal).

The importance of speech rate data in gauging treatment outcome is illustrated in a Sequential Modification procedure described by Williamson, Epstein, and Coburn (1981). They assessed a 39-year-old male stutterer during oral readings, conversations, role playing a social situation, and telephoning a clinician over an office intercom and found 16 to 46% words "dysfluent" at a mean of 24.6 words per minute (WPM) during once or twice weekly base rate sessions. Azrin and Nunn's (1974) regulated breathing treatment was then introduced to the oral reading and conversation tasks, and then to the role playing and telephone tasks. With each introduction of treatment, the percentage of dysfluencies decreased and remained at less than 10% during eight sessions over a

TABLE 21-1. Assessment procedure data from across treatment conditions reported by Ryan (1979, p. 156)

	Preestablishment SW/M Mean ($n = 40$)	Postestablishment SW/M Mean ($n = 39$)	Posttransfer SW/M Mean ($n = 27$)
Criterion Test	7.2	1.0	0.8
Fluency Interview	7.4	3.7	1.0
Natural Speech Sample	7.5	3.8	1.6

3-month period. However, the subject's speech rate improved only to around 45 WPM. The treatment was then extended to home sessions by training the subject's wife to model regulated breathing and to use this speaking method in the home. Two 30-minute audio recordings, obtained at the end of the second and third month of this training, showed a final measure of 2% words dysfluent, but at only 33.2 WPM. Listener judgments of the subject's speech indicated that it was understandable, from a person with whom the listener would interact, and socially acceptable. Despite this, it is difficult to understand how such an extremely slow speech rate was not debilitative.

James (1981a) and Ingham (1982) also reported introducing sequential treatment strategies to previously base rated beyond-clinic settings. These were self-managed treatment programs that are reviewed in a subsequent section as examples of "mediated generalization," but they also constitute two of the few data-based studies of sequential modifications.

Introduce to Natural Maintaining Contingencies

The introduce-to-natural-maintaining-contingencies procedure relies on naturally occurring reinforcers in a client's environment to generalize/maintain a target behavior(s). In some instances the client is taught additional behaviors that will activate critical reinforcing agents, or the client's environment is restructured to provide contrived "natural" reinforcers.

Despite much speculation there is no evidence that a treated stutterer's environment is rich with fluency-maintaining contingencies. It is often presumed, for example, that parent reactions or (for adults) job demands might help sustain treatment benefits. At best, it seems that such potential reinforcers may operate primarily during contrived conditions.

An interesting example of this is Griffin and Van Kirk's (see Ryan, 1974) report on a previously treated lecturer's stuttering during class presentations. In some classes students were organized to cough contingent on stuttering and to smile or be attentive "during periods of fluency." This resulted in reduced stuttered words per minute in lectures. Thereafter, students were scheduled to converse with the lecturer in different locations, where it was claimed that his stuttering continued at a low level. But no supportive (nor reliability) data were provided. Browning (1967) used a similar principle in treating a hospitalized 9-year-old schizophrenic stutterer. After treatment by reciprocal inhibition and reinforcement for fluency, hospital staff were trained to ensure that the subject repeated a statement fluently whenever he stuttered. This procedure was associated with reduced stuttering in conversational speech and oral reading probes. Unfortunately, neither reliability nor post-treatment data were collected and, at best, the results show that this improvement only continued while the social environment remained programmed.

Other attempts to recruit natural contingencies have been described by Johnson (1980) and Howie et al. (1981). Johnson described a parent-managed treatment for preschool stutterers. The parents of seven children (3–6 years) were trained to "speak at a slowed speech rate of 160 to 190 syllables per minute while maintaining an effortless, smooth, continuous breathflow and short five- to six-word phrases to help maintain slower rate" (Johnson, 1980 p. 303). They were also taught not to attend to "abnormally disfluent utterances and to increase attention to fluency" (p. 303). Three months to 6 years later five children had reduced their percentage of disfluent syllables, and the parents of four judged their child to be normally fluent. But Johnson provided insufficient data to determine the relationship between such interventions and outcome.

Howie et al. (1981) reported an extensive outcome evaluation of a variation of the Ingham and Andrews (1973b) therapy program. Some of their groups' mean score data from 3-minute telephone calls made immediately before treatment, immediately after completing a transfer phase, and then 12 to 18 months later showed that speech improvement was relatively well sustained (13.0% SS at 140.2 SPM before treatment, and 3.9% SS at 207.1 SPM 12–18 months post-transfer). These data were also consistent with those obtained from ostensibly covert telephone calls made close to the final assessment occasion. But these data should not be considered a measure of post-treatment performance. For in addition to follow-up clinic practice sessions, there were home speech practice tasks, and most subjects attended weekly self-help groups managed by former subjects. This organization, known as "speakeasy," arranges social activities, "booster" programs, and regular assessments along the lines of the Weight Watchers organization. This organization's contribution to the authors' final assessment data is unclear, but it is an inventive use of planned natural contingencies.

Thus far there is no evidence that Natural Maintaining Contingencies aid generalization/maintenance in stuttering therapy. There exist some useful examples of how *significant others* may be organized to control beyond-clinic performance, but no convincing data that show improved generalization or maintenance.

Train Sufficient Exemplars

The Train Sufficient Exemplars procedure assumes that relatively few generalizing interventions may be required before a treatment's effects spread. This notion is conceptually and clinically appealing, but it has yet to be investigated carefully. In practice it means that a client's speech is monitored across settings to determine when direct intervention in some settings produces generalization in untreated settings.

One example of the spread of generalization from one *intervened* setting to another is described in a study by Ingham (1982). At the end of prolonged-speech treatment a 20-year-old male stutterer was trained to self-evaluate (or score) his speech performance and then, on the basis of his scores, systematically reduce the frequency of self-assessments. Self-evaluation training was first introduced to family conversations, but the resulting gains failed to generalize to conversations with relatives or telephone conversations. However, when self-evaluation training was introduced to conversations with relatives, the covertly recorded telephone conversations also became stutter-free, and virtually remained so over the following 6 months.

The most likely reason for the limited use of this procedure is the infrequency with which treatment studies report evaluations over time within selected beyond-clinic situations. In short, the procedure may be effective but few studies are designed to discover this.

Train Loosely

One method for reducing the tight control that certain environmental conditions may exert over post-treatment performance is to use variable stimulus conditions during treatment. Stokes and Baer argue that relatively standardized therapy conditions may lead to stimulus discrimination which restricts generalization/maintenance. It seems self-evident that when treatment is conducted in one setting, and with one clinician, that such circumstances probably result in discrimination training, and that the simplest way to reduce this problem is to vary settings, methodology, and, if possible, clinicians during treatment. Nevertheless, there are no examples of the systematic use of this procedure in stuttering therapy.[2] However, later phases of many therapy programs probably involve a considerable amount of loose training—subjects are frequently required to speak with strangers, make various telephone calls, and so forth. Since stuttering variability is subject to discrimination control (see, for example, Martin & Siegel, 1966; Reed & Lingwall, 1980), there is ample reason why the "train loosely" principle should be practiced more commonly.

Use of Indiscriminable Reinforcers

An alternative to continuous delivery of treatment agents, or contingencies, for generalization/maintenance is a schedule of noncontinuous or intermittent use of such agents. Such intermittent schedules are often claimed to aid generalization, but, as Stokes and Baer noted, they are infrequently investigated in treatment. The purpose of such schedules is to reduce discrimination control by delivering contingencies only after a fixed or variable number of target behaviors. Discrimination may also diminish if contingencies are delayed relative to the target behavior.

Intermittent contingency schedules are rarely investigated in connection with stuttering, despite their frequently recommended use for generalization (see Hanna & Owen, 1977; Ingham, 1975a; Ryan, 1974; Shames, 1975; Shames & Egolf, 1976). Nevertheless, many treatment procedures probably use intermittent contingencies. Martin, Kuhl, and Haroldson (1972), for example, used time out contingent only on stutterings of 2 sec or more in duration and produced beneficial effects on one child's stuttering. Crowder and Harbin (1971) treated a 21-year-old male stutterer (a prisoner) with response contingent shock "once for every five stutters" during part of each treatment session. Data from the untreated parts of each session show that his stutterings declined from about 40 to less than 5 over the course of therapy. Beattie (1973) delivered shock contingent on every third appearance of certain categories of stuttering during a 20-year-old female stutterer's treatment, but insufficient data were provided to judge the procedure's merits. Other examples probably occur among therapy programs that use decreasingly frequent client contacts during maintenance (Ryan, 1974; Ingham, 1980), although the target behavior is rarely shown to have been maintained between such contacts. However, some studies have shown that covert

---

[2] Costello (1982) has suggested that the notion of organizing a relatively unprogrammed pattern of treatment is contrary to the common practice of behavioral treatments.

data obtained between these contacts often resemble overt or client contact data (Ingham, 1980, 1981, 1982). In turn, these findings suggest that improved performance is probably sustained by an intermittent schedule. While there is some evidence that intermittent schedules have been useful in some treatment programs, there is no clear evidence that they have helped to generalize or maintain treatment benefits.

Program Common Stimuli

An alternative to controlling stimulus discrimination is to exploit its effects by increasing the resemblance between relevant environmental stimuli and those of the treatment setting. This principle is evident in stuttering therapies that incorporate other persons, physical settings, or specific speaking tasks in their treatment format. These tasks are often ordered to help reduce the difference between a client's clinic and nonclinic environment, and thereby aid generalization.

Such procedures are described in many therapy programs (Boberg, 1976; Brady, 1971; Ingham & Andrews, 1973a, 1973b; Perkins, 1973; Ryan, 1971; Shames & Florance, 1980), but there are few data which demonstrate its contribution to generalization/maintenance. Some suggestive data appear in Resick, Wendiggensen, Ames, and Meyer's (1978) treatment of six adult stutterers by a combination of *slowed speech* and systematic desensitization. Their subjects were assessed on oral reading, conversation, and telephone tasks immediately before and after treatment, plus on three occasions over 6 months. But their treatment involved the use of oral reading and conversational tasks, and *not* conversations with strangers or telephone conversations with strangers. The beyond-clinic data show the group's performance on all assessment tasks was improved after treatment, but in their conversations with strangers and telephone calls they showed much less improvement, which also failed to maintain over the following 6 months. Similar factors may have operated in Ingham and Packman's (1977) single-subject investigation on the effects of within-clinic treatment on beyond-clinic performance. Their subject's within-clinic stutter-free speech completely failed to generalize to beyond-clinic conditions. Other relevant data occur in Ryan's (1974) report on the treatment progress of 39 children and adult stutterers. During the treatment's transfer phase, the subjects completed beyond-clinic tasks which incorporated the stimulus conditions used in two treatment assessment procedures—the fluency interview and the natural speech sample. Group results indicate much improved performance on these assessments after the transfer phase was completed.[3] Similar claims might be made for maintenance, except that

[3] This improvement may also be confounded by a 31% drop in the number of subjects who completed the transfer stage (see Table 21-1).

many subjects received additional therapy during the treatment's maintenance stage.

There are many ways in which common stimuli might be programmed to aid generalization. One method, which has received only limited consideration, is exemplified by Adamczyk's (1963) use of the telephone to provide remote access to DAF treatment. This procedure showed how treatment may be paired with a stimulus condition that is often associated with higher-than-usual frequencies of stuttering (Resick et al., 1978; Ryan, 1974). Another example occurs in Peters' (1977) report of response contingent treatment of two children. During treatment each child conversed with his school friend who, ostensibly, could serve as a useful generalization agent.

The practice of programming common stimuli in stuttering treatment is almost commonplace. Nevertheless, it is assumed to promote generalization despite surprisingly few data which demonstrate it achieves that goal. The need for such data is obvious, particularly in order to identify functionally powerful common stimuli.

Mediate Generalization

The essence of the Mediate Generalization procedure is to establish a response during treatment that will be used in other settings to aid generalization. As Stokes and Baer argue, these procedures are exemplified by self-control and self-management training. The purpose of these procedures is to provide a readily available technique for generalizing/maintaining a behavior change—or to establish a response which will maintain that change.

A number of studies have shown that self-managed procedures may modify stuttering. Goldiamond (1965) was the first to document that self-counting stutterings could reduce stuttering. Later, La Croix (1973) arranged for two stutterers to count their disfluencies on a golf counter while conversing with a clinician during 30-minute sessions. The procedure's effects were quite pronounced—both subjects reduced their disfluencies by approximately 80% over a number of sessions. Less spectacular findings were reported by Hanson (1978) and Ingham, Adams, and Reynolds (1978) who found that while some subjects markedly reduced stuttering by simply activating a handswitch or counting each stuttering, others failed to show similar benefits. One intriguing finding from these studies was that the accuracy with which subjects counted stutterings was unrelated to their responsiveness to the procedure. Indeed, a group study by James (1981b) showed that the *least* accurate self-recorders of stuttering (least agreement with the experimenter's counts) were generally those who showed most reductions in stuttering under this procedure. Nelson and Hayes (1981) observed a similar phenomenon in relation to self-monitoring of other problem behaviors. In other words, the beneficial effects of self-monitoring or self-counting stuttering probably involve some inconspicuous mediational factors.

The potential generalizing effects of self-management procedures were also demonstrated in a group experiment by Martin and Haroldson (1982). They compared the effects of either experimenter- or self-administered time out contingent on stuttering. Both groups reduced stuttering during an initial period of treatment and then showed extinction effects on a subsequent assessment. But after another interval of time out treatment, assessment showed that the self-administered treatment group retained much of their improved performance, while the experimenter-administered time out group virtually returned to pretreatment stuttering levels.

A related method for mediating generalization is to use instructions to highlight trained behaviors. Guitar's (1975) previously mentioned report on treating an adult stutterer with EMG biofeedback nicely illustrates this practice. After the subject substantially reduced stuttering during conversational speech, it was found that his frequency of stuttering during telephone conversations was unaltered. He was then instructed to use his muscle relaxation skills (without biofeedback) during telephone calls. Almost immediately his stuttering ceased and remained absent over a number of daily assessments. Costello (1975) reported that response contingent procedures were effective in substantially reducing the disfluencies of three stutterers, but these reductions stabilized across treatment and nontreatment conditions only after the subjects were instructed "to remain fluent."

A number of therapy programs that use prolonged speech or its variants (Ingham, 1984), also use self-management of specific speaking skills (mediating responses) in order to promote generalization and maintenance. Perkins (1973) recommends a package of such procedures in order to aid generalization and maintenance of aspects of his breath stream management treatment. Included are self-assessments on dimensions such as fluency, rate, breath flow, prosody, and self-confidence to determine a subject's speech performance in various nonclinic situations. Ryan (1974) also reported that adult stutterers were trained to self-monitor or self-count stuttering during their performance in transfer tasks, although their therapy progress was determined by clinician scores. Webster (1974a, 1980) has described a variety of mediational techniques for aiding generalization and maintenance from the Hollins program. His most recent description of treatment techniques includes careful training in how to gently initiate phonation, connect unvoiced consonants with "correct" phonatory activity, and slightly increase the duration of most speech sounds. The client's skill in using these target behaviors in the clinic is then regularly tested in various nonclinic settings to form what Webster refers to as a "parallel transfer process."

The "regulated breathing" treatment program devised by Azrin and Nunn (1974) employs a number of procedures that are assessed by stutterers' self-counts of stuttering in daily speech (Azrin, Nunn, & Frantz, 1979). It is impossible to determine the value of this activity for generalization or maintenance. However, the self-count procedure may have a substantial functional role since later investigations that have failed to yield comparable results have also failed to have subjects self-count their stutterings during the following regulated breathing treatment (Andrews & Tanner, 1982; Cote & Ladouceur, 1982; Ladouceur, Boudreau, & Theberge, 1981; Ladouceur, Cote, Leblond, & Bouchard, 1982; Williamson, Epstein & Coburn, 1981).[4]

Only two treatment studies have provided independently gathered beyond-clinic data when evaluating self-managed treatments. The first, by James (1981a), used self-managed time out to treat an 18-year-old male stutterer. The subject was repeatedly assessed in the clinic (alone and in conversation) and beyond the clinic (at home, on the telephone, and in shopping or business conversations). Initially, the subject was trained to pause briefly (2 sec) contingent on stuttering, a technique that substantially reduced stuttering in the clinic. Instructions to use this procedure in "all day-to-day speaking situations" then produced reduced stuttering in beyond-clinic assessments (without an overall reduction in speech rate). But these gains were lost after the subject was instructed to cease using time out. A response cost procedure was added to improve the subject's "accuracy" in delivering time out, and treatment was reintroduced to clinic and beyond-clinic conditions. The subject's stuttering reduced to near zero over the following 4 to 5 weeks. When the response cost procedure was removed, improved performance was sustained with only a slight reduction in speech rate. Follow-up data collected 6 and 12 months after treatment was formally ended (although it is uncertain that the subject ceased using such a useful treatment) show near zero stuttering. However, this measure excluded *interjections* which increased substantially during follow-up and the subject's accuracy in delivering time out was also found to have decreased considerably.

---

[4] Most of these studies also failed to employ the extensive telephone contact that Azrin and Nunn used to check their clients' daily stuttering counts. These phone calls may have also been powerful treatment agents that promoted generalization and maintenance.

The second study, conducted by Ingham (1982), amalgamated two generalization techniques; mediation and training "to generalize." Two young adult male stutterers were treated initially by a slight variation on Ingham and Andrews's (1973b) procedure involving prolonged speech. Following the transfer stage, each subject proceeded through a performance-contingent maintenance schedule in which successful speech performance earned decreasingly frequent clinic assessments. But concurrent measures in various beyond-clinic conditions revealed some continuing stuttering. Each subject was then taught to score his speech for stutterings and speech rate. When the clinician's and client's scores agreed, the subject made his own clinic assessments, but with intermittent checks by the clinician. When these checks agreed, each subject began to manage his maintenance schedule in beyond-clinic conditions. Concurrent covert recordings showed that introduction of self-evaluation and self-managed maintenance each resulted in generally sustained target behaviors (zero stuttering at 170–210 syllables per minute) in beyond-clinic conditions. One subject's data show generalization to covertly recorded telephone conversations. The most significant finding was that, in both cases, the beyond-clinic gains (as assessed by covert recordings with parents, relatives, and over the telephone) were sustained for at least 6 months during self-managed maintenance schedules.

Both of these studies demonstrated that self-managed procedures may be extremely effective in obtaining generalized and maintained treatment gains. At the same time it is not clear that either study's procedures were entirely self-managed since both incorporated a considerable amount of external control. For example, subjects were obliged to record their speech in self-managed treatment conditions and were aware that these recordings would be heard (if not evaluated) by the experimenter/clinician. Nevertheless, in the case of the Ingham study, the numerous covert recordings during intervals when subjects were not obliged to self-evaluate suggests the findings had substantial clinical validity.

Another variable that has been considered to mediate maintenance is the stutterer's attitude toward communication (Andrews, Guitar, & Howie, 1980; Guitar & Bass, 1978; Perkins, 1981). This notion gained impetus from Guitar and Bass's (1978) report that post-treatment performance was influenced by the status of stutterers' communication attitudes at the end of their treatment. These findings, however, have been challenged by the lack of evidence that the S24 communication attitudes scale (Andrews & Cutler, 1974), which was used in this study, measures a variable that is independent of a stutterer's speech performance (Ingham, 1979). In fact, subsequent analyses of the relationship between scores on the S24 Scale and beyond-clinic measures of stuttering show that the scale's scores are probably influenced by beyond-clinic speech performance (Ulliana & Ingham, 1984).

The use of mediators to generalize therapy benefits has shown exceptional promise. There is now considerable evidence that one particular mediational technique, self-recording, may modify stuttering—and some carefully gathered data have also shown that it may aid generalization and maintenance. The use of training to retain certain types of speech motor skills, such as the many variants of prolonged speech, probably produces the most commonly used mediating technique for aiding generalization and maintenance.

Train "To Generalize"

The main principle of training to generalize is that the appearance of generalization or maintenance may be treated as a response that can be modified by consequences. Stokes and Baer suggest, for example, that any verbal praise that a clinician offers when generalization occurs may also reinforce a subject's ability to generalize. This principle may well be functionally relevant in treatments that use setting hierarchies to systematically introduce increasingly complex or "real life" situations. In many programs it is often presumed that when the target behavior is practiced in increasingly complex situations, then this raises the probability of generalization. In such programs, of course, it is equally conceivable that each successful step in the hierarchy reinforces generalization, although there is no direct evidence to support this notion. Indirect evidence, such as that provided by Ryan (1974), does suggest that generalization may follow completion of such a program's setting hierarchy.

This principle may also be functionally effective in treatments that seek to produce maintenance by systematically withdrawing or reintroducing treatment contact contingent upon maintained performance. Several studies have yielded findings consistent with this possibility. For example, a treatment described by Ingham and Andrews (1973b) included a maintenance phase in which decreasingly frequent clinic-based assessments were contingent on maintained target speech behavior in the clinic. Under this performance-contingent schedule, subjects were assessed in the clinic 1 and 2 weeks after completing the transfer phase. If, at each visit, they completed six speaking tasks (three conversations and three telephone calls) with zero stuttering at between 170 and 210 syllables per minute, the next clinic assessment was scheduled for 2 weeks later and, if successful, after a further 2 weeks. Successful completion of the clinic tasks, then, earned a 4-week break between clinic assessments, and so on, until two 32-week-apart visits were passed successfully. If a subject failed to achieve target behavior during any clinic assessment, the schedule was restarted; that is, the subject returned to once weekly clinic assessments.

Three studies sought to determine whether a performance-contingent maintenance procedure sustains generalized improved performance. Ingham (1980) had nine stutterers (9–23 years) enter either an ABA or BAB experimental design maintenance program in which the B condition was 32 weeks of performance-contingent maintenance and the A condition was an equivalent period using a non-performance-contingent schedule (if a subject failed to obtain the target behavior the schedule was not restarted). Regular within- and beyond-clinic assessments were supplemented by irregular covert assessments via telephone. Data collected over 96 weeks indicated that the performance-contingent schedule did produce maintained and generalized reductions in stuttering. The clinical value of this procedure was demonstrated by the complete absence of stuttering in six subjects across all assessment conditions at the final assessment. However, for two subjects covert recordings at the final assessment revealed that substantial stuttering still occurred during telephone conversations. Another study (Ingham, 1981) described treating beyond-clinic performance deterioration in a 15-year-old female stutterer. She had achieved criterion performance during within-clinic conditions; yet recordings made with her family, friends, and at school showed that stuttering remained. When these recordings were integrated with a performance-contingent maintenance schedule in a multiple-baseline experimental design, her stuttering was reduced almost immediately and remained close to zero for over 30 weeks. The clinical validity of these overt recordings was supported by two covert recordings made in the family setting. A third study (Ingham, 1982), which was described earlier, was conducted with two male stutterers (18 and 20 years) and assessed the efficacy of using a self-evaluation procedure with a self-managed maintenance schedule versus a clinician-managed maintenance schedule. Whenever the self-evaluation procedure was introduced to a situation, there were almost immediate reductions in stuttering during overt *and* covert recordings in those situations. For both subjects, across all five speaking situations assessed, stuttering remained at virtually zero for 6 months following self-evaluation training. The results from all studies show that maintenance and generalization can be modified by either a clinician-managed, or largely self-managed, performance-contingent schedule. They also demonstrate that successful maintenance of target behaviors may be a response that is modifiable by contingencies.

SUMMARY OF INVESTIGATIONS ON
GENERALIZATION/MAINTENANCE IN STUTTERING TREATMENT

The preceding review has identified a burgeoning generalization/maintenance technology within stuttering therapy. There are relatively few investigations of this technology, but they yield heartening signs of some clinically useful procedures.

This review found some evidence that even Train and Hope techniques may have merit in producing generalization/maintenance, particularly with children. More predictable findings, however, have tended to emerge when specific procedures have been used in order to achieve generalization/maintenance. It is clear, for instance, that modifying stuttering in sequentially different settings may yield benefits, although such benefits may rely upon the conjoint use of self-managed procedures. There are also some interesting reports on the use of natural contingencies, such as parents or spouses, to control beyond-clinic performance, but these reports lack careful documentation. Unfortunately, few studies have used multibaseline data to identify beyond-clinic therapy effects. The lack of such data limits the possibilities of determining which beyond-clinic interventions may be sufficient to promote generalization/maintenance.

One useful feature of Stokes and Baer's review is that it highlights certain approaches that could benefit stuttering treatment. For example, it has highlighted the complete absence of reports on the use of the "train loosely" principle in stuttering treatment. This principle is probably practiced when subjects are exposed to various settings, but its clinical value needs investigation. The use of indiscriminable contingencies in the form of intermittent schedules are frequently advocated to aid maintenance, but again, there is virtually no evidence that such schedules achieve this purpose. And despite encouraging experimental demonstrations, the same is true of procedures that program stimuli commonly found in nontherapy settings.

Some promising findings are emerging from procedures embraced by Stokes and Baer's latter two categories. The benefits of mediating generalization by training subjects to self-evaluate motor skills and to self-manage treatment is evident from some recent studies that have also employed multibaseline and multidimensional methods of evaluation. This is also true of some recent attempts to train stutterers to generalize, or more specifically, to train them to maintain therapy benefits.

As mentioned earlier the search for techniques that promote generalization/maintenance in stuttering therapy has been mainly directed to the general area of behavior therapy literature. While this was a restricted search for such techniques, it is evident that many behavioral techniques have yet to be tried in stuttering treatment. In fact, many procedures, such as sequential modification, training sufficient exemplars, training loosely, and the use of indiscriminable contingencies clearly warrant investigation.

There is a promising increase in the number of small scale investigations or procedures that might enhance generalization/maintenance. While it can be claimed that such analog studies have limited clinical value (Kazdin & Wilson, 1978), the daunting demands of large scale clinical studies on generalization/maintenance procedures might be approached with more enthusiasm if suitably designed analog studies yielded positive results. In the interim, clinicians have available a variety of procedures that appear capable of enhancing stutterers' therapy outcomes.

Finally, this review indicates that clinicians and researchers should be aware of at least three considerations in designing generalization/maintenance strategies for stuttering therapy. The first is the type of behavior(s) needed to modify stuttering and the extent to which all or part of that behavior must be continued in order to sustain improved fluency. Second, environmental contingencies should be arranged to link up with treatment procedures and/or the behavior(s) required for improved fluency. Third, self-management principles should be utilized, when possible, in order to maximize a stutterer's capacity to manage and evaluate beyond-clinic performance. Over and above these considerations, however, there is now ample indication that the value of any procedure can only be determined if therapy is conducted under circumstances in which speech performance is systematically evaluated to identify the durability (or otherwise) of treatment benefits (Ingham & Costello, 1984).

REFERENCES

Adamczyk, B. Correction of speech in stutterers by means of a telephone with the use of an artificial echo. *Otolaryngologia Polska*, 1963, *17*, 482–484.

Andrews, G., & Cutler, J. Stuttering therapy: The relation between changes in symptom level and attitudes. *Journal of Speech and Hearing Disorders*, 1974, *39*, 312–319.

Andrews, G., Guitar, B., & Howie, P. Meta-analysis of the effects of stuttering treatment. *Journal of Speech and Hearing Disorders*, 1980, *45*, 287–307.

Andrews, G., & Tanner, S. Stuttering treatment: An attempt to replicate the regulated-breathing method. *Journal of Speech and Hearing Disorders*, 1982, *47*, 138–140.

Azrin, N. H., & Nunn, R. G. A rapid method of eliminating stuttering by a regulated breathing approach. *Behaviour Research and Therapy*, 1974, *12*, 279–286.

Azrin, N. H., Nunn, R. G., & Frantz, S. E. Comparison of regulated-breathing versus abbreviated desensitization on reported stuttering episodes. *Journal of Speech and Hearing Disorders,* 1979, *44,* 331–339.

Baer, D. M., Wolf, M. M., & Risley, T. R. Some current dimensions of applied behavior analysis. *Journal of Applied Behavior Analysis,* 1968, *1,* 91–97.

Beattie, M. S. A behaviour therapy programme for stuttering. *British Journal of Disorders of Communication,* 1973, *8,* 120–130.

Bloodstein, O. *A handbook on stuttering* (3rd ed.). Chicago: National Easter Seal Society, 1981.

Boberg, E. Intensive group therapy program for stutterers. *Human Communications,* 1976, *1,* 29–42.

Boberg, E. Intensive adult therapy program. *Seminars in Speech, Language and Hearing,* 1980, *1,* 365–373.

Boberg, E. *Maintenance of fluency.* New York: Elsevier, 1981.

Boberg, E., Howie, P., & Woods, L. Maintenance of fluency: A review. *Journal of Fluency Disorders,* 1979, *4,* 93–116.

Boberg, E., & Sawyer, L. The maintenance of fluency following intensive therapy. *Human Communication,* 1977, *2,* 21–28.

Brady, J. P. Metronome-conditioned speech retraining for stuttering. *Behavior Therapy,* 1971, *2,* 129–150.

Browning, R. M. Behaviour therapy for stuttering in a schizophrenic child. *Behaviour Research and Therapy,* 1967, *5,* 27–35.

Costello, J. M. The establishment of fluency with time-out procedures: Three case studies. *Journal of Speech and Hearing Disorders,* 1975, *40,* 216–231.

Costello, J. M. Generalization across settings: Language intervention with children. In D. Yoder, J. Miller, & R. Schiefelbusch (Eds.), *Language intervention.* New York: Thieme-Stratton, 1982.

Cote, C., & Ladouceur, R. Effects of social aids and the regulated breathing method in the treatment of stutterers. *Journal of Consulting and Clinical Psychology,* 1982, *50,* 450.

Crowder, J. E., & Harbin, R. The effect of punishment on stuttering: A case study. *Psychotherapy: Theory, Research and Practice,* 1971, *8,* 179–180.

Curlee, R. F., & Perkins, W. H. Conversational rate control therapy for stuttering. *Journal of Speech and Hearing Disorders,* 1969, *34,* 245–250.

Erickson, R. L. Assessing communication attitudes among stutterers. *Journal of Speech and Hearing Research,* 1969, *12,* 711–724.

Goldiamond, I. Stuttering and fluency as manipulatable operant response classes. In L. Krasner & L. P. Ullmann (Eds.), *Research in behavior modification.* New York: Holt, Rinehart & Winston, 1965.

Goldstein, A. P., & Kanfer, F. H. (Eds.). *Maximizing treatment gains.* New York: Academic Press, 1979.

Gregory, H. H. (Ed.). *Controversies about stuttering therapy.* Baltimore, MD: University Park Press, 1979.

Guitar, B. Reduction of stuttering frequency using analog electromyographic feedback. *Journal of Speech and Hearing Research,* 1975, *18,* 672–685.

Guitar, B., & Bass, C. Stuttering therapy: The relationship between attitude change and long-term outcome. *Journal of Speech and Hearing Disorders,* 1978, *43,* 392–400.

Hanna, R., & Owen, N. Facilitating transfer and maintenance of fluency in stuttering therapy. *Journal of Speech and Hearing Disorders,* 1977, *42,* 65–76.

Hanson, B. R. The effects of a contingent light-flash on stuttering and attention to stuttering. *Journal of Communication Disorders,* 1978, *11,* 451–458.

Hersen, M., & Barlow, D. H. *Single-case experimental designs.* New York: Pergamon Press, 1976.

Howie, P. M., Tanner, S., & Andrews, G. Short- and long-term outcome in an intensive treatment program for adult stutterers. *Journal of Speech and Hearing Disorders,* 1981, *46,* 104–109.

Ingham, R. J. Operant methodology in stuttering therapy. In J. Eisenson (Ed.), *Stuttering: A second symposium.* New York: Harper & Row, 1975. (a)

Ingham, R. J. A comparison of covert and overt assessment procedures in stuttering therapy outcome evaluation. *Journal of Speech and Hearing Research,* 1975, *18,* 346–354.(b)

Ingham, R. J. Comment on "Stuttering therapy: The relation between attitude change and long-term outcome." *Journal of Speech and Hearing Disorders,* 1979, *44,* 397–400.

Ingham, R. J. Modification of maintenance and generalization in stuttering treatment. *Journal of Speech and Hearing Research,* 1980, *23,* 732–745.

Ingham, R. J. Evaluation and maintenance in stuttering treatment: A search for ecstasy with nothing but agony. In E. Boberg (Ed.), *Maintenance of fluency.* New York: Elsevier, 1981.

Ingham, R. J. The effects of self-evaluation training on maintenance and generalization during stuttering treatment. *Journal of Speech and Hearing Disorders,* 1982, *47,* 271–280.

Ingham, R. J. *Stuttering and behavior therapy: Current status and experimental foundations.* San Diego: College-Hill Press, 1984.

Ingham, R. J., Adams, S., & Reynolds, G. The effects on stuttering of self-recording the frequency of stuttering or the word "the." *Journal of Speech and Hearing Research,* 1978, *21,* 459–469.

Ingham, R. J., & Andrews, G. An analysis of a token economy in stuttering therapy. *Journal of Applied Behavior Analysis,* 1973, *6,* 219–229.(a)

Ingham, R. J., & Andrews, G. Details of a token economy stuttering therapy programme for adults. *Australian Journal of Human Communication Disorders,* 1973, *1,* 13–20.(b)

Ingham, R. J., & Costello, J. M. Stuttering treatment outcome evaluation. In J. M. Costello (Ed.), *Recent advances: Speech disorders in children.* San Diego: College-Hill Press, 1984.

Ingham, R. J., & Packman, A. Treatment and generalization effects in an experimental treatment for a stutterer using contingency management and speech rate control. *Journal of Speech and Hearing Disorders,* 1977, *42,* 394–407.

Ingham, R. J., & Packman, A. C. Perceptual assessment of normalcy of speech following stuttering therapy. *Journal of Speech and Hearing Research,* 1978, *21,* 63–73.

James, J. E. Behavioral self-control of stuttering using time-out from speaking. *Journal of Applied Behavior Analysis,* 1981, *14,* 25–37.(a)

James, J. E. Self-monitoring of stuttering: Reactivity and accuracy. *Behaviour Research and Therapy,* 1981, *19,* 291–296.(b)

Johnson, L. J. Facilitating parental involvement in therapy of the disfluent child. *Seminars in Speech, Language and Hearing,* 1980, *1,* 301–309.

Johnson, W., Darley, F. L., & Spriestersbach, D. C. *Diagnostic methods in speech pathology.* New York: Harper & Row, 1963.

Jones, R. J., & Azrin, N. H. Behavioral engineering: Stuttering as a function of stimulus duration during speech synchronization. *Journal of Applied Behavior Analysis,* 1969, *2,* 223–229.

Karoly, P., & Steffen, J. J. *Improving the long-term effects of psychotherapy.* New York: Gardner Press, 1980.

Kazdin, A. E., & Wilson, G. T. *Evaluation of behavior therapy.* Cambridge: Ballinger, 1978.

La Croix, Z. E. Management of disfluent speech through self-recording procedures. *Journal of Speech and Hearing Disorders,* 1973, *38,* 272–274.

Ladouceur, R., Boudreau, L., & Theberge, S. Awareness training and regulated-breathing method in modification of stuttering. *Perceptual and Motor Skills,* 1981, *53,* 187–194.

Ladouceur, R., Cote, C., Leblond, G., & Bouchard, L. Evaluation of regulated-breathing method and awareness training in the treatment of stuttering. *Journal of Speech and Hearing Disorders,* 1982, *47,* 422–426.

Leach, E. Stuttering: Clinical applications of response-contingent procedures. In B. B. Gray & G. England (Eds.), *Stuttering and the conditioning therapies.* Monterey, CA: Monterey Institute of Speech and Hearing, 1969.

Luper, H. L. Consistency of stuttering in relation to the goal gradient hypothesis. *Journal of Speech and Hearing Disorders,* 1956, *21,* 336–342.

Martin, R. R. Direct magnitude-estimation judgments of stuttering severity using audible and audible–visible speech samples. *Speech Monographs,* 1965, *32,* 169–177.

Martin, R. R., & Haroldson, S. K. Contingent self-stimulation for stuttering. *Journal of Speech and Hearing Disorders,* 1982, *47,* 407–413.

Martin, R. R., Haroldson, S. K., & Triden, K. A. Stuttering and speech naturalness. *Journal of Speech and Hearing Disorders,* 1984, *49,* 53–58.

Martin, R. R., Kuhl, P., & Haroldson, S. K. An experimental treatment with two preschool stuttering children. *Journal of Speech and Hearing Research,,* 1972, *15,* 743–752.

Martin, R. R., & Siegel, G. M. The effects of response contingent shock on stuttering. *Journal of Speech and Hearing Research,* 1966, *9,* 340–352.

Mowrer, D. An instructional program to increase fluent speech of stutterers. *Journal of Fluency Disorders,* 1975, *1,* 25–35.

Nelson, R. O., & Hayes, S. C. Theoretical explanations for reactivity in self-monitoring. *Behavior Modification,* 1981, *5,* 3-14.

Perkins, W. H. Replacement of stuttering with normal speech: II. Clinical procedures. *Journal of Speech and Hearing Disorders,* 1973, *38,* 295–303.

Perkins, W. H. Measurement and maintenance of fluency. In E. Boberg (Ed.), *Maintenance of fluency.* New York: Elsevier, 1981.

Perkins, W. H., Rudas, J., Johnson, L., Michael, W. B., & Curlee, R. F. Replacement of stuttering with normal speech: III. Clinical effectiveness. *Journal of Speech and Hearing Disorders,* 1974, *39,* 416–428.

Peters, A. D. The effect of positive reinforcement on fluency: Two case studies. *Language, Speech and Hearing Services in Schools,* 1977, *8,* 15–22.

Reed, C. G., & Godden, A. L. An experimental treatment using verbal punishment with two preschool stutterers. *Journal of Fluency Disorders,* 1977, *2,* 225–233.

Reed, C. G., & Lingwall, J. B. Conditioned stimulus effects on stuttering and GSRs. *Journal of Speech and Hearing Research,* 1980, *23,* 336–343.

Resick, P. A., Wendiggensen, P., Ames, S., & Meyer, V. Systematic slowed speech: A new treatment for stuttering. *Behaviour Research and Therapy,* 1978, *16,* 161–167.

Ryan, B. P. An illustration of operant conditioning therapy for stuttering. In *Conditioning in stuttering therapy* (Publication No. 7). Memphis: Speech Foundation of America, 1970.

Ryan, B. P. Operant procedures applied to stuttering therapy for children. *Journal of Speech and Hearing Disorders*, 1971, *36*, 264–280.

Ryan, B. P. *Programmed therapy for stuttering in children and adults*. Springfield, IL: Thomas, 1974.

Ryan, B. P. Stuttering therapy in a framework of operant conditioning and programmed learning. In H. H. Gregory (Ed.), *Controversies about stuttering therapy*. Baltimore, MD: University Park Press, 1979.

Shames, G. H. Operant conditioning and stuttering. In J. Eisenson (Ed.), *Stuttering: A second symposium*. New York: Harper & Row, 1975.

Shames G. H., & Egolf, D. B. *Operant conditioning and the management of stuttering*. Englewood Cliffs, NJ: Prentice–Hall, 1976.

Shames, G. H., & Florance, C. L. *Stutter-free speech: A goal for therapy*. Columbus, OH: Merrill, 1980.

Shelton, J. L. The elimination of persistent stuttering by the use of homework assignments involving speech shadowing: A case report. *Behavior Therapy*, 1975, *6*, 392–393.

Silverman, F. H. Long-term impact of a miniature metronome on stuttering: An interim report. *Perceptual and Motor Skills*, 1976, *42*, 1322.

Silverman, F. H. Dimensions of improvement in stuttering. *Journal of Speech and Hearing Research*, 1980, *23*, 137–151.

Silverman, F. H. Relapse following stuttering therapy. In N. J. Lass (Ed.), *Speech and language: Advances in basic research and practice* (Vol. 5). New York: Academic Press, 1981.

Stokes, T. F., & Baer, D. M. An implicit technology of generalization. *Journal of Applied Behavior Analysis*, 1977, *10*, 349–367.

Trotter, W. D., & Lesch, M. M. Personal experiences with a stutter-aid. *Journal of Speech and Hearing Disorders*, 1967, *32*, 270–272.

Ulliana, L., & Ingham, R. J. Behavioral and non-behavioral variables in the measurement of stutterers' communication attitudes. *Journal of Speech and Hearing Disorders*, 1984, *49*, 83–93.

Webster, R. L. Stuttering: A way to eliminate it and a way to explain it. In R. Ulrich, T. Stachnik, & J. Mabry (Eds.), *Control of human behavior* (Vol. 2). Glenview, IL: Scott, Foresman, 1970.

Webster, R. L. A behavioral analysis of stuttering: Treatment and theory. In K. S. Calhoun, H. E. Adams, & K. M. Mitchell (Eds.), *Innovative treatment methods in psychopathology*. New York: Wiley, 1974.(a)

Webster, R. L. *The precision fluency shaping program: Speech reconstruction for stutterers*. Roanoke, VA: Hollins Communication Research Institute, 1974.(b)

Webster, R. L. Evolution of a target-based behavioral therapy for stuttering. *Journal of Fluency Disorders*, 1980, *5*, 303–320.

Williamson, D. A., Epstein, L. H., & Coburn, C. Multiple baseline analysis of the regulated breathing procedure for the treatment of stuttering. *Journal of Fluency Disorders*, 1981, *6*, 327–339.

Author Index

A

Abbs, J., 140, 150
Abramson, A., 90
Adamczyk, B., 460
Adams, J., 245, 250, 278
Adams, M. R., 15, 20, 26, 65, 95, 96, 99, 100, 101, 102, 109, 110, 111, 191, 202, 245, 313, 314, 315, 322, 324, 340, 349, 351, 378, 388, 389, 390, 437
Adams, S., 201, 202, 442, 460
Adler, J., 98
Agnello, J., 92, 93, 249, 250
Ahuja, Y. R., 155, 159
Alfonso, P., 93, 99
Alfrey, A. C., 38
Ainsworth, S., 345, 366, 376
Al-Issa, I., 297
Allen, G., 249
Allen, J. D., 261, 287
Ames, S., 459, 460
Anderson, S., 250
Andrews, G., 38, 39, 40, 41, 59, 154, 159, 160, 180, 187, 193, 204, 283, 284, 290, 294, 305, 308, 318, 343, 367, 387, 390, 416, 425, 426, 428, 429, 431, 433, 435, 436, 439, 441, 450, 453, 459, 462, 463, 464
Andrews, J. G., 3, 5, 6, 8, 9, 10, 75
Appel, J. B., 192
Arend, R., 35
Arnold, G. E., 38
Aronson, A. E., 33
Aschenback, K., 76
Asp, C. W., 82
Austin, W. T., 79
Avari, D. N., 178
Azrin, N. H., 194, 204, 205, 244, 315, 425, 434, 435, 450, 462

B

Backus, O., 79
Baer, D. M., 447, 448, 449, 451, 457, 458, 460, 466
Bakker, D., 56
Bandura, A., 203, 347, 397, 401, 405, 409, 414, 415
Bar, A., 15, 19, 379
Baratz, R., 43, 44
Barber, V., 320
Barlow, D. H., 188, 206, 305, 388, 439, 450
Barocas, V. S., 197, 203, 205
Barr, D. F., 276
Basili, A., 106, 109
Basmajian, J. V., 105
Bass, C., 324, 390, 463
Bates, E., 238, 245, 246, 251, 254
Baumgartner, J., 99
Beattie, M. S., 458
Bell, J., 262, 275, 293, 387
Benguerel, A., 116
Benigni, L., 238
Benignus, V., 177
Benson, D. F., 30, 39, 41, 74
Berger, K., 223
Berlin, C. I., 17, 56, 287, 359
Berlin, S., 359
Bernard, J. R. L., 313
Berndt, L. A., 190, 320
Bernstein, N., 139
Bernstein, N. E., 294, 389
Berry, M. F., 180, 181, 343
Berson, J., 59
Berwick, N., 398
Besozzi, T. E., 313
Biggs, B., 193, 194, 204
Blood, G. W., 180, 321, 367
Bloodstein, O., 8, 9, 10, 15, 22, 23, 64, 138, 175, 178, 179, 181, 182, 187, 198, 228, 237, 241, 242, 244, 247, 252, 254, 294, 304, 308, 313, 339, 342, 343, 357, 359, 368, 398, 400, 449

Subject Index